AF822622

Medical Terminology for the Health Professions

Medical Terminology
for the Health Professions

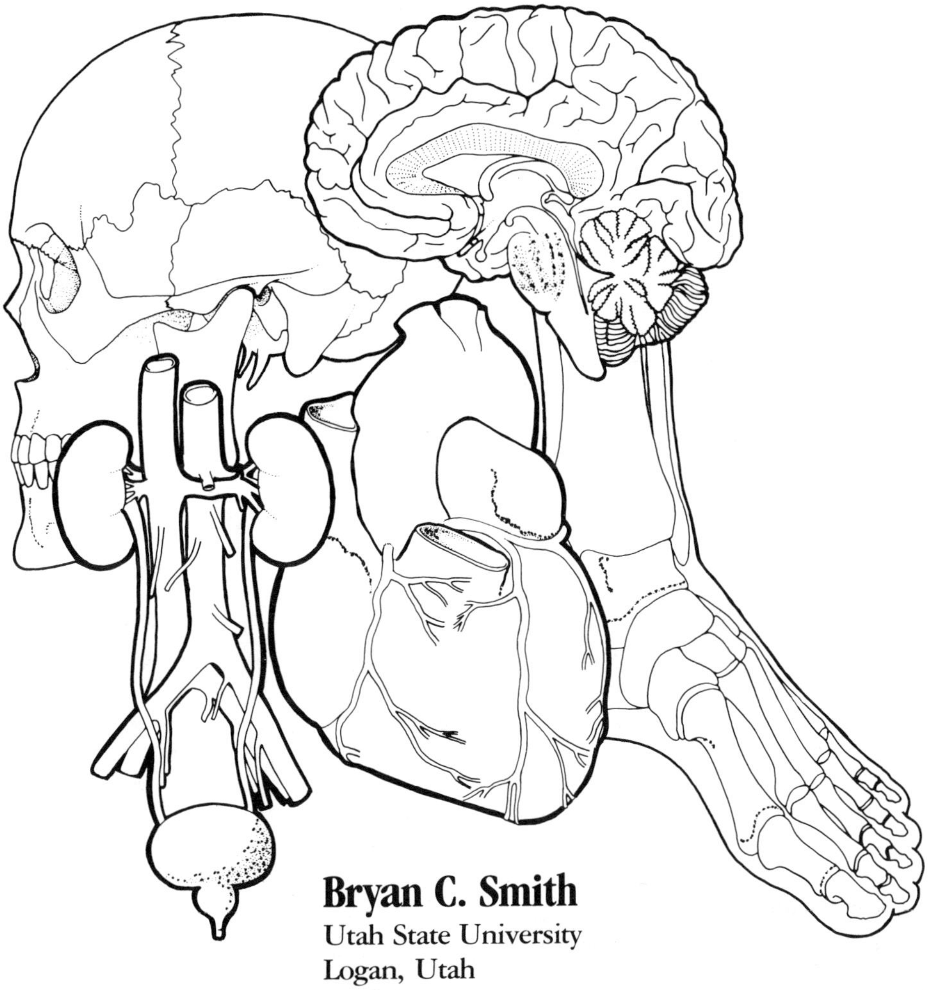

Bryan C. Smith
Utah State University
Logan, Utah
Bentley E. Smith, M.D.

HBJ

Harcourt Brace Jovanovich, Inc.
(and it's subsidiary, Academic Press)
San Diego New York Chicago Austin Washington, D.C.
London Sydney Tokyo Toronto

Illustrations by Cecile Duray-Bito

ISBN: 0-15-557881-2
ISBN: 0-15-557884-7 Software Package
Library of Congress Catalog Card Number: 85-71003
Printed in the United States of America

Contents

PREFACE

The purpose of *Medical Terminology for the Health Professions* is to enable students of health-related fields to communicate and understand the language of medicine. Although each profession and specialty area has its own precise terminology, most health workers share a single vocabulary. This vocabulary is the focus of our writing.

Sound learning principles and a thorough study of medical terminology have guided the writing of this book. At the same time, we have tried to be sensitive to the needs and abilities of the reader. Students who field-tested earlier drafts of this book expressed enthusiasm for the quality and combination of materials in this learning package. They applauded our approach and expressed relief that the drudgery of memorization, so often found in other language-learning experiences, was absent. They also appreciated the illustrations that enhanced the written materials and found that "Terminology Trivia" lightened the content in a pleasant, yet functional, way. They found the Glossary to be a comprehensive reference for definitions and pronunciations and the Index to be extensive and precise.

The organization of the book was formed from certain fundamental principles of medical terminology. One such principle is that the rules of medical word construction are based on Latin and Greek origins. From this, students can learn a few frequently used word elements and be able to recognize literally hundreds of medical words. For example, the term **osteochondroma** is composed of the elements *osteo, chondr,* and *oma.* Combining these elements, we can interpret the term to mean a tumor (*oma*) made up of bone (*osteo*) and cartilage (*chondr*). These three elements are used with other common prefixes and suffixes to form over fifty medical words. **Osteoma** and **chondroma** are only two of the medical words constructed with these elements. The Glossary describes over 1300 medical terms, and more than 1400 medical words are listed in the Index. These words represent only a part of the reader's potential vocabulary. The ability of the medical terminology student to build a medical vocabulary exceeds the limits of the words found in this book.

The *Apple Software* version of *Medical Terminology for the Health Professions* offers the reader a motivating opportunity to use the latest technological tools in combination with an exciting learning package. Ability and confidence in the use of medical terminology is reinforced by the many self-test exercises as well as the multiple choice, spelling, and flash word tests available on the diskette. The software is personalized and gives users a record of their progress.

Medicine is continually changing. Research and clinical experiences broaden the base of medical knowledge, which eventually leads to changes in health care. With these changes come new words and abbreviations to describe materials, procedures, and instruments. Despite these dynamics, the authors and the publisher have made every effort to ensure the information contained here is accurate and of the highest standard.

The authors wish to express their appreciation to Diane Carlson and her students at Northern Illinois University for their assistance in field testing. Appreciation is also extended to Sheila Korman of Academic Press for her editorial excellence and to other employees for their attention to detail. The quality of this publication is a tribute to their efforts.

B.C.S. and B.E.S.
1986

One
Introduction

The Eskimo language has over a dozen words for "snow"—one refers to falling snow, another to new-fallen snow, another to hard-packed snow, still others to soft snow, iced snow, and so on. To most of us for whom snow is simply snow, the specificity of that language for describing snow must seem redundant or superfluous. To the Eskimos, however, an accurate description that conveys the character of the snow is critical to their very survival.

To the layperson, the fact that there are thousands of technical terms that deal only with the heart must stagger the imagination. If you have ever seen a medical dictionary with its practically endless columns of complex terms, you might think that the medical vocabulary is redundant and a plot to perpetuate the doctor–as–God myth. After all, anyone who could master or even comprehend such a large amount of information must be superhuman. To the medical community, however, an accurate description that conveys the character of the condition or event is critical both to good medical care and to life itself.

In actuality, most medical terms are combinations of a relatively small core of word roots that are derived from Latin and Greek. While the list of word roots presented in this book represents only a basic foundation of medical terminology, it still demonstrates how the vast medical language is built through a combination of word roots, prefixes, suffixes, and terminals. Medical terminology is an exact vocabulary used by health care professionals. Most terms are compound words consisting of prefixes + word root(s) + combining form + suffix or a word terminal. All of the various word components you will be learning, except word roots, cut across anatomical systems.

It is crucial in the medical field to describe accurately the minute characteristics and changes that occur. For example, an accurate diagnosis often necessitates taking a cell sample from an organ. This procedure is called a biopsy and is used to confirm or refute the existence of a malignancy (cancer). One such procedure is the Pap test (an abbreviation for the Papanicolaou test), used by a physician to detect precancerous uterine cells. A sample of cells is first gathered from the cervix—the neck of the uterus—and is then sent to a laboratory where a pathologist examines it under a microscope. It is the job of the pathologist to describe the status of each cell sample. Because normal cells exhibit certain characteristics, even the most minute variations described by the pathologist can help the physician in making an accurate diagnosis. For this purpose, pathologists must have at their disposal an inexhaustible and precise storehouse of words and phrases to communicate their findings.

In addition to refining communication between pathologists and examining physicians, this precision of terms also aids communication between health care providers through the medium of professional journals. The information presented in journals must be precise so that professionals are able to understand and update their techniques. It is obviously essential that health science, dedicated to the improvement and preservation of human life, have a language exact enough to encompass the immense scope of the human organism.

Method of Study

The method of study presented in this book involves learning both to reduce medical terms into their components—root or roots, prefixes, and suffixes—and to translate these components from their Greek or Latin origins into English. In this manner, you will learn to determine the definition of a medical term by analyzing its components.

The first step in building a medical vocabulary is mastery of prefixes, suffixes, and word roots. These elements are combined to create medical words. The second step in the process involves learning the basic anatomy and physiology of each of the body's systems. The third step, then, is to connect terms with meanings and associate them with the medical language. The principle used here connects both new knowledge and old knowledge, making retention easier.

The principal method of building a medical vocabulary consists of breaking down a word by identifying its root (roots, in compound words), suffix, and prefix. Except for those used in anatomy, most medical terms are not derived from a single Greek or Latin word, but rather are a combination of two or more roots or word elements. The identification of a word through structural analysis involves a search for the meaning of each of its units or components. When translated separately and then incorporated into a whole word, the components give the word its essential meaning. For example, in the word rhinitis, *rhin*, meaning nose, is the root, and *itis*, meaning inflammation, is the suffix. Translated as a whole, rhinitis means inflammation of the nose.

Your ability to divide medical terms into components or to recognize a complete word depends on your mastery of several facets: the combining forms (a word root with an *i*, *o*, or *u* attached), the word roots that appear in medical terms, and the prefixes and suffixes that alter or modify meaning and usage. Treat each medical word as though it is a puzzle to solve and you will see how enjoyable and rewarding it is to define it without referring to the glossary or a medical dictionary.

Components of Medical Terms

Understanding what the various components of medical terms mean is essential to building a medical vocabulary. You will find this basic understanding an enormous help throughout the book.

A **medical term** is a word or phrase composed of elements and used to express a specific idea. An **element** is a word part used to form a medical term. All elements in a medical word are essential to its meaning.

For example:

Element +	Element +	Element	= Medical Term
chole-	lith	-iasis	cholelithiasis
(bile)	(stone)	(condition of)	(gall stone)

A **word root** is the main element within a medical term and it is always the subject or main topic of the term—often a body part. A term may contain more than one root element. For example, in the word nephradenoma, *nephr-* and *aden-* are both word roots and *-oma* is a suffix.

A **prefix** is an element used at the beginning of a medical term that changes the meaning of the term or makes it more specific. For example:

Prefix +	Word Root =	Medical Term
hydro-	cele	hydrocele
(water)	(hernia)	(water hernia)

or:

Prefix +	Word Root =	Medical Term
hemi-	plegia	hemiplegia
(half)	(paralysis)	(paralysis of one-half of the body)

A **suffix** is an element at the end of a medical term (after the root element) that usually describes a condition or an action. For example:

Prefix +	Word Root +	Suffix	= Medical Term
hemi-	gastr	-ectomy	hemigastrectomy
(half)	(stomach)	(excision)	(surgical removal of half of the stomach)

A term may contain more than one element of each type.

A **word terminal** is a suffix that denotes the term's part of speech (noun, verb, adjective) or that changes it to singular or plural. The following examples of word terminals are used in your everyday vocabulary:

Adjective Terminals	Noun Terminals
-ic	-y
-al	-ia
-ical	-um
-ac	-is
	-a (ae-plural)

Pronunciation of Medical Terms

At the end of each chapter you will find a list of some phonetically spelled words that have been introduced in that chapter. A composite list can be found in the glossary. Correct pronunciation will help you to learn and remember these words. Most are easy to figure out, but there are a few that are illogical and that require memorization. Refer to the pronunciation list or glossary often while studying each chapter. Not only will this aid your pronunciation skills, but you also will benefit from becoming familiar with your newly learned medical vocabulary.

Medical terms may be difficult to pronounce, particularly if you have never before heard them spoken. The following are some general rules of pronunciation you should keep in mind:

ch is sometimes pronounced like *k*. Examples: chromatin, chronic.
ps is pronounced like *s*. Examples: psychiatry, psychology.

pn is pronounced with only the *n* sound. Examples: pneumonia, pneumothorax.
c and **g** are given the soft sound of *s* and *j*, respectively, before *e*, *i*, and *y* in words of both Greek and Latin origins. Examples: cycle, cytoplasm, giant, generic.
c and **g** have a harsh sound before other letters. Examples: cast, cardiac, gastric, gonad.
ae and **oe** pronounce only the second vowel. Examples: aerosol, bursae, roentgen, gastroenteritis.
i at the end of a word (to form a plural) is pronounced eye. Examples: alveoli, glomeruli, fasciculi.
e and **es**, when forming the final letter or letters of a word, are often pronounced as separate syllables. Examples: rete (ree' tee), nares (nare' ez).

There are also some general rules concerning phonetic spelling you should heed when referring either to the glossary at the end of the book or to the pronunciation list contained within each chapter. The following should aid you in interpreting phonetic spelling:

1. An unmarked vowel at the end of a syllable is long.
2. An unmarked vowel in a syllable ending in a consonant is short.
3. A long vowel that is followed by a consonant is marked with a macron (*e.g.*, sāt).

Word Building and Word Interpreting

You will be able to build suitable words expressing medical concepts from your knowledge of the word parts. Sometimes you will have a choice of two or more parts that mean the same thing. For example, the suffixes *-dynia* and *-algia* both mean pain. So, which do you use? Familiarity is the guide to your decision. Build the word, sound it out and, if it does not sound right or cannot be spelled without dropping some vowels, try it another way. The following rules should assist you in word building:

1. *Define the word you are building*. For example, suppose you want a word that means a condition of the blood characterized by increased sugar.
2. *Choose an appropriate suffix*. For example, a suffix that means a condition of the blood is *-emia*.
3. *Choose one or more suitable prefixes*. For example, a prefix that means increased is *hyper-*, and a word root that means sugar is *glyco-*.
4. *Arrange prefixes in order of increasing importance and put the suffix after the last prefix or word root*. For example, since the word sugar is more important than the word increased, *glyco-* follows *hyper-*; thus, *glyco-*, *hyper-*, and *-emia* are arranged as *hyper-glyco-emia*.
5. *Drop all hyphens, and, if the suffix begins with a vowel, drop the final vowel of the last prefix*. For example, since *-emia* begins with a vowel, *hyper-glyco-emia* becomes hyperglycemia.
6. *To check the word, look it up in the glossary*. For example, hyperglycemia is listed and fits our earlier definition.

Knowing definitions of word elements enables the medical terminology student to interpret most medical words. For example, the word gastroenterostomy can be interpreted as: *gastro-*, pertaining to the stomach, *enter-*, pertaining to the intestines, and *-ostomy*, which means a surgical opening; Hence, the word gastroenterostomy means a surgical opening between the stomach and the intestines.

The student will find word interpretation an easy process by following these basic rules:

1. Determine the meaning of the suffix first. For example, the suffix *-itis* means inflammation, so the word appendicitis refers to an inflammation of the appendix.
2. Sometimes an *o* or *h* is omitted from a word, so adding either of them to the root might help you recognize the word. For example, the word anemia means without blood (cells), *an-* means without, and, *hemia* with the *h* dropped, means blood.
3. Be aware that a consonant is sometimes changed to make a word easier to pronounce. For example, the word immobile literally means *in*mobile (not mobile).
4. See how the word is used in the context of the sentence. Read the sentence and insert your interpreted meaning to see if it makes sense. For example, *sclera-* has two meanings: hard, and, the dense white covering of the eye. The word arteriosclerotic refers to hardened arteries, not to the eye. The sentence should cue you as to which meaning is intended.

Problems of Literal Interpretation

When you first begin learning medical terminology or when you are in doubt concerning pronunciation or meaning, always refer to the glossary or to a medical dictionary to ensure that you are accurately interpreting a medical term. Failure to verify its meaning may result in an inaccurate interpretation; an error that may haunt you for a long time. For example, in the word cardiectomy, cardi = heart and ectomy = surgical removal of all or part. From this, one might assume that cardiectomy means surgical removal of all or part of the heart. To quote one dictionary, however, cardiectomy means "surgical removal of the upper end of the stomach. . . ." The meaning of this medical term probably was derived from the fact that the upper end of the stomach is called the cardia; the end toward the heart. In any case, it clearly emphasizes the importance of referring to a medical dictionary rather than accepting the literal interpretation of a medical term.

Another difficulty in literal interpretation occurs when there is the possibility that something might be missing. For example, the letter *h* is retained when the element *hem-* appears at the beginning of a medical term:

hemangioma—tumor made up of blood vessels
hemic—pertaining to the blood
hematology—study of the blood

When the element *hem-* appears within the medical term, however, the letter *h* is dropped:

anemia—absence of blood (cells)
polyemia—excessive amount of blood in the body
cyanemia—bluish condition of the blood
hyperemia—excess (abnormal) amount of blood in a body part

The form *-emia* (which is *hemia* with the letter *h* dropped) appears often within medical terms. It means condition (*ia*) of the blood (*hem*).

So, to avoid confusion, be aware of the problems of literal interpretation. Remember these few rules and try to fit the word into the context of the sentence. Obviously, it must relate somehow to the subject, but if it doesn't seem logical, look it up in the glossary or in a medical dictionary.

Organization of the Text

The text chapters 2–17 are divided into five sections:

1. Overview
2. Word Elements and Examples
3. Terminology Trivia
4. Pronunciation
5. Self–test

Each chapter of the text begins with an overview and description of the chapter topic. Next, word elements are presented with their meanings and explanations of any unique aspects. At least three examples are given for each word part. Immediately following each example, the word (in parentheses) is divided into its elements, using slash ("/") marks, and is then defined.

At the end of each chapter is a section entitled "Terminology Trivia." This informative and light-hearted section is intended to be both entertaining and a source of interesting historical facts. Its purpose is to break up the monotony of reading and memorizing word elements; it also can serve as the source of interesting information the reader may relate to others not studying this new language.

Terminology Trivia is followed in each chapter by a pronunciation section. Both the pronunciation and the meaning of each new word presented in the chapter are listed. The last section of each chapter presents a self-test containing a sampling of the words or word elements just learned. This section may also draw on word elements presented in previous chapters by creating new words for you to interpret. A score of 90 percent or better on each of the self-tests indicates a mastery of the information. We suggest you write your answers in the spaces provided since writing tends both to reinforce your learning and to involve you actively in the process. The answers to the self-tests are listed by chapter number in the back of the book.

Using the Learning Package

This learning package is designed for use either as a self-learning module or as part of a course in medical terminology. Since the content of the package pertains to a number of different disciplines and professions, the reader might need to emphasize one area over another or to learn the topics in a different order.

It is very important that everyone read Chapters 1–4 as they are critical to the concepts of word building and interpretation. Chapters 5–15, on the other hand, contain word roots based on body systems, some of which may not be considered as important to your field of study. Chapters 16–17 similarly are relevant only to certain professions.

The sequence of topics pursued should correlate with your sequence of study. By the time the first four chapters are read, the student is sufficiently prepared to learn body systems; the focus of study in a companion course in anatomy and physiology. This type of collateral learning experience enhances acquisition of the language and aids in retention of necessary information. For persons in those fields that require they spend more time on one system than on another, this book can serve as a reference for medical words or elements not frequently used by those specialties.

The following is a selection of specialty areas within the health field and a suggested sequential reading list for each. If the sequence does not fit your course of study, be guided by the recommendation that the best sequence is the one that correlates with other subjects you are studying, particularly anatomy and physiology.

Emergency Medical Technology

Chapters	1–4	(required)
	5	Body Structure
	9	Respiratory System
	10	Cardiovascular System
	11	Skeletal System
	6	Digestive System
	8	Nervous System
	7	Genitourinary System
	14	Special Senses
	15	Endocrine System
	13	Integumentary System
	16–17	(required)

Health Education—should study the chapters in the order they are presented (1–17).

Medical Records Personnel—should study the chapters in the order they are presented (1–17).

Medical Technology (Medical Laboratory Technicians)

Chapters	1–5	(required)
	9	Cardiovascular System
	7	Genitourinary System
	15	Endocrine System
	11	Skeletal System
	12	Muscular System
	8	Nervous System
	10	Respiratory System
	6	Digestive System
	13	Integumentary System
	14	Special Senses
	16–17	(required)

Physical Therapy

Chapters	1–5	(required)
	8	Nervous System
	11	Skeletal System
	12	Muscular System
	9	Cardiovascular System
	10	Respiratory System
	6	Digestive System
	13	Integumentary System
	7	Genitourinary System
	15	Endocrine System
	14	Special Senses
	16–17	(required)

Preprofessional (Prepharmacy, Premedicine, Prenursing)—should study the chapters in the order they are presented (1–17).

Radiological Technology

Chapters	1–5	(required)
	11	Skeletal System
	12	Muscular System
	6	Digestive System
	10	Respiratory System
	9	Cardiovascular System
	8	Nervous System
	7	Genitourinary System
	15	Endocrine System
	13	Integumentary System
	14	Special Senses
	16–17	(required)

Respiratory Therapy

Chapters	1–5	(required)
	10	Respiratory System
	9	Cardiovascular System
	8	Nervous System
	11	Skeletal System
	12	Muscular System
	6	Digestive System
	7	Genitourinary System
	15	Endocrine System
	13	Integumentary System
	14	Special Senses
	16–17	(required)

Surgical Technology

Chapters	1–5	(required)
	13	Integumentary System
	6	Digestive System
	7	Genitourinary System
	10	Respiratory System
	14	Special Senses
	9	Cardiovascular System
	11	Skeletal System
	12	Muscular System
	8	Nervous System
	16–17	(required)

The most important ingredient that will ensure your success in learning medical terminology is your desire to learn. This attitude will help you have a good academic experience, especially when you remember that you will learn, in a very short time, what has taken others years of difficult and frustrating study to accomplish.

Two
Prefixes

Prefixes are elements used at the beginning of medical terms that change the meanings of the terms or make them more specific. They are never used alone, but rather as parts of other words. Most are used in ordinary speech and so do not specifically refer to medical terminology.

Sets of Prefixes

The prefixes that follow have been grouped in sets both for your convenience and to help you identify other words. For example, the prefix *prim-* means first and is found in the set of prefixes relating to time and place. The prefix *uni-* means one and is found in the set relating to number. Using our examples, primary means first in order, while unilateral means on one side.

Prefixes are presented either in their basic form or in their combining form followed by a vowel placed in parentheses. For example, *angi-* is a prefix that means vessel, while *angi(o)* is its combining form.

The prefixes in this chapter are presented as follows:

1. Prefixes Relating to Time and Place
2. Prefixes Relating to Size
3. Prefixes Relating to Type
4. Prefixes Describing Position
5. Prefixes Describing Direction
6. Prefixes Describing Number
7. Prefixes Denoting Color

Prefixes Relating to Time and Place

2.1 **ante-** before; forward

EXAMPLES:

anteflexion (ante/flexion)—abnormal bending forward
antenatal (ante/natal)—occurring before birth
antepartum (ante/partum)—before delivery

2.2 **gen-** original; originate; production; produce; formation; bring forth; arise in; be the source of; the beginning of

This is an important prefix having many applications both in medicine and in common speech.

EXAMPLES:

gene (gen/e)—the basic producer (generator) of heredity

genital (genit/al)—pertaining to reproduction or to the organs of reproduction (genit/al/ia—organs of reproduction)
genitoplasty (genit/o/plast/y)—surgical repair of the genital organs

It is also used in the form of a suffix with many medical terms;
-gen, that which produces a producer (generator) or that which is produced:

carcinogen (carcin/o/gen)—cancer producer; any cancer-producing substance
allergen (aller/gen)—allergy producer
pathogen (path/o/gen)—disease producer

2.3 **meta-** beyond; change; transformation

EXAMPLES:

metabolic (meta/bol/ic)—sum of all chemical and physical changes in the body
metacarpal (meta/carp/al)—bones of the hand (beyond the wrist)
metachrosis (meta/chr/osis)—change of color

2.4 **noct(i)-** night

EXAMPLES:

noctiphobia (noct/i/phobia)—fear of the night
nocturia (noct/uria)—urination occurring at night
nocturnal (noct/urnal)—occurring at night

2.5 **nyct-** night

EXAMPLES:

nyctalgia (nyct/algia)—pain during the night
nyctalopia (nyct/al/opia)—night blindness
nyctaphonia (nyct/a/phonia)—hysterical loss of voice occurring at night

2.6 **post-** after; behind in time; situated behind; following

EXAMPLES:

postpneumonia (post/pneumon/ia)—following pneumonia
postoral (post/or/al)—situated behind the mouth
postnatal (post/natal)—following the occurrence of birth
posterior (poster/ior)—situated in the back part of or affecting the back part of an organ
posteriad (poster/i/ad)—toward the posterior part of the body
posterolateral (poster/o/later/al)—situated behind and to one side

2.7 **pre-** in front of; before; situated before or in front of; occurring before; prior to; earlier than

EXAMPLES:

prerenal (pre/ren/al)—situated in front of the kidney
prepartal (pre/part/al)—occurring before, or just previous to, labor
prenatal (pre/nat/al)—existing or occurring before birth
preoperative (pre/operative)—preceding an operation

2.8 **prim-** first

EXAMPLES:

primary (prim/ary)—first in time or in order
primate (prim/ate)—first in the order of vertebrates belonging to the class Mammalia

primiparous (prim/i/par/ous)—having borne one child
primipara (prim/i/para)—woman with one child

2.9 **proto-** first

EXAMPLES:

protocol (proto/col)—clinical report made from first notes taken
protoplast (proto/plast)—first cells to form
prototrophic (proto/trophic)—first nourishment

2.10 **syn-, sym-** together

EXAMPLES:

syndactyly (syn/dactyl/y)—finger (digit) togetherness; the most common congenital defect of the hand—adjacent digits are more or less attached by a membranous web
symphysis (sym/phy/sis)—natural togetherness; type of joint in which the connected bones are firmly united, such as the joint formed by the various bones of the hip
synalgia (syn/algia)—pain together with; pain experienced in one area of the body as the result of soreness or injury in another area

Prefixes Relating to Size

2.11 **brachy-** short

EXAMPLES:

brachyphalangia (brachy/phal/ang/ia)—short fingers
brachypnea (brachy/pnea)—shortness of breath
brachystasis (brachy/stasis)—contracted muscle maintaining its shortened length

2.12 **lepto-** small; slender; soft; thin

EXAMPLES:

leptodermic (lepto/derm/ic)—having thin skin
leptophonia (lepto/phon/ia)—weak or soft voice
leptosome (lepto/some)—thin person

2.13 **macro-** large; enlargement

This prefix means large in the sense of abnormal size or length. The form indicating abnormal size or length usually is either macr/_____/ia or macr/_____/y.

EXAMPLES:

macropsia (macr/ops/ia)—large vision; a disturbance wherein objects are seen as larger than they really are
macrophthalmia (macr/opthalm/ia)—large eyes; abnormal enlargement of the eyeballs
macrostomia (macro/stom/ia)—large mouth; greatly exaggerated width of the mouth

2.14 **megalo-** enlarged

The form indicating abnormal condition of enlargement is megal/o/_____/ia.

EXAMPLES:

megalocardia (megal/o/card/ia)—abnormal enlargement of the heart

megalogastria (megal/o/gastr/ia)—abnormal enlargement of the stomach
megalohepatia (megal/o/hepat/ia)—abnormal enlargement of the liver

The suffix *-megaly* is more commonly used, but has the same meaning:

hepatomegaly (hepat/o/megaly)—enlarged liver
splenomegaly (splen/o/megaly)—enlarged spleen

2.15 micr- small; small size; minute, as in microscopic

This prefix is frequently used in medical terms to convey the idea of smallness. Micr/_____/ia or micr/_____/y are forms used to designate abnormally small body structures.

EXAMPLES:

microblepharia (micr/o/blephar/ia)—small eyelids
microcephaly (micr/o/cephal/y)—small head
microcardia (micr/o/card/ia)—small heart
microangi (micr/o/angi)—small blood vessels
microscopic (micr/o/scop/ic)—of extremely small size; visible only with the aid of a microscope
microsurgery (micr/o/surgery)—dissection of small structures under a microscope

This prefix illustrates some of the distinctions in the use of synonymous or related elements:

microphthalmia (micr/ophthalm/ia)—abnormally small eyes
micropsia (micr/ops/ia)—condition in which objects are seen as smaller than they really are
micrencephaly (micr/en/cephal/y)—abnormally small brain

2.16 olig(o)- small; few

EXAMPLES:

oliguria (olig/ur/ia)—small production of urine
oligocytosis (olig/o/cyt/osis)—deficiency of red blood corpuscles
oligodentia (olig/o/dent/ia)—fewer teeth than normal because of a developmental anomaly

Prefixes Relating to Type

2.17 ambly- dull

EXAMPLES:

amblyaphia (ambly/aphia)—dull sense of touch
amblyopia (ambly/opia)—dull vision

2.18 an-, a- without; not; lacking; weakness; deficiency

This is a frequently used prefix that can be attached to a word to indicate its negative or opposite aspect. It is most often used to mean without, either in the sense of a lack, a deficiency, or a weakness.

Note: An- is the form of the prefix used before vowels (a,e,i,o,u and usually h); the form used before all other letters (the consonants) is *a-*.

EXAMPLES:

anemia (an/em/ia)—deficiency of red blood cells
anesthesia (an/esthesia)—lack of feeling; unconsciousness
atrophy (a/trophy)—lacking development of growth; wasting away or

diminution in the size of a cell, tissue, organ, or part due to a nutritional defect

2.19 **andro-** male; man; masculine

EXAMPLES:

androgen (andro/gen)—male sex hormone
androgynous (andro/gyn/ous)—without definite sexual characteristics (*andro* refers to male, while *gyn* refers to female)

2.20 **angi(o)-** vessel; duct; blood vessel

EXAMPLES:

angiocarditis (angi/o/card/itis)—inflammation of the heart's large blood vessels
angiodermatitis (angi/o/dermat/itis)—inflammation of cutaneous vessels
angiospasm (angio/spasm)—contraction of a blood vessel

2.21 **ankyl(o)-** crooked; bent; fusion or a growing together

EXAMPLES:

ankylosed (ankyl/o/sed)—fused joint
ankylosis (ankyl/osis)—fixation of a joint due to disease
ankylotia (ankyl/otia)—closure of external ear

2.22 **auto-** self

EXAMPLES:

autodiagnosis (auto/dia/gnosis)—self-diagnosis of disease
automatic (auto/matic)—spontaneous or self-acting
autonomic (auto/nomic)—self-controlling

2.23 **basi-** base; the thing or part on which something rests; lowest part or bottom; foundation

EXAMPLES:

basal (bas/al)—pertaining to or situated near a base; fundamental
basilysis (basi/lysis)—the crushing of the base of the fetal skull to facilitate delivery

2.24 **brady-** slow; slowness; abnormally slow physical or mental process

This prefix is descriptive and usually can be interpreted either as slowness or abnormal slowness.

EXAMPLES:

bradycardia (brady/card/ia)—slow heartbeat (usually less than 60 beats per minute)
myobradia (my/o/brad/ia)—slow, sluggish reaction of muscle to electrical stimulation

Brady- is an interesting illustration of the use of a single prefix to describe different causes of similar symptoms:

bradyglossia (brady/glossia)—abnormal slowness of mechanical speech (the forming of sounds to express speech)
bradylogia (brady/log/ia)—abnormal slowness of speech due to slowness of thinking, as in a mental disorder

Note that physical difficulty in forming words is conveyed by the use of *gloss-* (tongue), the principal organ used in the formation of speech sounds, while the use of *log-* (*-ology* or study of) implies difficulty with a mental process. The application of the element *log-* for the mental process makes sense when we remember that the original meaning of *log-* was "discourse" or "speaking on." An *-ologist*, a student of a subject, had the ability to speak on the subject.

2.25 **co-, com-, con-** with; together

Note: The consonant that follows *co-* usually is determined by which consonant begins the word root.

EXAMPLES:

commissure (com/missure)—coming together of two structures
conception (con/ception)—joining together of sperm and ovum; fertilization
congenital (con/genital)—born together; present at birth

2.26 **cryo-** cold

EXAMPLES:

cryotherapy (cryo/therap/y)—therapeutic use of cold
hematocryal (hemat/o/cry/al)—cold blooded
cryosurgery (cryo/surgery)—destruction of tissue by the application of extreme cold in, for example, the treatment of malignant skin tumors

2.27 **dura, scirrh-, scler-** hard

All three elements refer to hardness. Dura is used principally as a shortened name for the dura mater, the hard outer covering of the brain and spinal cord. An important exception to this usage is the word induration (in/dur/ation), which refers to hardness or the process of hardening. The word scirrhous is most usually used in reference to a hard, cancerous tumor. The word sclerotic can mean hardness, while sclera refers to the white part of the eye.

2.28 **dys-** difficult; painful; bad

EXAMPLES:

dysentery (dys/entery)—inflammation of the intestines caused by a variety of bacterial or viral agents
dyslexia (dys/lexia)—difficulty in reading, writing, and learning
dysmenorrhea (dys/men/o/rrhea)—painful or difficult menstruation

2.29 **eu-** healthy; normal; good; well

EXAMPLES:

eugenics (eu/gen/ics)—improvement of the human race through genetic control
euphonia (eu/phon/ia)—having a clear voice
euthanasia (eu/than/asia)—dying quietly and peacefully

2.30 **gyno-, gyneco-** woman; female

EXAMPLES:

gynecology (gynec/ology)—study of women's health problems
gynecopathy (gynec/o/pathy)—diseases peculiar to women
gyniatric (gyn/i/atric)—treatment of women's diseases

2.31 **heter-, hetero-** relationship to another; different

EXAMPLES:

heterosexual (hetero/sexual)—belonging to the other sex

heterotopia (hetero/top/ia)—development of normal tissue in an unusual area of the body

heterotopy (hetero/topy)—displacement of an organ or a part of the body

2.32 **homeo-** unchanged; resemblance

EXAMPLES:

homeoplastic (homeo/plast/ic)—resembling the structure of adjacent parts

homeostasis (homeo/stasis)—state of equilibrium

2.33 **homo-** likeness; same

EXAMPLES:

homologous (hom/o/log/ous)—same fundamental structure

homosexual (homo/sexual)—same sex

homotonic (homo/tonic)—same or uniform tension

2.34 **hydra-, hydro-** water; fluid, particularly the accumulation of fluid in a body part

Note: The prefix *hydro-* may also appear as either *hidr-* when referring to a sweat gland or as *hygr-* when referring to moisture.

EXAMPLES:

hydric (hydr/ic)—pertaining to water

hidrocystoma (hidro/cyst/oma)—cyst (pouch, bag) of the sweat gland consisting of retained (nonsecreted) sweat

hydrocyst (hydro/cyst)—cyst (pouch, bag) filled with water

hydremia (hydr/em/ia)—watery state of the blood

2.35 **iso-** equal; alike; the same

This prefix is frequently used to indicate sameness.

EXAMPLES:

isocellular (iso/cell/ul/ar)—composed of cells of the same size and kind

isopia (is/op/ia)—equality of vision in the two eyes

The prefix *iso-* also can be combined with the prefix *an-*, meaning not, to indicate an inequality:

anisodont (an/is/odont)—having teeth of unequal size or length

anisopia (an/is/op/ia)—inequality of vision in the two eyes

anisomastia (an/iso/mast/ia)—inequality in the size of the breasts

2.36 **mal-** bad; irregular; abnormal; faulty; poor (in the sense of inadequate or insufficient)

EXAMPLES:

maldigestion (mal/digestion)—faulty or impaired digestion

malformation (mal/formation)—defective or abnormal formation; deformity

malpractice (mal/practice)—improper or injurious practice; unskillful and faulty medical or surgical treatment

2.37 **neo-** new; recent

EXAMPLES:

neonatal (neo/natal)—new born; pertaining to the first four weeks after birth

neopathy (neo/path/y)—new disease; a new condition or the complication of disease in a patient

neoplasm (neo/plasm)—any new and abnormal growth, such as a tumor

Both *plast-* and *-plasia* contain the root element *plas-*, which denotes a forming or formation. The suffix *-plasm* indicates formative or formed material. The reference in medical terminology usually is to the formation of cells or tissues.

2.38 **orth(o)-** straight; normal

EXAMPLES:

orthodontic (ortho/dont/ic)—straight teeth

orthograde (orth/o/grade)—walking upright; a normal stance

2.39 **path-, path(o)-** disease; suffering; feeling

EXAMPLES:

pathic (path/ic)—pertaining to disease or feeling

pathosis (path/osis)—condition of disease

pathologic (path/o/logic)—diseased

The suffix *-pathy* can be combined with various parts of the body to denote any disease:

adenopathy (aden/o/path/y)—any disease of a gland

angiopathy (angi/o/path/y)—any disease of a blood vessel

arthropathy (arthr/o/path/y)—any disease of a joint

2.40 **phag-, phag(o)-** eat; consume; ingest

EXAMPLES:

phagocyte (phag/o/cyte)—cell that can ingest

phagomania (phag/o/mania)—abnormal craving to eat

2.41 **pseudo-** false

EXAMPLES:

pseudocyst (pseudo/cyst)—dilation resembling a cyst

pseudoesthesia (pseudo/esthes/ia)—imaginary or false sensation

pseudotyphoid (pseudo/typhoid)—condition resembling typhoid but one not caused by the typhoid bacteria

2.42 **steno-** narrow; contracted; constricted; close

This prefix can be applied to any body structure term when indicating less than normal width.

EXAMPLES:

stenocephalous (steno/cephal/ous)—having a narrow head

stenocephalia (steno/cephal/ia)—excessive narrowness of the head

stenostomia (steno/stom/ia)—narrowing of the mouth

Stenosis (steno/sis) refers to the constriction of a passage in the body, such as a duct or canal, causing interference with the flow of material:

stenosis, -stenosis (steno/sis, -steno/sis)—narrowing of a duct or canal

angiostenosis (angi/o/steno/sis)—narrowing of the diameter of a vessel
enterostenosis (enter/o/steno/sis)—narrowing of the intestine

Stricture refers to the abnormal narrowing of a canal, duct, or passage. This results either from the accumulation of healing tissue (such as scar tissue), from the deposit of normal tissue, from inflammation (swelling), or from a spasm.

2.43 **tachy-** fast; swift; rapid

EXAMPLES:

tachycardia (tachy/cardia)—rapid heart action
tachyphagia (tachy/phag/ia)—rapid eating
tachypnea (tachy/pnea)—rapid respiration

2.44 **terat(o)-** malformed fetus

EXAMPLES:

teratoid (terat/oid)—resembling a malformed fetus
teratoma (terat/oma)—unusual tumor composed of malformed tissues, none of which is native to the area in which it occurs
teratophobia (terato/phobia)—abnormal fear of giving birth to a malformed fetus

2.45 **therm(o)-** hot; heat; warmth

EXAMPLES:

thermocautery (therm/o/caut/ery)—cauterization by means of heat application
thermogenesis (therm/o/genesis)—production of heat
thermometer (therm/o/meter)—an instrument for measuring heat (temperature)

2.46 **toxic-** poison

EXAMPLES:

toxicoderma (toxic/o/derm/a)—skin disease resulting from poison
toxicosis (toxic/osis)—disease condition resulting from poison
toxigenic (toxi/genic)—producing poisons

Prefixes Describing Position

2.47 **acro-** extremities; tip; end; top or peak; extremity of the body; outermost portion

The word extremity is a general medical term used to designate an end portion of an organ or body part; a part located away from the center of the body or away from a point of attachment.

In skeletal anatomy (bone parts and structures), the extremities technically include: bones of the shoulders and hips; bones of the wrists and ankles; and, bones of the hands and feet. In general usage, extremity or extremities may refer to: arms and legs; wrists and ankles; feet and hands; toes and fingers. No matter its reference, extremity (*acro-*) always points to the farthest end(s) or to parts leading to the farthest end(s).

EXAMPLES:

acrodermatitis (acro/dermat/itis)—inflammation of the skin of the hands or feet

acromegaly (acro/megal/y)—enlargement of the extremities of the skeleton—the fingers, toes, nose, and jaw (also megal/acr/ia)

acrocyanosis (acro/cyan/osis)—blue discoloration of the extremities—the fingers, toes, wrists, and ankles

2.48 **anti-** against; opposing; counteracting (acting against); inhibiting; preventing; neutralizing; destroying

This prefix is most often used to mean against.

EXAMPLES:

antigen (anti/gen)—substance that, when introduced into the body, stimulates the production of an opposing substance called an antibody (anti/body)

antibody (anti/body)—physical substance, either in the body or produced by the action of an antigen, that prevents, relieves, or destroys infections or poisonous substances in the blood or tissues

anticoagulant (anti/coagulant)—substance that suppresses or opposes the coagulation of blood

2.49 **contra-** against; counter; in opposition to; a thing opposite to or against another

This prefix may be attached to a word or stem to mean either opposite to or against some action or thing.

EXAMPLES:

contraction (contr/action)—acts against; a shortening (a muscle contraction, for example)

contraception (contra/ception)—that which acts against conception; the prevention of pregnancy

contrastimulant (contra/stimulant)—that which acts against stimulation; a medicine or action intended to overcome or alleviate stimulation

The prefix *counter-* carries the same meanings as the prefix *contr-* (against or opposite to). It is also used to indicate an opposite direction:

counteropening, counterincision (counter/opening, counter/incision)—second incision made opposite to an earlier one to promote drainage in, for example, an abscess

counterirritation (counter/irritation)—irritation that is intended to relieve some other irritation

2.50 **ecto-** situated on the outside; outside

EXAMPLES:

ectosteal (ect/oste/al)—pertaining to or situated on the outside of a bone

ectocytic (ecto/cyt/ic)—outside the cell

ectopic (ecto/p/ic)—outside the expected place, such as an ectopic pregnancy outside the uterus

2.51 **en-** in; within; inside

The prefix *em-* is the form usually used when the word part following it begins with any one of the letters *b*, *m*, or *p*.

EXAMPLES:

empathy (em/path/y)—entering into the feelings of another person

encephal- (en/cephal-)—within the head; usually refers to the brain; however, the reference may be to other conditions within the head, such as encephalalgia (pain within the head, or headache)

enostosis (en/ost/osis)—abnormal bony growth that develops within the cavity of a bone

2.52 **end-, ent-** inside; within; inner

This prefix is generally used to indicate the inside of some body part. For example, it may refer to the inner lining (usually a membrane) of a structure, taking the form end/o/____/ium.

EXAMPLES:

endometrium (end/o/metri/um)—inner lining of the uterus

endocardium (end/o/cardi/um)—inner membrane of the heart

It may also refer to the inside of a structure or organ taking the form end/o/____/al:

endarterial (end/arter/i/al)—within an artery

endocardial (end/o/cardi/al)—situated or occurring within the heart; pertaining to the endocardium

Additionally, it may indicate a state or condition, taking the form end/o/____/itis or end/o/____/osis:

endangiitis (end/angi/itis)—inflammation of the inner lining of a blood vessel

endocarditis (end/o/card/itis)—inflammation of the lining of the heart

entostosis (ent/ost/osis)—abnormal bony growth within the hollow interior of a bone

2.53 **epi-** upon; in addition

This prefix is used extensively to name tissue structures or regions of the body in relation to other body parts.

EXAMPLES:

epidermis (epi/derm/is)—outer skin; the outermost layer of skin; also called epiderm

epicyst- (epi/cyst-)—over the bladder; the structures above the bladder

epigastrium (epi/gastr/ium)—over the stomach; the upper middle region of the abdomen

2.54 **ex-** out; away; from; out of; outside of

EXAMPLES:

exostosis (ex/ost/osis)—condition (bony growth) projecting outward from the surface of a bone

extensor (ex/tens/or)—that which stretches (extends); for example, a muscle that extends a joint

2.55 **exo-** outside; outward; outer

EXAMPLES:

exogenic (exo/gen/ic)—produced outside; developing or originating from some cause outside the body

exopathy (exo/path/y)—outside disease; a disease originating from some cause outside the body

2.56 extra- outside of; beyond

EXAMPLES:

extracardial (extra/cardi/al)—outside the heart
extrahepatic (extra/hepat/ic)—situated or occurring outside the liver

2.57 fore- before; in front of

EXAMPLES:

forebrain (fore/brain)—anterior portion of the brain
foregut (fore/gut)—first part of the embryonic gut
forehead (fore/head)—anterior part of the head

2.58 hyper- above; excessive; more than normal

EXAMPLES:

hyperalgia (hyper/algia)—excessive pain; excessive sensitivity to pain
hyperemia (hyper/em/ia)—excessive blood in a body part
hypernormal (hyper/normal)—in excess of what is normal

2.59 hypo- under; beneath; deficient

This prefix is used most frequently to mean deficient in or less than normal.

EXAMPLES:

hypoadenia (hypo/aden/ia)—abnormally diminished glandular activity (also hypo/glandular)
hypohepatia (hypo/hepat/ia)—deficient functioning of the liver
hypotension (hypo/tension)—diminished tension; lowered blood pressure; low blood pressure

The prefix *hypo-* may also be used to mean underneath or beneath in space:

hypodermic (hypo/derm/ic)—underneath the skin; for example, a hypodermic needle is one inserted below the skin
hypogastrium (hypo/gastr/ium)—lowest part of the abdomen.

2.60 infra- beneath

EXAMPLES:

inframammary (infra/mamm/ary)—beneath the mammary gland
inframandibular (infra/mandibu/lar)—beneath the jaw
infracostal (infra/cost/al)—beneath rib or ribs

2.61 inter- between

This prefix is frequently used to identify an area between or among the parts or structures named in the second word element.

EXAMPLES:

interlabial (inter/labi/al)—between lips
intermuscular (inter/muscul/ar)—between muscles
interdigital (inter/digit/al)—between adjacent fingers or toes

2.62 intra- within; situated within; occurring within

EXAMPLES:

intraspinal (intra/spin/al)—situated or occurring within the vertebral column
intraoperative (intra/operative)—occurring within the course of a surgical operation

A variation of *intra-* is the prefix *intro-*, which means either into or insertion into.

2.63 **later-** side

EXAMPLES:

lateral (later/al)—pertaining to a side; also, denoting a position farther from the middle or midline of the body or from a structure

laterad (later/ad)—toward a side

lateroposition (later/o/position)—displacement to one side

2.64 **medi-, meso-** middle

EXAMPLES:

medial (medi/al)—near the midline of the body

mesoaortitis (meso/aort/itis)—inflammation of the aortic artery's middle coat

mesoderm (meso/derm)—middle layer of skin

2.65 **para-** beside; by the side; at the side of; to one side; side by side; beyond; wrong; faulty

EXAMPLES:

paracystitis (para/cyst/itis)—inflammation of the tissues around the urinary bladder

paralysis (para/lysis)—faulty or lost power of movement in a part of the body

2.66 **peri-** about; around

This prefix is used to designate the area or space around a body part.

EXAMPLES:

periodontal (peri/odont/al)—situated or occurring around a tooth

periosteoma (peri/oste/oma)—morbid bony growth surrounding a bone

periadenitis (peri/aden/itis)—inflammation of the tissues around a gland

It can also be used to identify a tissue that covers, surrounds, or encloses a part of the body. When used in this sense, the term takes either the peri/o/____/ium or peri/o/____/eum form:

periosteum (peri/oste/um)—specialized connective tissue covering all bones of the body

pericardium (peri/card/ium)—fibrous sac surrounding the heart

2.67 **pro-** in front of; before

EXAMPLES:

prochondral (pro/chondr/al)—occurring before the formation of cartilage

prolabium (pro/labi/um)—prominent central part of the upper lip; the philtrum

prolapse (pro/lapse)—slipping forward (or out of place) of an organ or part of the body; a displacement (lapse means a fall)

proptosis (pro/ptosis)—forward displacement

2.68 **schisto-, schizo-** split; divide

EXAMPLES:

schistothorax (schisto/thorax)—surgically splitting or dividing the thorax

schizophrenia (schizo/phren/ia)—complex mental disorder, described as split personality
schizonychia (schizo/nych/ia)—split fingernails

2.69 **sub-** under; beneath; below

EXAMPLES:

subdermal (sub/derm/al)—situated or occurring under the skin
subnormal (sub/norm/al)—below or less than normal
sublingual (sub/lingu/al)—located beneath the tongue; also, subglossal

2.70 **supra-** above; over

EXAMPLES:

supracerebral (supra/cerebr/al)—situated above or on the surface of the cerebrum
supracostal (supra/cost/al)—situated above or on a rib or ribs
suprahepatic (supra/hepat/ic)—situated above the liver

There is a closely related prefix, *super-*, that means either over (usually in the sense of an upper part) or excessive:

supercerebral (super/cerebr/al)—in the upper part of the cerebrum (compare with supracerebral above)
superacute (super/acute)—extremely acute
superior (super/ior)—situated above; directed upward; used in anatomy to designate the upper surface of an organ or structure

2.71 **trans-** through; across; beyond

The use of the prefix *trans-* to mean through is encountered frequently in the description of operating techniques to describe the type of approach being made.

EXAMPLES:

transparent (trans/parent)—light passing through a substance
transdermic (trans/derm/ic)—through the skin

It is also used to mean across, in the sense of a movement across, a carrying across, or a transfer across:

transfusion (trans/fus/ion)—the introduction of blood from another source; a pouring across of blood (*fus-* means to pour)
transplant (trans/plant)—piece of tissue used for grafting, taken from another part of the patient's body or from a donor; planting across parts

Additionally, the prefix *trans-* can be used to mean beyond, in the sense of more than:

transnormal (trans/normal)—beyond the norm; more than normal

Prefixes Describing Direction

2.72 **ab-** away from

This prefix takes the form *a-* when the word part following it begins with any one of the letters *m*, *p*, or *v*; *abs-* is used before the letter *c* or *t*.

EXAMPLES:

abnormal (ab/normal)—away from the norm; departing from normal
avulsion (a/vuls/ion)—pulling away from a structure (vulsion means pulling)

2.73 **ad-** to; toward; increase

EXAMPLES:

adduct (ad/duct)—move toward the midline
adductor (ad/duct/or)—muscle that draws toward the midline

2.74 **de-** down; from; away from

EXAMPLES:

decay (de/cay)—waste away from normal
decontaminate (de/contamin/ate)—render free from a contaminating substance
dehydrate (de/hydr/ate)—take away water

2.75 **dextro-** right

EXAMPLES:

dextrocardia (dextro/card/ia)—heart located in the right side of the chest
dextrotropic (dextro/tropic)—turning to the right

2.76 **e-, ex-** out; away from

EXAMPLES:

enuncleate (e/nuncle/ate)—remove from
exhale (ex/hale)—breathe out
expel (ex/pel)—drive out

2.77 **in-, im-** in; inside; within; not

EXAMPLES:

inactive (in/active)—not working
incontinent (in/con/tin/ent)—not able to retain urine or feces
incorporate (in/corpor/ate)—combine into one

2.78 **ir-** against; into; toward

EXAMPLES:

irradiate (ir/radi/ate)—radiate (x-rays) into some thing
irrigate (ir/rig/ate)—wash into

2.79 **retro-** backward

EXAMPLES:

retraction (retr/action)—the act of drawing back
retractor (retr/actor)—instrument for drawing back the edges of a wound
retrocardiac (retro/cardi/ac)—behind the heart

2.80 **sinistr(o)-** left

EXAMPLES:

sinistrocular (sinistr/ocular)—having stronger vision in the left eye
sinistrous (sinistr/ous)—awkward or clumsy; the opposite of dexterous

Prefixes Describing Number

The prefixes in this section are presented in ascending order.

2.81 **null(i)-** none

EXAMPLES:

nullipara (null/i/para)—woman with no children
nulliparity (null/i/parity)—never having given birth

2.82 **demi-** half

EXAMPLES:

demilune (demi/lune)—half-moon shaped serous cells
demibain (demi/bain)—half a bath; sitz bath

2.83 **hemi-** half; relating to or affecting one half or one side; part of

EXAMPLES:

hemialgia (hemi/algia)—pain affecting one side of the body only
hemicrania (hemi/cran/ia)—pain or aching on one side of the head
hemihepatectomy (hemi/hepat/ectomy)—surgical removal of half the liver

2.84 **semi-** half; partially

EXAMPLES:

semicomatose (semi/coma/tose)—partially conscious; arousable
semilunar (semi/lunar)—resembling a crescent or half-moon
seminormal (semi/normal)—one half the normal strength

2.85 **mono-** one

EXAMPLES:

monorchid (mon/orchid)—having one testicle
monospasm (mono/spasm)—spasm of one limb or part
monovalent (mono/valent)—having the combining power of a single hydrogen atom

2.86 **uni-** one

EXAMPLES:

unit (unit)—one of anything
unilateral (uni/lateral)—affecting only one side

2.87 **bi-** two; double; both

EXAMPLES:

bigeminy (bi/gemin/y)—the condition of occurring in pairs, such as the occurrence of two beats of the pulse in rapid succession
bipedal (bi/ped/al)—with, or pertaining to, both feet
bifurcate (bi/furc/ate)—divide into two branches

This prefix may also appear in the form *bin-*, meaning two or both:

binaural (bin/aur/al)—pertaining to both ears; a synonym for binotic (bin/ot/ic)
binocular (bin/ocul/ar)—pertaining to both eyes

2.88 **gemin-** twin; double; pair

EXAMPLES:

geminate (gemin/ate)—paired; occurring in pairs; a synonym for bigeminal (bi/gemin/al)
geminus (gemin/us)—twin
gemini (gemin/i)—twins

2.89 **tri-** three; having, combining, or involving three; triply; in three ways or directions; three times; every three; every third

EXAMPLES:

trifurcation (tri/furc/ation)—division into three parts; literally, three forks

trilateral (tri/later/al)—pertaining to or having three sides

trilobate (tri/lob/ate)—having three lobes

2.90 **tetr(a)-** four

EXAMPLES:

tetrad (tetr/ad)—group of four with something in common

tetragenous (tetra/genous)—organisms that divide into groups of four

tetrasomic (tetra/somic)—having four chromosomes where ordinarily there would be two

2.91 **quadr(i)-** four

EXAMPLES:

quadrant (quad/rant)—one of four regions

quadriplegia (quadr/i/plegia)—paralysis of all four limbs

2.92 **pan-** all

EXAMPLES:

panhysterectomy (pan/hyster/ectomy)—surgical removal of the entire uterus and cervix

pancarditis (pan/card/itis)—inflammation of the entire heart, involving the outer covering (peri/card/itis), the muscular wall (my/o/card/itis), and the linings of the cavities (end/o/card/itis)

pantalgia (pant/algia)—pain over the entire body

pancytopenia (pan/cyto/pen/ia)—decreased numbers of all cells in the blood

2.93 **poly-** many; much

EXAMPLES:

polyacoustic (poly/acoust/ic)—much sound; increasing or intensifying sound

polycythemia (poly/cyt/hem/ia)—excessive number of cells in the blood

polyemia (poly/em/ia)—excessive amount of blood in the body

This prefix may be used to indicate a single condition involving many similar body parts or organs:

polyadenitis (poly/aden/itis)—inflammation of several or many glands; synonyms are polyadenoma (poly/aden/oma), polyadenopathy (poly/aden/o/path/y), and polyadenosis (poly/aden/osis)

polydysplasia (poly/dys/plas/ia)—faulty development in several types of tissues or several organs or systems

Prefixes Denoting Color

2.94 **alb-** white

EXAMPLES:

albino (alb/in/o)—an individual affected with white skin due to an hereditary lack of pigment

albicans (albi/cans)—whitish
albinuria (alb/in/uria)—white or colorless urine

2.95 chloro- green

EXAMPLES:

chloroma (chlor/oma)—green-colored tumor
chloropsia (chlor/opsia)—vision defect in which all objects appear to be tinted green
chloroplast (chloro/plast)—green body found in cells of plants

2.96 cirrh- yellow

EXAMPLES:

cirrhosis (cirrh/osis)—yellowing (jaundiced) chronic liver condition
cirrhotic (cirrh/otic)—affected with cirrhosis

2.97 cyano- blue; dark blue

EXAMPLES:

cyanomycosis (cyano/myc/osis)—pus colored blue due to a fungus infection
cyanopathy (cyano/pathy)—blue skin
cyanosis (cyan/osis)—bluish discoloration due to low oxygen

2.98 erythro- red

EXAMPLES:

erythema (eryth/ema)—eruption of the skin marked by redness and swelling
erythralgia (erythr/algia)—condition marked by pain and redness of the skin

The term erythrocyte (erythr/o/cyte), meaning red blood cell, is a frequently used combination:

erythrocytopenia (erythr/o/cyt/o/penia)—deficiency in the number of red blood cells; a synonym for erythropenia (erythr/o/pen/ia)
erythrocythemia (erythr/o/cyt/hem/ia)—increase in the number of red blood cells

2.99 leuk- white

EXAMPLES:

leukemia, leukocythemia (leuk/em/ia, leuk/o/cyt/hem/ia)—frequently fatal condition in which there is an overproduction of white blood cells in the tissues
leukocyte (leuk/o/cyt/e)—white (colorless) blood cell

Because there are so many conditions characterized by an increase in the number of leukocytes in the blood, a variety of suffixes may be attached to the leukocyt- stem:

leukocytosis (leuk/o/cyt/osis)—slight increase in the number of leukocytes in the blood
leukocytoma (leuk/o/cyt/oma)—tumor-like mass of leukocytes

2.100 melan- black

EXAMPLES:

melanin (melan/in)—black or dark brown pigment found in the skin and hair

melanocyte (melan/o/cyt/e)—cell responsible for the production of black pigment
melanodermic, melanous (melan/o/derm/ic, melan/ous)—having dark skin
melanemia (melan/em/ia)—condition in which the blood contains a black or dark brown pigment

2.101 rube- red

EXAMPLES:
rubedo (rube/do)—temporary redness of the skin
rubescent (rube/scent)—becoming red or flushed
rubor (rub/or)—redness caused by inflammation

2.102 xantho- yellow

EXAMPLES:
xanthocyte (xantho/cyte)—cell with yellow pigment
xanthoderma (xantho/derma)—yellow skin
xanthopsis (xanth/opsis)—yellow pigment seen in some cancers and degenerating tissues

Terminology Trivia

Early Medical Theories

In the days of Pliny, Cicero, and Caesar (100 B.C.–20 A.D.), the practice of medicine was considered a profession only for slaves; Roman patricians, or nobles, were forbidden by law to participate. Early East Indian medicine held fever to be the cause of all diseases, resulting from the anger of the god, Siva. According to ancient Greek physiology, diseases resulted from disturbances in the red, yellow, black, and white humors of the body.

The Miasmic (refers to noxious air) Theory of disease, popular in Pasteur's time, implicated odor as the main cause of disease, and certain fragrances were thought to have curative properties. Along this line, the current children's rhyme, ring-around-the-rosies, actually comes from the time of the Bubonic Plague in England when people tried to counteract the disease with the sweet fragrance of flowers. We place flowers on graves today as part of this tradition; an attempt to counter the effects of breathing air fouled by decomposition. Not coincidentally, malaria is a disease named for breathing "mal" (the French word for "bad") air, at one time thought to be its cause. It is, of course, a protozoan-caused disease transmitted by the mosquito.

Pronunciation and Meaning of New Terms

acrodermatitis (ak″ ro der″ mah ti′ tis) Inflammation of the skin on the hands or feet.

adductor (ad duk′ tor) Any muscle responsible for adduction, or drawing toward the midline of the body.

adenopathy (ad″ ē nop′ ah the) Enlargement of glands, especially of the lymph nodes.

anatomy (ah nat′ o me) The science of the structure of living organisms.

anemia (ah ne′ me ah) A condition in which the blood is deficient in red blood cells and/or hemoglobin.
aplastic a., anemia caused by a disease of the bone marrow, characterized by absence of regeneration of red blood cells.
sickle cell a., a genetically caused defect of hemoglobin synthesis, occurring almost exclusively in blacks, characterized by the presence of sickle-shaped erythrocytes in the blood and homozygosity for S hemoglobin. Other symptoms include arthralgia, acute abdominal pain, and ulcerations of the legs.

angiospasm (an′ je o spazm″) Spasmodic contraction of the blood vessels.

antenatal (an″ te na′ tal) Occurring or formed before birth; prenatal.

antibody (an′ tī bod″ e) An immunoglobulin molecule that interacts only with the specific antigen that induced its synthesis or with a closely related antigen.

cirrhosis (sir ro′ sis) A chronic liver disease characterized by marked degeneration of liver cells with eventual increased resistance to flow of blood through the liver.

contraception (kon″ trah sep′ shun) Prevention of conception or impregnation.

cyanosis (si″ ah no′ sis) Blue discoloration of the skin.

dysentery (dis′ en ter″ e) Any of a number of disorders marked by inflammation of the intestine, especially the large intestine, with abdominal pain and frequent stools.

erythrocyte (ē rith′ ro sīt) A red blood cell.
e. count, enumeration of the number of red blood cells in a blood sample.

erythrocytopenia (ē rith″ ro si″ to pe′ ne ah) A deficiency in the number of red blood cells; anemia.

epididymis (ep″ ī did′ ī mis) The elongated cordlike structure along the posterior border of the testis, which provides for storage, transit, and maturation of spermatozoa and is continuous with the ductus deferens.

hyperalgia (hi per al′ je ah) Excessive sensitivity to pain.

lateral (lat′ er al) Pertaining to a side; denoting a position farther from the median plane or midline of the body or of a structure.

mesoderm (mes′ o derm) In embryology, the middle layer of cells in the blastoderm.

metacarpal (met″ ah kar′ pal) Pertaining to the metacarpus; one of the bones of the metacarpus.

orthodontics (or″ tho don′ tiks) That branch of dentistry concerned with irregularities of teeth and malocclusions, and associated facial problems.

orthopedic (or″ tho pe′ dik) Pertaining to the correction of deformities of the musculoskeletal system.

phagocytize (fag′ o sīt″ iz) To eat or ingest by phagocytosis.

phagomania (fag″ o ma′ ne ah) An abnormal craving for food; obsessive preoccupation with eating.

posterior (pos tēr′ e or) Situated behind.

posteroexternal (pos″ ter o ek ster′ nal) Situated on the outside of a posterior part.

prenatal (pre na′ tal) Referring to the time period before birth.

prolapse (pro laps′) Dropping or sagging of a body part.

retrocardiac (ret″ ro kar′ de ak) Behind the heart.

sublingual (sub ling′ gwal) Situated under the tongue.

subnormal (sub nor′ mal) Below normal.

superior (soo pe′ re or) Situated above, or directed upward.

supracostal (soo″ prah kos′ tal) Above or outside the ribs.

suprahepatic (soo″ prah he pat′ ik) Above the liver.

tachycardia (tak″ e kar′ de ah) Fast heart beat; fast pulse.

tachyphagia (tak″ e fa′ je ah) Rapid eating.

tachypnea (tak″ ip ne′ ah) Rapid breathing.

thermometer (ther mom′ ē ter) Instrument used for measuring temperature.

toxicosis (tok″ sī ko′ sis) Any disease condition due to poisoning.

xanthoderma (zan″ tho der′ mah) A yellow coloration of the skin.

xanthosis (zan tho′ sis) A yellow condition, especially of the skin.

Self-test

1. Match Column A with Column B. Items in Column B may be used more than once.

Column A	*Column B*
___ ante-	a. beyond, over, between, change
___ gen-	b. night
___ meta-	c. together, union
___ noct(i)-	d. before
___ nyct-	e. first
___ post-	f. after
___ pre-	g. beginning, origin
___ prim-	
___ proto-	
___ sym-	
___ syn-	

2.

Column A	*Column B*
___ acro-	a. on, upon, over
___ anti-	b. within
___ contra-	c. above, excessive, beyond
___ ecto-	d. extremity, tip
___ endo-	e. opposite, against
___ epi-	f. before, in front of
___ fore-	g. outside, misplaced
___ hyper-	h. against

3.

Column A	*Column B*
___ infra-	a. around
___ inter-	b. excessive, extreme
___ intra-	c. between parts
___ medi-, meso-	d. beside, beyond
___ para-	e. below
___ peri-	f. excessive
___ schisto-	g. within a part
___ sub-	h. beneath
___ super-	i. middle
___ supra-	j. above, over
___ trans-	k. split, divided
	l. across, through
	m. situated, formed or occurring between

4.

Column A	*Column B*
___ a-, an-	a. dull
___ ambly-	b. self
___ andro-	c. without
___ angi(o)-	d. slow
___ ankyl(o)-	e. crooked, bent
___ auto-	f. cold
___ brady-	g. with
___ co-, com-, con-	h. male
___ cryo-	i. difficult, abnormal
___ dys-	j. vessel, duct
	k. dullness

5.

Column A	*Column B*
___ eu-	a. other, different
___ gyno-	b. good, normal
___ hetero-	c. female
___ homo-	d. bad
___ hydra-, hydro-	e. peculiar to the individual
___ iso-	f. new, strange, separate, distinct
___ mal-	g. water
___ neo-	h. same
___ ortho-	i. equal
	j. broad, wide
	k. straight, normal

6.

Column A	*Column B*
___ path(o)-	a. disease
___ phag(o)-	b. fast
___ pseudo-	c. malformed, monster
___ scler-	d. eat, consume
___ steno-	e. rough
___ tachy-	f. heat, warmth
___ terato-	g. false
___ thermo-	h. hard
___ toxic-	i. behind, backward
___ trachy-	j. straight, erect
	k. contracted, narrowing
	l. poison

7.

Column A	*Column B*
c ab-	a. away, not, down
e ad-	b. forward, anterior
a de-	c. away from
f dextro-	d. against, into, toward
k e-	e. to, toward
g ex-	f. right
h im-, in-	g. away from, out
d ir-	h. in, inside, within
i levo-, sinistro-	i. left
l pro-, proso-	j. behind, backward
j retro-	k. out
	l. before, in front of

8. Fill in the meaning of the prefix.

Prefix	*Meaning*
a. demi-	one half
b. mono-	one
c. pan-	all
d. bi-	two
e. tetr(a)-	four
f. semi-	half
g. null(i)-	none
h. quadr(i)-	four
i. poly-	many
j. uni-	one
k. tri-	three
l. hemi-	half
m. brachy-	short
n. lepto-	thin
o. micr-	small
p. macro-	large
q. olig(o)-	few
r. alb-	white
s. xantho-	yellow
t. leuko-	white
u. rube-	red
v. cyano-	blue
w. erythro-	red
x. melan-	black
y. chloro-	green
z. cirrh-	yellow

Three
Suffixes

Suffixes are elements added to the end of word roots (parts that express essential meaning) that alter the meaning of the roots or indicate their intended part of speech. Most suffixes find common usage in the English language; some, however, are unique to medical science. For example, the suffixes most commonly used to indicate disease are: *-itis*, meaning inflammation; *-oma*, meaning tumor; and *-osis*, meaning condition. Suffixes used in medical terminology usually denote conditions or actions.

Sets of Suffixes

To facilitate learning, word endings are divided in to two groups: suffixes and word terminals. Word terminals are presented and explained in the next chapter. The suffixes in this chapter are presented in the following sets:

1. Suffixes Denoting State or Condition
2. Suffixes Relating to Medical Actions
3. Suffixes Associated with Small Size

In order to make medical words easier to pronounce, it is sometimes necessary to change the last letter or letters of the word roots. In some words, for example, the last vowel of the root is changed to an *o*; in others, an *o* is inserted between the root and the suffix when the suffix begins with a consonant, as in the word cardi*o*logy. Also, words that contain suffixes beginning with vowels, such as neur*i*tis, may drop the final vowel of the root part for ease of pronunciation.

Suffixes Denoting State or Condition

3.1 **-agra** severe pain

EXAMPLES::

myagra (my/agra)—severe muscle pain
podagra (pod/agra)—severe foot pain
mentulagra (mentul/agra)—painful involuntary erection of the penis

3.2 **-algia** pain caused by an injury and transmitted through the nervous system

The suffix *-algia* can be combined with words indicating parts of the body containing nerves to denote the exact location of pain.

EXAMPLES:

cerebralgia, cephalalgia (cerebr/algia, cephal/algia)—headache; (although cerebr- refers to brain and cephal- refers to head, both forms may be used to denote headache—cephalalgia, though, is more commonly used)

myalgia (my/algia)—muscle pain

gastralgia (gastr/algia)—stomachache

The element *-algia* itself may be divided into parts: *-ia*, meaning condition of, and, *alg-*, meaning pain. Their combined form, the suffix *-algia*, is the most frequently used form to express pain. However, *alg-* is also a word root meaning pain and can appear in various forms, such as *algesi-*, *algo-*, *algeo-*, and *algio-*:

algesia (alges/ia)—sensitivity to pain

hyperalgesia (hyper/alges/ia)—excessive sensitivity to pain

hypoalgesia (hypo/alges/ia)—abnormally low sensitivity to pain

algesic (alges/ic)—pertaining to pain; painful

algospasm (alg/o/spasm)—painful involuntary contraction; painful cramp

The alternate forms of *alg-* are used to avoid confusion with algae, the name for a group of water plants.

3.3 **-asthenia** weakness

This suffix is formed from three useful elements: the prefix *a-*, meaning not or lacking; the root *sthen-*, meaning strength; and, the word ending *-ia*, meaning morbid (diseased) condition. Their combination can be translated as: a condition of lacking strength (weakness).

EXAMPLES:

adenasthenia (aden/asthenia)—weakness in glandular secretion; deficient glandular activity

gastric adenasthenia (gastr/ic aden/asthenia)—deficient glandular secretion in the stomach

3.4 **-atresia** abnormal closure

EXAMPLES:

biliary atresia (bil/iary atr/esia)—abnormal closure of liver and gall bladder to the small intestine

proctatresia (proct/atr/esia)—closed anus

3.5 **-cele** hernia

The suffix *-rrhexis* names a condition of breaking, bursting, or rupturing. The physical evidence of such a rupture or break is a hernia; a balloon-like protrusion of an organ through its containing wall. *-cele* is the suffix used to denote a hernia.

EXAMPLES:

myocele (myo/cele)—muscle hernia; muscle protrusion

cystocele (cyst/o/cele)—protrusion of the bladder through the vaginal wall

hydrocele (hydr/o/cele)—collection of fluid in a swelling, especially in male genitals

3.6 **-cyst** bladder–like sac

EXAMPLES:

cholecyst (chole/cyst)—gallbladder

hydrocyst (hydro/cyst)—sac containing watery solution

3.7 **-dynia** pain

EXAMPLES:

cephalodynia (cephal/o/dynia)—headache
pleurodynia (pleuro/dynia)—pain on the side of the chest
scapulodynia (scapul/o/dynia)—pain in the shoulder muscles

3.8 **-ectasis** expansion; enlargement

This suffix denotes an enlargement caused by stretching; the condition of being stretched beyond normal dimensions (*ec-* is a variation of *ex-*, meaning out and *-tasis* means stretching).

EXAMPLES:

angiectasis (angi/ectasis)—blood vessel stretched beyond normal
nephrectasis (nephr/ectasis)—stretching (distention) of the kidney
bronchiectasis (bronch/i/ectasis)—stretching of bronchi

Use of the word dilation is another way to express the idea behind ectasis. Dilate means to expand or stretch.

3.9 **-edema** swelling

Edema can be used as a word in terms such as "edema of ___" or "___ edema." Pulmonary edema is swelling and fluid in the air sacs of the lungs. It is also used as a suffix to indicate location or kind of fluid accumulation.

EXAMPLES:

cephaledema (cephal/edema)—excess cranial fluid
pneumonedema (pneumon/edema)—abnormal quantities of fluid in the lungs
dactyledema (dactyl/edema)—abnormal swelling of the fingers or toes due to fluid accumulation

3.10 **-ema** swelling; distention

EXAMPLES:

emphysema (emphys/ema)—distention of air sacs in the lungs
erythema (eryth/ema)—swelling and redness of a body area

3.11 **-emesis** vomiting

Eme- is a root meaning vomit. The ending *-osis* refers to a condition with the (o) dropped to form the suffix *-sis*.

EXAMPLES:

emesis (eme/sis)—vomiting
emetic (eme/tic)—that which causes vomiting, such as a drug
hematemesis (hemat/eme/sis)—vomiting of blood

3.12 **-esis** condition; process

EXAMPLES:

enuresis (en/ur/esis)—condition of involuntary urination
genesis (gen/esis)—process of producing or originating

3.13 **-esthesia** sensation; feeling

This suffix deals both with physical sensations, particularly the sense of pain, and with the general state of the senses (consciousness, perception).

An important derivative of *esthes-* is its opposite, *anesthes-*, meaning a lack or absence of feeling.

EXAMPLES:

-esthetic (-esthet/ic)—pertaining to feeling
optesthesia (opt/esthesia)—ability to see; ability to perceive visual stimuli
anesthesiology (an/esthesi/ology)—branch of medical science that is concerned with sensation-reducing techniques, particularly those used in conjunction with pain-causing therapeutic procedures such as surgery.

3.14 **-grad(e)** walk; take steps; progression of steps

EXAMPLES:

retrograde (retr/o/grad/e)—going backward
digitograde (digit/o/grad/e)—characterized by walking on the toes

3.15 **-ia** disease; unhealthy state or condition

This suffix is most frequently used to name diseases, such as diptheria, pneumonia, and leukemia. It may also be used to denote an unhealthy (morbid) condition.

EXAMPLES:

amnesia (amnes/ia)—loss of memory
anesthesia (anesthes/ia)—loss of consciousness
phobia (phob/ia)—abnormal fear

3.16 **-iasis** condition; formation of; presence of

This suffix denotes a disease process or the condition resulting from disease. Literally, it means illness condition or sick condition.

EXAMPLES:

lithiasis (lith/iasis)—condition characterized by the formation of stones
elephantiasis (elephant/iasis)—condition characterized by enlargement of body parts, and thickening and discoloration of the skin covering these parts due to blockage of the lymph system.

3.17 **-itic** pertaining to or affected by inflammation

This suffix combines *-itis* and *-ic* (which means pertaining to) and is used to refer to a condition of inflammation.

EXAMPLES:

gastritic (gastr/itic)—affected by stomach inflammation
arthritic (arthr/itic)—affected by inflamed joints
nephritic (nephr/itic)—affected by inflamed kidneys

3.18 **-itis** inflammation

This suffix can be added to words denoting practically all body parts to indicate a condition, the symptoms of which are pain or discomfort, redness, heat, and swelling.

EXAMPLES;

gastritis (gastr/itis)—inflammation of the stomach
carditis (card/itis)—inflammation of the heart
dermatitis (dermat/itis)—inflammation of the skin

3.19 **-lysis** loosening; set free; destruction; release; breaking down; decomposition; dissolving

EXAMPLES:

litholysis (lith/o/lysis)—dissolving of stones found in the urinary bladder
hemolysis (hem/o/lysis)—breaking down and dissolving of red blood cells
gastrolysis (gastr/o/lysis)—surgical procedure in which the stomach is loosened from adhesions
autolysis (auto/lysis)—destruction of body tissues or cells from internal causes

3.20 **-malacia** soft condition; softness; softening

EXAMPLES:

adenomalacia (aden/o/malacia)—softening of a gland
cardiomalacia (cardi/o/malacia)—softening of the heart
hepatomalacia (hepat/o/malacia)—softening of the liver

In hollow structures, such as blood vessels or stomachs, *-malacia* would indicate a softening of the walls:

angiomalacia (angi/o/malacia)—softening of the walls of a blood vessel
gastromalacia (gastr/o/malacia)—softening of the walls of the stomach

3.21 **-megaly** enlarged

Body parts have a normal size according to age, sex, body type, and so on. Abnormal increases in size are indicated by the suffix *-megal*.

EXAMPLES:

adenomegaly (aden/o/megal/y)—enlargement of a gland
angiomegaly (angi/o/megal/y)—enlargement of a blood vessel
cardiomegaly (cardi/o/megal/y)—enlargement of the heart

3.22 **-oma** tumor; swelling on some part of the body

Most applications of this suffix relate to the composition of the tumor; that is, the kind of tissue forming the tumor.

EXAMPLES:

cerebroma (cerebr/oma)—abnormal mass of brain tissue
dermatoma (dermat/oma)—abnormal growth of skin tissue

It is also used to describe structural features:

adenoma (aden/oma)—tumor with a gland-like structure
angioma (angi/oma)—tumor that tends to consist of blood vessels
blepharadenoma (blephar/aden/oma)—tumor of the eyelid consisting of gland-like structures; glandular tumor of the eyelid

Additionally, *-oma* is used to indicate the location of the tumor:

hepatoma (hepat/oma)—tumor of the liver

3.23 **-osis** condition or disease

The suffix *-ism* is similar in meaning to *-osis* and is used in such words as alcoholism, morphinism, and mongalism.

EXAMPLES:

acidosis (acid/osis)—condition of acidity in the body
gastrosis (gastr/osis)—condition of the stomach
dermatosis (dermat/osis)—condition of the skin

3.24 **-penia** decrease; deficiency of; less than; less than usual

EXAMPLES:

-penic (-pen/ic)—pertaining to a state of deficiency
hematopenia (hemat/o/penia)—deficiency of blood in the body
lipopenia (lip/o/penia)—deficiency of lipids (fatlike chemicals) in the body

3.25 **-philia** love of; craving for

EXAMPLES:

pedophilia (ped/o/philia)—abnormal sexual craving for children
necrophilia (necro/philia)—a craving for or violation of dead bodies

3.26 **-plasia** development; growth

EXAMPLES:

hyperplasia (hyper/plasia)—abnormal growth increase; usually relates to abnormal increase in the cells composing tissues
hypoplasia (hypo/plasia)—incomplete or defective development
mastoplasia (mast/o/plasia)—development of breast tissue

3.27 **-plegia** paralysis; loss of power

EXAMPLES:

panplegia (pan/plegia)—total paralysis
hemiplegia (hemi/plegia)—paralysis of one side of the body

3.28 **-ptosis** falling; sagging; drooping; downward displacement

EXAMPLES:

hepatoptosis (hepat/o/ptosis)—displacement of the liver
cystoptosis (cyst/o/ptosis)—downward displacement of the urinary bladder
hysteroptosis (hyster/o/ptosis)—downward displacement of the uterus
blepharoptosis (blephar/o/ptosis)—drooping of upper eyelid

3.29 **-rrhage, -rrhagia** bursting forth; abnormal discharge

EXAMPLES:

pyorrhagia (pyo/rragia)—profuse flow of pus
hemorrhage (hemo/rrhage)—bursting forth of blood

3.30 **-rrhea** flow; discharge

EXAMPLES:

menorrhea (men/o/rrhea)—flow of menses
diarrhea (dia/rrhea)—flow of feces
gonorrhea (gon/o/rrhea)—discharge of gonococcal organism
pyorrhea (pyo/rrhea)—discharge of pus

3.31 **-rrhexis** breaking; bursting; forcible tearing; rupture

EXAMPLES:

cardiorrhexis (cardi/o/rrhexis)—rupture of the heart
angiorrhexis (angi/o/rrhexis)—rupture of a blood vessel
hysterorrhexis (hyster/o/rrhexis)—rupture of the uterus

3.32 **-stasis** stopping; standstill

EXAMPLES:

hemostasis (hemo/stasis)—stagnation of blood
homeostasis (homeo/stasis)—state of equilibrium

3.33 **-tonia** stretching; tension

EXAMPLES:

hypertonia (hyper/tonia)—excessive tension
myotonia (myo/tonia)—tonic muscle spasm

3.34 **-trophy** development; growth; nutrition; nourishment; nutritional growth

EXAMPLES:

trophic (troph/ic)—pertaining to nutrition, development, and growth
trophopathy (troph/o/path/y)—any disease caused by faulty nutrition
trophotherapy (troph/o/therap/y)—treatment of disease by nourishment (dietetic) measures

The suffix *-trophy* is used in some important combinations that frequently appear at the ends of medical words or phrases:

hypertrophy (hyper/trophy)—overdevelopment
atrophy (a/trophy)—wasting away or diminution in the size of a cell, tissue, organ, or body part
dystrophy (dys/trophy)—bad development; any disorder arising from faulty nutrition

Suffixes Relating to Medical Actions

3.35 **-centesis** puncture; surgical puncture or incision, usually for the purpose of drainage

EXAMPLES:

arthrocentesis (arthr/o/centesis)—surgical puncture of a joint
cardiocentesis (cardi/o/centesis)—surgical puncture or incision of the heart
pericardiocentesis (peri/cardi/o/centesis)—surgical puncture of the tissues surrounding the heart (the pericardium)

3.36 **-desis** binding; fixation; surgical union

EXAMPLES:

iridesis (iri/desis)—surgical binding to form an iris
arthrodesis (arthr/o/desis)—surgical fusion of a joint

The suffix *-pexy* is used more often than *-desis* when denoting surgical fixation.

3.37 **-ectomy** partial or total surgical removal (excision) of a body part

EXAMPLES:

adenectomy (aden/ectomy)—surgical removal of a gland
angiectomy (angi/ectomy)—surgical removal of a vessel
arthrectomy (arthr/ectomy)—surgical removal of a joint

3.38 **-ostomy** create an opening; provide a new opening to the outside of the body

The suffix *-ostomy* is used to denote the creation of a new opening or passage between two functionally related organs.

EXAMPLES:

gastroenterostomy (gastr/o/enter/ostomy)—surgical creation of an artificial passage between the stomach and the intestines

enterocholecystostomy (enter/o/chole/cyst/ostomy)—surgical creation of an artificial passage between the intestines and the gallbladder

It is also used to denote a surgical operation in which an artificial opening is created in an organ or structure for the purposes of draining body fluids or waste. Some examples are: enterostomy, gastrostomy, cholecystostomy, arthrostomy. The root element in the suffix *-ostomy* is *stom-*, meaning mouth. Because the mouth is the most prominent of the body openings, it was adopted as the designation for all openings.

3.39 **-otomy** surgical incision

EXAMPLES:

adenotomy (aden/otomy)—surgical incision of a gland

arthrotomy (arthr/otomy)—surgical incision of a joint

enterotomy (enter/otomy)—surgical incision of the intestines

3.40 **-pexy** suspension; fixation; surgical act of fastening

The surgical operation performed to restore a displaced organ to its proper place is called fixation or suspension. The suffix *-pexy* is used to denote this procedure and may be interpreted as a surgical fixation of some body part.

EXAMPLES:

nephropexy (nephr/o/pexy)—surgical fixation of the kidney

gastropexy (gastr/o/pexy)—surgical fixation of the stomach

hysteropexy (hyster/o/pexy)—surgical fixation of the uterus

3.41 **-plasty** molding; shaping; rebuilding by surgery

EXAMPLES:

osteoplasty (osteo/plasty)—bone rebuilding

rhinoplasty (rhino/plasty)—nose rebuilding or reshaping

mastoplasty (masto/plasty)—breast rebuilding

3.42 **-rrhaphy** suture; suturing; joining the edges of a rupture, wound, or incision by stitching

EXAMPLES:

myorrhaphy (my/o/rrhaphy)—suture of a muscle

proctorrhaphy (proct/o/rrhaphy)—suture of the rectum

cardiorrhaphy (cardi/o/rrhaphy)—suture of the heart muscle

3.43 **-scope** look; observe; reveal

EXAMPLES:

telescope (tele/scope)—instrument used for observing distant things (the root *tele-* means distant)

microscope (micr/o/scope)—instrument used for observing small things (the prefix *micr-* means small)

stethoscope (steth/o/scope)—instrument applied to the chest, back, and abdomen to determine the condition of the internal organs, such as the heart, lungs, and so on (*steth-* is a word root meaning chest)

3.44 **-tome** cutting instrument

EXAMPLES:

dermatome (derma/tome)—instrument used in cutting skin for skin grafts

craniotome (cranio/tome)—instrument for cutting into the skull

3.45 **-tripsy** surgical crushing

EXAMPLES:

neurotripsy (neuro/tripsy)—surgical crushing of a nerve

lithotripsy (lith/o/tripsy)—crushing of a calculus (stone)

Suffixes Associated with Small Size

The following table lists suffixes that indicate small size. They are presented in their singular forms.

Suffix	Example	Meaning
-cle	particle	small part
-cule	molecule	smallest part of an atom
-culum	tuberculum	small nodule or knot
-culus	calculus	small stone.
-et	facet	small plane surface
-ium	bronchium	small bronchial tube
-ole	arteriole	small artery
-olum	mesenteriolum	small mesentery
-olus	bronchiolus	smallest subdivision of a bronchus
-ule	veinule	small vein

Terminology Trivia

Alcohol Consumption

While most of us believe the sunny "light wine" countries, such as France and Italy, consume less per capita alcohol than do the "hard liquor" countries, such as the United States, England, and Sweden, this simply is not the case. Reliable figures are scarce, but data from the 1960s—which exclude most iron curtain countries—show that France had the highest total per capita consumption of alcohol, consuming nearly three times as much per person as people in the United States. Surprisingly, Italy was number two in total per capita consumption of alcohol, eighty percent of which was wine. The United States was eighth on the list of twenty countries in per capita consumption of alcohol, but was second only to France in its use of distilled liquors. The United Kingdom, famous for its production of Scotch whiskey and commonly thought to be high on the list in the consumption of spirits, actually drank less liquor per capita than did any other country on the list.

Another alcohol-related fallacy surrounds the idea that in Germany "they just drink beer." While it is true that, per capita, Germany drank the most liters of beer, its per capita intake of all types of alcohol combined put it behind Australia on the list. Also, West Germany was number four in its total use of liquor; number five in per capita consumption of wine. Switzerland was number three. Guess who was number four—Japan, with its consumption of sáke! The United States was the number nine consumer of beer, the number eight consumer of wine, and, the number one consumer of water.

Pronunciation and Meaning of New Terms

acidosis (as″ ī do′ sis) An abnormal condition resulting from accumulation of acid or loss of base from the body.

adenectomy (ad″ ē nek′ to me) Surgical removal of a gland.

angiectasis (an″ je ek′ tah sis) The dilatation of a blood vessel.

angiectomy (an″ je ek′ to me) Removal or resection of a vessel.

anesthesiology (an″ es the″ ze ol′ o je) The science that deals with loss of feeling or sensation.

arthrectomy (ar threk′ to me) Surgical removal of a joint.

arthrocentesis (ar″ thro sen te′ sis) Surgical puncture of a joint.

arthrotomy (ar throt′ o me) Incision of a joint.

cardiomegaly (kar″ de o meg′ ah le) Enlarged heart.

cardiorrhexis (kar″ de o rek′ sis) Rupture of the heart.

carditis (kar di′ tis) Inflammation of the heart.

cephalodynia (sef″ ah lo din′ e ah) Pain in the head; headache.

cystocele (sis′ to sēl) Herniation of the urinary bladder into the vagina.

dermatosis (der″ mah to′ sis) Any skin condition.

diarrhea (di″ ah re′ ah) Abnormal frequency and softness of fecal discharge.

elephantiasis (el″ ē fan ti′ ah sis) A disease caused by a parasitic infestation and characterized by inflammation and obstruction of the lymphatics and increased size of nearby tissue.

emphysema (em″ fī se′ mah) A pulmonary disease characterized by destruction of many of the alveolar walls.

gastric (gas′ trik) Pertaining to the stomach.

gastritis (gas tri′ tis) Inflammation of the stomach.

gastropexy (gas′ tro pek″ se) Surgical fixation of the stomach to the abdominal wall.

gonorrhea (gon″ o re′ ah) A sexually transmitted disease characterized by a discharge and painful urination.

hematemesis (hem″ ah tem′ ē sis) Vomiting of blood.

hemiplegia (hem″ e ple′ je ah) Paralysis of one side of the body.

hemophilia (he″ mo fil′ e ah) A hereditary hemorrhagic disorder due to deficiency of antihemophilic factor VIII.

hemorrhage (hem′ or ij) Bleeding; the escape of blood from the vessels.

hemostasis (he″ mo sta′ sis, he mos′ tah sis) The checking of the flow of blood either by coagulation or surgical means; interruption of blood flow through any vessel or to any part of the body.

hypoglossal (hi″ po glos′ al) Beneath the tongue.

hysteropexy (his′ ter o pek se) Surgical fixation of the uterus.

hysterorrhexis (his″ ter o rek′ sis) Rupture of the uterus.

lipopenia (lip″ o pe′ ne ah) A deficiency of fats in the body.

lithiasis (lī thi′ ah sis) A condition marked by formation of stones.

lithotripsy (lith′ o trip″ se) Surgical crushing of a stone.

myocele (mi′ o sēl) Hernia of the muscle.

nephropexy (nef′ ro pek″ se) Surgical fixation of a floating kidney.

neurotripsy (nu′ ro trip″ se) Surgical crushing of a nerve.

osteoplasty (os′ te o plas″ te) Plastic surgery of the bones.

otolaryngology (o″ to lar″ in gol′ o je) Study of the ear as well as the throat and its associated parts.

pharyngomycosis (fah ring″ go mi ko′ sis) Any fungal infection of the pharynx.

pleurodynia (ploor″ o din′ e ah) Pain of the pleura; pleurisy.

proctorrhaphy (prok tor′ ah fe) Suture of the rectum for the purpose of repair.

trophopathy (tro fop′ ah the) Any abnormal state of the nutrition.

Self-test

1. Match Column A with Column B. Items in column B may be used more than once.

Column A	*Column B*
___ -centesis	a. setting free, dissolution
___ -ectomy	b. creation of a mouth or opening
___ -lysis	c. fixation
___ -ostomy	d. an instrument for cutting
___ -otomy	e. puncture of a cavity
___ -pexy	f. looking at, examining
___ -plasty	g. cut into
___ -rrhaphy	h. closure by suturing, repair
___ -scope, -scopy	i. rubbing, crushing
___ -tome	j. looking at, examining
___ -tripsy	k. to mold or shape
	l. excision, cutting out

2. Fill in the meaning of the suffix.

Suffix	*Meaning*
a. -agra	___
b. -algia	___
c. -atresia	___
d. -cele	___
e. -cyst	___
f. -dynia	___
g. -ema	___
h. -ia	___
i. -iasis	___
j. -itis	___
k. -malacia	___
l. -oma	___
m. -osis	___
n. -pathy	___
o. -penia	___
p. -philia	___
q. -phobia	___
r. -ptosis	___
s. -rrhage	___
t. -rrhea	___
u. -stasis	___
v. -tonia	___

Four
Word Terminals

Sets of Word Terminals

There are a special set of suffixes that are called word terminals. These are word endings that change word roots to nouns or adjectives and that change singular forms to plural forms. Knowledge of word terminals lends quality to the use of medical words.

The word terminals in this chapter are presented as follows:

1. Terminals that change Word Roots to Nouns
2. Terminals that change Word Roots to Adjectives or Verbs
3. Terminals that change Singular Words to Plural Words

Terminals that change Word Roots to Nouns

4.1 **-a** names a thing when used with the word root

EXAMPLES:

derma (derm/a)—the skin
gingiva (gingiv/a)—the gum
costa (cost/a)—a rib

4.2 **-ac** affected by; having; frequently, one who is affected by

The element *-ac* is also used as a suffix that means pertaining to.

EXAMPLES:

cardiac (cardi/ac)—having heart disease
maniac (mani/ac)—person acting wildly or violently insane

4.3 **-an, -ian** of; belonging to; pertaining to

EXAMPLES:

Freudian (Freud/ian)—pertaining to Sigmund Freud or his psychoanalalytic doctrines
European (Europe/an)—of or belonging to Europe

4.4 **-ance, -ancy** state or condition; act of

EXAMPLES:

elegance (eleg/ance)—state or condition of being elegant
assistance (assist/ance)—act of assisting
resistance (resist/ance)—act of resisting

The terminal *-ence* is a form of *-ance* that carries the same meaning; that is, it refers either to a state or condition, or to an action.

4.5 **-form** having the same form; shaped like; resembling

EXAMPLES:

dentiform (denti/form)—shaped like a tooth

uniform (uni/form)—having the same form as others of its kind (the element *uni-* means one)

4.6 **-genesis** process or condition leading to production

EXAMPLES:

carcinogenesis (carcin/o/genesis)—production of cancer

hypergenesis (hyper/genesis)—excessive development or excessive production

autogenesis (auto/genesis)—self generation; originating within the body

agenesis (a/genesis)—lack of development

4.7 **-gram, -graphy** record; write

This terminal is used to denote the drawn or written record made by some instrument. The terminal denoting the instrument itself is *-graph.*

EXAMPLES:

cardiogram (cardi/o/gram)—record made by an instrument (cardi/o/graph) that shows heartbeats

myogram (my/o/gram)—tracing made by an apparatus (my/o/graph) that records the effects of muscular contractions

radiography (radi/o/graph/y)—act of making records (principally photographs) through the use of x-rays (radi means ray)

4.8 **-ician** person belonging to or associated with

EXAMPLES:

technician (techn/ician)—person skilled in the technicalities of a field

pediatrician (pediatr/ician)—person associated with the medical care of children

4.9 **-ics** the art or science of; the study of

EXAMPLES:

optics (opt/ics)—science that deals with light and vision

politics (polit/ics)—science of government

The element *-ology* carries a meaning identical with that for *-ics*. There is, however, a subtle distinction between them in medical usage. When *-ics* or *-ology* is used to denote a body of medical knowledge, the *-ology* ending refers to the knowledge as it applies to physicians, while the *-ics* form refers to the knowledge as it applies to nonmedical personnel. For example, while anesthesiology is the broad field of knowledge held by physicians, anesthetics refers to knowledge held by technicians. Similarly, ophthalmology is the field of study covered by physicians, while optics is the same field as covered by nonmedical personnel. This is far from a hard and fast rule, however. Orthopedics, pediatrics, and obstetrics are medical fields of study that carry *-ic* endings.

4.10 **-ion** action; condition resulting from action

EXAMPLES:

incision (incis/ion)—act or result of cutting into flesh

action (act/ion)—result of acting

4.11 **-ior** more toward

This terminal indicates a higher degree of something and corresponds to many common English words ending in *-er*. For example:

-er	-ior	Meaning
high/er	super/ior	more above
inn/er	inter/ior	more toward the inside
out/er	exter/ior	more toward the outside

4.12 **-is** names a thing when used with the word root

EXAMPLES:

glottis (glott/is)—sound-producing apparatus of the larynx
dermis (derm/is)—skin

4.13 **-ist** one who practices or is concerned with

EXAMPLES:

chemist (chem/ist)—one who practices the science of chemistry
internist (intern/ist)—one who practices internal medicine

4.14 **-ite** of the nature of

EXAMPLES:

cellulite (cellu/lite)—having the nature of cellulose
dendrite (dendr/ite)—part of a nerve characterized by branching that appears to be in the nature of a tree

4.15 **-ition, -ation** process; action; condition

EXAMPLES:

addition (add/ition)—process of adding
prohibition (prohib/ition)—act of denying or prohibiting
ambition (amb/ition)—state of striving for achievement

4.16 **-ium** place; region; lining or covering tissue

EXAMPLES:

medium (med/ium)—place used for the cultivation of bacteria
auditorium (auditor/ium)—place for a public gathering
podium (pod/ium)—place for standing; platform

4.17 **-ologist** specialist

EXAMPLES:

gastrologist (gastr/ologist)—specialist in the study of the stomach
cardiologist (cardi/ologist)—specialist in the study of the heart
dermatologist (dermat/ologist)—specialist in the study of the skin

4.18 **-ology** study of; knowledge of; science of

This terminal is used to name the field in which a physician limits his or her practice.

EXAMPLES:

dermatology (dermat/ology)—branch of medicine dealing with the skin and its disorders

pathology (path/ology)—branch of medicine that deals with the nature of disease

Internal medicine names a branch of medical study that deals with diagnosis and nonsurgical treatment of disease. Within this branch are specialized fields, termed subspecialties. These include:

cardiology (cardi/ology)—study of the heart and its functions
nephrology (nephr/ology)—study of the kidney and its functions
gastroenterology (gastr/o/enter/ology)—study of the digestive system (may be further broken down to the specialties of gastrology and enterology)

4.19 **-on** names a thing when used with the word root

EXAMPLES:

nephron (nephr/on)—function unit of the kidney
encephalon (en/cephal/on)—the brain

4.20 **-or** thing that commits some act

EXAMPLES:

elevator (elevat/or)—that which elevates or raises
flexor (flex/or)—that which flexes or bends
incisor (incis/or)—that which incises or cuts into

It is also used to indicate a person who commits some act. Some examples are: inventor, objector, sailor, and vendor

4.21 **-um** names a thing when used with the word root

EXAMPLES:

cementum (cement/um)—thin layer of modified bone on the roots of teeth
addendum (addend/um)—something added
momentum (moment/um)—something moving; a force

4.22 **-ure** result of an action; means of an action; device

EXAMPLES:

exposure (expos/ure)—result of being exposed
pressure (press/ure)—result of pressing
legislature (legislat/ure)—means for legislating or passing laws

4.23 **-us** names a thing when used with the word root

EXAMPLES:

viscus (visc/us)—any internal organ of the body
discus (disc/us)—any disc of the spinal column

Terminals that change Word Roots to Adjectives or Verbs

4.24 **-ad** toward; in the direction of

EXAMPLES:

cephalad (cephal/ad)—toward or in the direction of the head
retrad (retr/ad)—toward the back

This terminal is rarely used since it also serves as a prefix with the same meaning:

adnerval (ad/nerval)—toward a nerve
adaxial (ad/axial)—toward an axis

4.25 **-ant** pertaining to; having the characteristic of

EXAMPLES:

pleasant (pleas/ant)—having a pleasing characteristic
malignant (malign/ant)—having the characteristic of badness

4.26 **-ar** pertaining to; having a connection with

EXAMPLES:

palmar (palm/ar)—pertaining to the palms
polar (pol/ar)—pertaining to the poles

This terminal is most frequently used with words ending in either *l* or *le* and becomes in these cases the form, *-ular*. Some examples are: triangular; circular; muscular; singular.

4.27 **-ary** pertaining to; having connection with

EXAMPLES:

budgetary (budget/ary)—pertaining to a budget
honorary (honor/ary)—pertaining to honor

4.28 **-ate** perform; bring about

EXAMPLES:

expectorate (ex/pector/ate)—bring up mucus secretions from the bronchial membranes
intoxicate (intoxic/ate)—bring about a state of drunkenness or intoxication
fixate (fix/ate)—fix
vacate (vac/ate)—make vacant

4.29 **-ation** process; action; condition

This terminal is a combination of the elements *-ate* (to put in to action) and *-ion* (condition resulting from an action).

EXAMPLES:

inspiration (inspir/ation)—draw air into the lungs
hyperventilation (hyper/ventil/ation)—increase the amount of air as a result of increased rate and depth of respiration

4.30 **-genic, -genous** producing; originating; giving rise to

EXAMPLES:

endogenous (end/o/gen/ous)—originating from within
carcinogenic (carcin/o/gen/ic)—producing cancer; pertaining to a carcinogen
myogenic (my/o/gen/ic)—giving rise to or forming muscle tissue

4.31 **-ic, -al, -ac, -ical** pertaining to; belonging to; connected with

EXAMPLES:

cranial (crani/al)—pertaining to the skull
cardiac (cardi/ac)—pertaining to the heart; one with heart disease
manic (man/ic)—pertaining to mania
mathematical (mathemat/ical)—pertaining to mathematics

4.32 **-id** pertaining to; added to the cause; in some state

EXAMPLES:

frigid (frig/id)—pertaining to cold
rigid (rig/id)—in a stiffened state
tuberculid (tubercul/id)—pertaining to tuberculosis

4.33 **-ive** of; relating to; having the nature or quality of

EXAMPLES:

sedative (sedat/ive)—having the nature of a pain or tension reliever
substantive (substant/ive)—relating to substance

4.34 **-oid** like; resembling; having the form or shape of

The terminal *-oid* is used to signify resemblance to the thing specified by the stem to which it is affixed.

EXAMPLES:

adenoid tumor (aden/oid)—tumor consisting of glandular or gland-like material; adenoma
dermoid tumor (derm/oid)—tumor containing skin-like elements
fibroid tumor (fibr/oid)—tumor containing fiber-like structures; fibroma
cystoid (cyst/oid)—soft mass resembling a cyst but lacking an enclosing capsule
lipoid (lip/oid)—like or resembling fat
myoid (my/oid)—like or resembling muscle

4.35 **-ous** full of; abounding in; having

EXAMPLES:

poisonous (poison/ous)—full of poison
famous (fam/ous)—having fame
nervous (nerv/ous)—nerve filled

4.36 **-tic** pertaining to

EXAMPLES:

emetic (eme/tic)—pertaining to an emesis
diagnostic (diagnos/tic)—pertaining to diagnosis
hypnotic (hypnot/ic)—pertaining to hypnosis

4.37 **-trophic** pertaining to nutrition, growth, or development

EXAMPLES:

dystrophic (dys/trophic)—progressively weakening muscle; growth difficulty
atrophic (a/trophic)—without growth

4.38 **-tropic** turned toward; changing

EXAMPLES:

hydrotropic (hydro/tropic)—turned toward water
phototropic (photo/tropic)—turned toward light

4.39 **-ular** pertaining to

EXAMPLES:

tubular (tub/ular)—pertaining to a tube
valvular (valv/ular)—pertaining to a valve

Some confusion may arise when determining whether the *-ular* terminal combines the meanings of both *-ul* (small) and *-ar* (pertaining to), or whether it simply means pertaining to. One hint to remember is when the main part of the word ends in *-l* or *-le*, the terminal *-ular* only means pertaining to. Context should also clarify meaning. For example, it makes no sense to define the word singular (sing/ular) as a small single.

4.40 **-y** act or result; condition or quality

EXAMPLES:

dreamy (dream/y)—characterized by dreams
inquiry (inquir/y)—act of questioning

Terminals that change Singular Words to Plural Words

The terminal used in converting a singular word to its plural form, or vice versa, depends on the word's Latin or Greek origin. There are no simple rules to follow, so it is suggested that you memorize the examples given for future reference.

Singular	Plural	Example
-a	-ae	bursa, bursae
-en	-ina	lumen, lumina
-ex	-ices	index, indices
-ies	-ietes	paries, parietes
-is	-es, -ides	psychosis, psychoses epididymis, epididymides
-ium	-ia	bacterium, bacteria
-ma	-mata	carcinoma, carcinomata
-nx	-nges	phalynx, phalynges
-on	-a	ganglion, ganglia
-s	-tes	pons, pontes
-u	-ua	cornu, cornua
-um	-a	atrium, atria
-us	-era, -i	viscus, viscera bacillus, bacilli
-x	-ces	appendix, appendices

Terminology Trivia

Plurals of Proper Names

A look around any middle-class suburb reveals a variety of misinformation regarding what happens to be one of the simplest rules of grammar: forming plurals of proper names. Embellishing many a mailbox, or suspended proudly beneath them in wrought iron, are such identifying signs as: The Robinson's; or, The Smith's; or even, The Jone's. Rather than indicating the plural forms of the names, however, these signs indicate possession, clearly not the owners' true intent.

Few grammatical processes in the English language are simpler than pluralizing proper nouns. All one needs to do is add the letter *s* to the end of the name; or *es* if the name already ends in *s*, *ch*, *sh*, or *x*. Thus, the signs would read properly as: The Robinsons; The Smiths; The Joneses. It may be argued that

The Robinsons' is not an incorrect plural, but rather a plural possessive: The Robinsons' (place or house). So, if you must use an apostrophe to indicate possession, add it to the end of the noun after first forming the proper plural.

Pronunciation and Meaning of New Terms

cardiac (kar′ de ak) Pertaining to the heart.
- *c. arrest*, ceasing of heart activity.
- *c. arrhythmia*, irregular heart action or irregular pulse.
- *c. block*, interferences with the heart's contractions due to failure of the impulses to pass through the conductile tissue.
- *c. catheterization*, passage of a small plastic tube into the heart through a blood vessel for the purpose of diagnosis of heart disorders.
- *c. insufficiency*, inadequate functioning of the heart.

cardiologist (kar de ol′ o jist) A physician who is specially trained in the study and treatment of heart disease.

dermatologist (der″ mah tol′ o jist) A specialist in skin diseases.

dermis (der′ mis) The layer of skin that lies under the epidermis.

dislocation (dis lo ka′ shun) Displacement of a bone from a joint.

flexor (flek′ sor) Any muscle that flexes a joint.

incision (in sizh′ un) A cut or wound produced by a sharp instrument; the act of cutting.

incisor (in si′ zer) Any of the four anterior teeth in either jaw.

internist (in ter′ nist) A specialist in internal medicine.

malignant (mah lig′ nant) Tending to grow worse and threatening to produce death.

pediatrician (pe″ de ah trish′ an) A physician who specializes in the treatment of children

Self-test

1. Define the italicized terminal in the following list of words.

Terminal	*Meaning*
pyro*genic*	a. ______________
circ*ular*	b. ______________
flacc*id*	c. ______________
lymph*oid*	d. ______________
osteo*genesis*	e. beginning

curat*ive*	f. ______
compli*ance*	g. ______

2. The following section relates to word endings that form plurals. The singular endings are given. Write in their plural forms.

Singular	*Plural*	*Singular*	*Plural*	*Singular*	*Plural*
-a	a. ae	-en	f. ina	-ex	j. ______
-ies	b. ______	-is	g. ______	-ma	k. ______
-nx	c. ______	-on	h. ______	-s	l. ______
-u	d. ______	-um	i. ______	-us	m. ______
-x	e. ______				

Five
Body Structure

Components of Body Structure

The human body is composed of basic elements that build in this way:

cells ⟶ tissues
tissues ⟶ organs
organs ⟶ systems
systems ⟶ function

Cells

Cells are the smallest units of life and are the building blocks from which tissues, organs, and systems are constructed. Specialized cells similar in structure and function are assembled into a mass called a tissue.

5.1 **cellular** cell

EXAMPLES:

intracellular (intra/cellular)—inside the cell
extracellular (extra/cellular)—outside the cell
interstitial (inter/stitial)—space between cells

5.2 **cyte** cell

EXAMPLES:

cytology (cyt/o/logy)—study of cells
leukocyte (leuko/cyte)—white blood cell
blastocyte (blast/o/cyte)—developing cell not yet differentiated

5.3 **plasm** substance of a cell

EXAMPLES:

plasma (plasm/a)—liquid part of lymph and blood
protoplasm (prot/o/plasm)—first living substance of a cell

Tissues

Tissues are collections of cells organized for special functions. The primary tissues are:

epithelial—tissue on the surface of an organ or part of the body; lining of an organ or cavity.

connective—tissue that holds organs in place, holds the body together, and shapes the body.

muscle—tissues involved in motion. There are three types: striated—those muscles controlled by the person, usually attached to the skeletal system; smooth—those muscles that function automatically. They are found in the digestive, circulatory, and genitourinary systems; and cardiac—the muscles of the heart.

nervous—tissues involved in muscle control, stimulation, perception, and body functions. There are two types of cells in these tissues—neurons and glial cells.

5.4 **fascia** sheet of fibrous tissue

The term fascia is used to denote connective tissues that form an outer layer for other tissues such as ligaments and tendons. Fascia also serves as an anchor to support or hold other tissue structures. Muscle bundles are held together and kept in place during movement.

EXAMPLES:

fasciculus (fasci/cul/us)—small bundle of nerve or muscle fibers
fasciodesis (fasci/o/desis)—suture of fascia to one of the tissues attached to the skeleton
fasciorrhaphy (fasci/o/rrhaphy)—suturing together of torn fascia

5.5 **histo-** tissue

EXAMPLES:

histology (hist/ology)—study of tissue
histolysis (histo/lysis)—breaking down of tissues
historrhexis (histo/rrhexis)—disintegration of tissue due to noninfectious agent

5.6 **lip-** fat

The root *lip-* denotes the oily or greasy substance that exists in many parts of the body.

EXAMPLES:

lipoid (lip/oid)—resembling fat
lipocardiac (lip/o/cardi/ac)—fatty heart
lipemia (lip/em/ia)—abnormal fat in the blood
lipoarthritis (lip/o/arthr/itis)—inflammation of the fatty tissue of a joint

Many tumors consist of fatty substances (lip/oma), or the tumor may contain other substances in addition to fat:

fibrolipoma (fibr/o/lip/oma)—tumor containing fiber-like (thread-like) structure and fat
myolipoma (my/o/lip/oma)—tumor composed of muscle and fat elements

Organs

Organs have specialized functions that together form body systems. The following word roots relate to the physical structure of organs:

ampulla: dilated portion of a canal or duct; small (*ulla*) area that resembles an oval-shaped storage jar (*ampu*).
aperture: opening in an organ.
apex: tip or point of an organ, usually an organ with a triangular shape.
base: part of an organ nearest its point of attachment; widest part.

collum: neck-like part of a body or an organ.
cortex: outer part of a structure; thick outer layer of a structure, usually found on the outer surface of the medulla of an organ.
duct: tube-like or canal-like structure that transports fluid or air from one part to another.
fascia: layer of connective tissue covering internal organs or parts.
foramen: opening or hole in an organ or in part of an organ.
fundus: part of an organ opposite an opening; body of an organ.
hilum: small place on an organ at which blood vessels, nerves, or ducts enter or leave; stalk of an organ.
lobe: roundish projection or roundish division of an organ.
meatus: opening or channel.
medulla: center of an organ; inside of the cortex.
node: small mass of tissue.
papilla: small nipple-like projection from a surface.
sinus: cavity, passageway, or channel; curved space.
stem: supporting structure or part of an organ.
tract: a definite region or area of the body; group, series, or systems of related parts or organs, especially nerves.
ventricle: hollow space; small (*icle*), belly-like (*ventr*) area in an organ.

5.7 **viscero-** organ

EXAMPLES:

visceral (viscer/al)—pertaining to an internal organ, especially one in the abdomen
viscera (viscer/a)—collective name for internal organs, especially those in the abdomen
viscerad (viscer/ad)—toward the viscera

Body Systems

Body systems are combinations of organs that serve particular functions. They are:

1. **Digestive System:** alters and absorbs food substances and excretes waste products.
2. **Genitourinary System:** a combination of three systems. One is the urinary system whose function is to excrete urine. The other two are male and female reproductive systems whose function is to produce and transport germ cells. The female reproductive system is active in the growth and development of the embryo and fetus.
3. **Nervous System** and **Special Senses:** both systems integrate the various intellectual and physical processes of the body and give it an awareness of its environment.
4. **Cardiovascular Lymphatic Systems:** the cardiovascular system produces and transports blood throughout the body. The lymphatic system is composed of vessels and glands that retrieve plasma and tissue fluids and furnish protective mechanisms for the body against pathogenic organisms.
5. **Respiratory System:** receives oxygen from the air, transfers it into the bloodstream, and gives off carbon dioxide produced by body tissues.
6. **Skeletal System:** provides the structural framework of the body, supports organs, and furnishes the muscles a place for attachment. Included in this system is the articular, or joint system that allows motion.

7. **Muscular System:** consists of all nonneurologic tissues permitting motion and movement.
8. **Integumentary System:** includes skin, breasts, hair, sweat and sebaceous glands. This system covers the body and protects it. It regulates temperature and has the functions of sensation and excretion.
9. **Endocrine System:** manufactures hormones responsible for metabolism, growth, and development.

Terms Relating to Body Structure

Medical records require explicit detail that enables the reader to locate the exact area of the body being described. Body positions, depth, regions, planes, directions, and cavities have a special place in medical language. Cavities of the body are shown in Figure 5-1.

Terms relating to the position of the body:

anatomical position: standing with the arms hanging to the side, palms facing forward.
erect: standing.
supine: horizontal position with the face up.

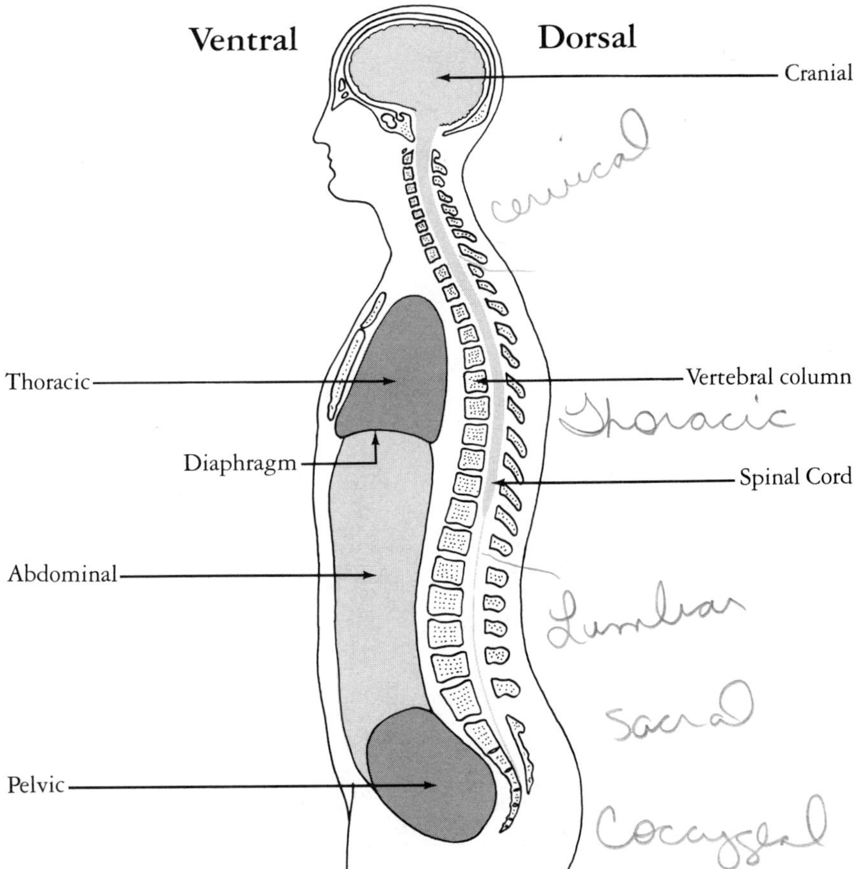

Figure 5–1 Body cavities.

prone: lying face down in a horizontal position.
laterally recumbent: lying horizontally on either the right or left side.

Terms relating to the surface and depth of body parts:

internal: inner part of the body; inner surface.
external: outer part of the body; outer surface.
deep: situated far beneath the surface.
superficial: situated close to the surface.
parietal: wall of a body part.

The back is divided into regions named in relation to the vertebrae of the spinal column. In descending order they are:

cervical: neck (seven cervical vertebrae).
thoracic: chest (twelve thoracic vertebrae).
lumbar: small of the back (five lumbar vertebrae).
sacral: sacrum (five sacral vertebrae that are fused in to one bone).
coccyx: tailbone (four coccygeal vertebrae that are fused in to one bone).

The abdomen as shown in Figure 5-2, is divided into four *quadrants* with lines radiating from the **umbilicus** that travel midline (or **sagittal**) from **xyphoid** to **pubic symphisis** and transversely from side to side. This makes four quadrants: right upper quadrant (*RUQ*), right lower quadrant (RLQ), left upper quadrant (*LUQ*) and left lower quadrant (*LLQ*). Three other areas are also noted in older literature: **epigastric**—midway between xyphoid and umbilicus; **paraumbilical**—around the umbilicus; and **suprapubic**—midway between umbilicus and pubic symphisis.

Terms relating to planes (flat surfaces) of the body (see Figure 5-3):

coronal plane: divides the body into front and back halves; frontal plane.

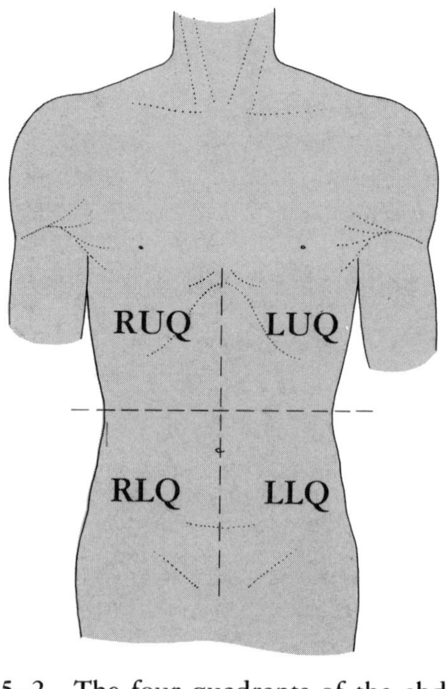

Figure 5–2 The four quadrants of the abdomen.

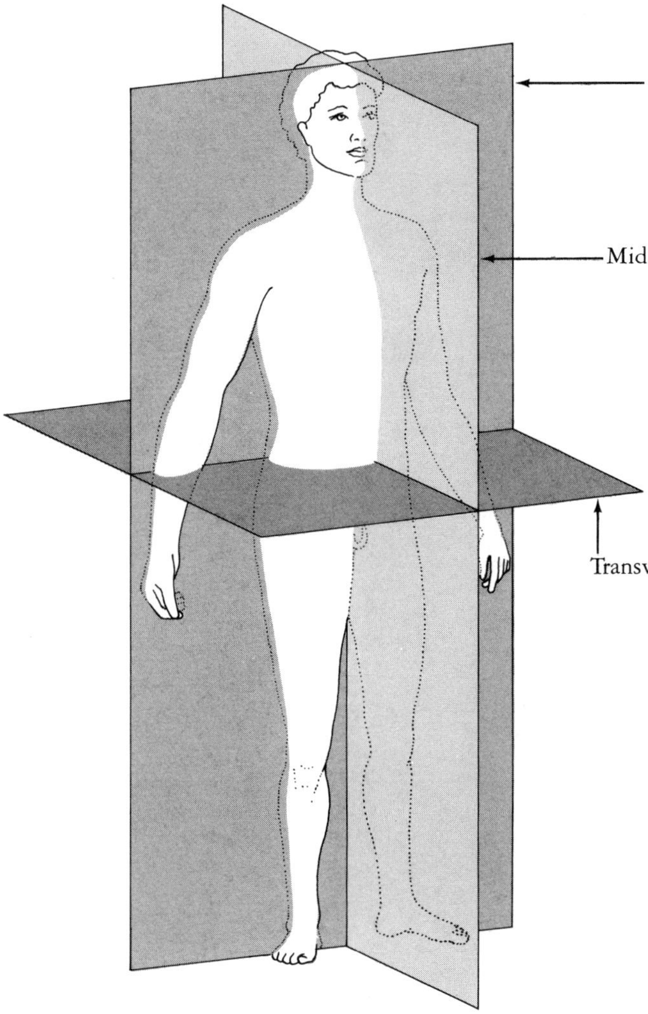

Figure 5–3 The body planes.

midsagittal plane: divides the body into right and left halves; median plane.
sagittal plane: any plane parallel to the midsagittal plane, vertically dividing the body into right and left portions.
transverse plane: plane cutting crosswise through the body at a right angle to the long axis of the body.

Terms relating to directional aspects of the body:

anterior, ventral: front (*ante*) surface.
caudad: toward (*ad*) the tail (*caud*).
cephalad: toward (*ad*) the head (*cephal*).
dextral, dextro: right.
distal: situated away from the center of a structure; distal (distant).
inferior: below or directed downward.
lateral: side of the body or point away from the midline.
medial: pertaining to the middle or midline of the body.
peripheral: *peri* (around) *pheral* (bear)—bearing around; circumference.
plantar: sole of the foot.
posterior, dorsal: back (post) surface.

proximal: point nearest the center; part in the area.
sinistral, sinistro: left; *levo* may also be used.
superior: above; directed upward.
valgus: bent outward.
varus: bent inward; angulation of a body part toward the midline.
volar: palm side of the hand; also called *palmar*.

Terms relating to body cavities:

cavum: hollow spaces.
ventral cavities: three cavities located in front part of the body—thoracic, abdominal, and pelvic.
thoracic cavity: chest cavity between the neck and diaphragm. The three sections of the thoracic cavity are: the *left pleural space*, the *mediastinum*, and the *right pleural space*.
abdominal cavity: belly cavity between the diaphragm and pelvic organs. Other terms relating to the abdomen are *celiac* (abdominal), *laparo* (loin or flank), and *flank* (wide upper part of the abdomen over the hipbone).
pelvic cavity: hollow space below the abdominal cavity.
dorsal cavities: hollow spaces located toward the back of the body.
cranial cavity: space containing the brain.
vertebral cavity: space containing the spinal cord that extends from the base of the cranial cavity to the bottom edge of the abdominal cavity.
torso, trunk: main part of the body to which the head and limbs are attached.

Terminology Trivia

Suntans

While many people believe a suntan is a sign of good health, it actually serves as a protective device against further damage from the ultraviolet rays of the sun which, like other forms of radiation, are dangerous. A suntan certainly is no indication of good health. In fact, during both the Renaissance and Elizabethan eras it was indicative of the lower classes, who were constantly outdoors and exposed to the sun. A suntan or sunburn, incidentally, can even be acquired on a fairly cloudy day, because clouds do not filter ultraviolet rays.

Pediatrics

The field of pediatrics concerns itself with the diseases of childhood. Surprisingly, it was not recognized as a separate branch of medicine until after the start of the twentieth century, even though prior to that time many physicians had already limited their practices to children.

Pronunciation and Meaning of New Terms

cytology (si tol′ o je) Study of cells.

leukocyte (loo′ ko sīt) A white blood cell.

lipoid (lip′ oid) Resembling fat.

intracellular (in″ trah sel′ u lar) Within a cell.

sagittal (saj′ ĭ tal) Shaped like an arrow; denotes a plane that is parallel to the midsagittal line vertically dividing the body into right and left portions.

thoracic (tho ras′ ik) Pertaining to the chest.

lumbar (lum′ ber) Pertaining to the lower back.

Self-test

1. Match Column A with Column B.

Column A

f histo
c cyto, cyte
d plasmo
e intracellular
b lipemia
a interstitial

Column B

a. space between the cells
b. fat in the blood
c. cell
d. cell substance
e. inside the cell
f. tissue

2. Write your answer in the space provided for each question.

1. The word root for a sheet of fibrous tissue is fascia.
2. Foramen is the word root meaning hole or opening.
3. The type of tissue that covers the body surfaces is called epithelial tissue.
4. The tissue that holds the body together is called connective.
5. The tissue of the body involved in movement is called muscle tissue.

3. For each set, match Column A with Column B.

Column A

d collum
f duct
c foramen
g hilum
h node
b sinus
a stem
e tract

Column B

a. supporting structure
b. cavity; passageway; curved space
c. opening or hole
d. neck-like part
e. definite region; series of related parts
f. tube-like structure that transports fluid or air
g. place where blood vessels, nerves, or ducts enter
h. small mass of tissue

4.

Column A	*Column B*
__d__ ampulla	a. body of an organ
__a__ fundus	b. middle or inner part
__e__ cortex	c. organ opening
__i__ fascia	d. dilated portion of a duct
__h__ aperture ✓ c	e. outside part; thick outer layer
__f__ meatus ✓ h	f. layer of connective tissue
__b__ medulla	g. small, belly-like space in an organ
__g__ ventricle	h. opening or channel
	i. sheet of fibrous tissue

5.

Column A	*Column B*
__c__ apex	a. body
__h__ base	b. roundish projection of an organ
__a__ corpus ✓	c. tip or point
__e__ fascicle ✓	d. mouth-like opening
__f__ labium	e. small bundle of tissue
__b__ lobe	f. lip-like part
__d__ orifice ✓	g. nipple-like projection from a surface
__g__ papilla	h. part of an organ nearest its attachment
__i__ viscera	i. organs of the body; usually abdominal organs

6.

Column A	*Column B*
__c__ anatomical	a. standing position
__a__ erect	b. lying horizontally on either the right or left side
__d__ supine	c. standing straight with arms to the side and palms facing forward
__e__ prone	d. lying horizontally face up
__b__ laterally recumbent	e. lying face down
__f__ internal	f. inner part or surface
__i__ external	g. far beneath the surface
__g__ deep	h. walls of a part
__j__ superficial	i. outer part or surface
__h__ parietal	j. close to the surface

7. List the regions of the back from the neck to the tail bone.

1. cervical
2. thoracic
3. lumbar
4. sacral
5. coccyx

8. Match Column A with Column B (some terms may be used more than once).

Column A	*Column B*
__c__ coronal	a. divides body into right and left sections
__a__ sagittal	b. divides body into top and bottom sections
__b__ horizontal	c. divides body into front and back sections
__c__ frontal	
__a__ median	
__b__ transverse	

9. **Identify the direction indicated by the terms.**

Term	*Direction*
superior	a. ________________
inferior	b. ________________
medial	c. ________________
lateral	d. ________________
peripheral	e. ________________
cephalad	f. ________________
caudad	g. ________________
proximal	h. ________________
distal cavity	i. ________________
ventral cavity	j. ________________
dorsal	k. ________________
volar	l. ________________
plantar	m. ________________
varus	n. ________________
valgus	o. ________________
dextral	p. ________________
sinistral	q. ________________
anterior	r. ________________
posterior	s. ________________

10. **Identify the system listed in Column B that is involved in Column A.**

Column A	*Column B*
___ lips	a. skeletal
___ nipple	b. cardiovascular and lymph
___ tendon	c. special senses
___ bronchi	d. integumentary
___ eye	e. respiratory
___ vein	
___ eyelash	

Six
Digestive System

Using Word Roots

The ten chapters that follow concentrate on word roots associated with the various body systems. It is important, therefore, to understand exactly what word roots are and how they are used.

Word roots are the main elements of words; in medical usage, word roots often stand for body parts. They combine with other word elements (prefixes, suffixes, and terminals) to give medical terms the specificity needed to accurately describe some condition or event. For example, the word root *tonsil-* stands for the anatomical part—the tonsils. By adding three different suffixes—*-itis*, meaning inflammation, *-ectomy*, meaning excision, and *-otomy*, meaning incision—we can form three very specific medical terms having different meanings: tonsillitis (inflammation of the tonsils), tonsillectomy (surgical removal of a tonsil or tonsils), and tonsillotomy (incision of a tonsil).

Unless already there, a combining vowel (*i*, *o*, or *u*) is inserted between the prefix and root of a term both to give the term a more pleasing sound and to make it easier to pronounce. The combining vowel may also be placed between the word root and the suffix or word terminal. Two vowels may appear together in a term when word roots are joined and the second one begins with a vowel; for example, the words electr*oe*ncephalogram, card*io*vascular, and gastr*oi*ntestinal have two vowels appearing together. A word root and a combining vowel, when used together in a word, are called a combining form.

When interpreting the medical terms presented in the following body system chapters, remember this simple formula: interpret the last element of the term first, the first element of the term next, and then interpret all the elements in between these two. Combine the meanings of the elements in this order and the meaning of the term should become clear. For example, the term tonsillitis is interpreted by taking the suffix *-itis*, meaning inflammation and the word root *tonsil-*, referring to the tonsils, and combining them to read: inflammation of the tonsils. Similarly, an electroencephalogram is a record or drawing (*-gram*) produced by electrical (*electr-*) impulses of the brain (*cephal-*).

Elements (prefixes, roots, suffixes, and terminals) may combine in many ways to give medical terms their needed specificity. The following are examples of the ways in which elements may combine:

Words formed with one word root:

word root +	suffix	= medical word
gastr	itis	gastritis

word root	+	word terminal				=	medical word
gastr		ic					gastric

prefix	+	word root	+	word terminal	=	medical word
epi		gastr		ic		epigastric

word root	+	combining vowel	+	suffix	=	medical word
gastr		o		dynia		gastrodynia

Words formed with two or more word roots:

word root	+	vowel	+	word root	+	vowel	+	suffix	=	medical word
electr		o		cardi		o		gram		electrocardiogram

word root	+	vowel	+	word root	+	terminal			=	medical word
gastr		o		intestin		al				gastrointestinal

root	+	vowel	+	root	+	vowel	+	suffix	=	medical word
cheil		o		stomat		o		plasty		cheilostomatoplasty

Keep these examples in mind as we turn first to an examination of the digestive system and later as we move through the other systems of the body.

Functions of the Digestive System

The digestive system consists of the alimentary canal, or tract, and its accessory organs (salivary glands, teeth, tongue, liver, pancreas, and gallbladder). It extends from the mouth to the anus and is a highly sophisticated energy-conversion system involving a wide variety of chemical processes. The entire digestive tract is shown in Figure 6–1.

The functions of the digestive system are twofold. It carries food for digestion and absorption and eliminates waste material. The accessory organs assist this process with secretions that prepare food for absorption and use by tissues.

A flowchart of the digestive pathway is shown in Figure 6–2. Food chewed in the mouth is swallowed, using the pharynx (throat) and esophagus (passageway to the stomach), and travels down through the neck and thorax into the abdomen. It is received by the stomach and there digested to a certain stage before it is passed to the small intestine for further digestion and absorption. The small intestine then passes the residue to the large intestine, where it is retained until it is excreted through the anus. The liver and the pancreas modify the food into forms suitable for storage and assimilation by the tissues. All the organs of the digestive tract are located in the abdominal cavity with the exception of the pharynx and esophagus, found in the first eighteen inches of the tract.

Word Roots Relating to the Digestive System

6.1 **alveol-** cavity; socket; small cavity, pit, or hollow

This word root is used to refer to sockets of the jaw in which roots of teeth are embedded.

EXAMPLES:

alveolectomy (alveol/ectomy)—surgical excision of the tooth socket's bony structure as a preparatory measure for dentures

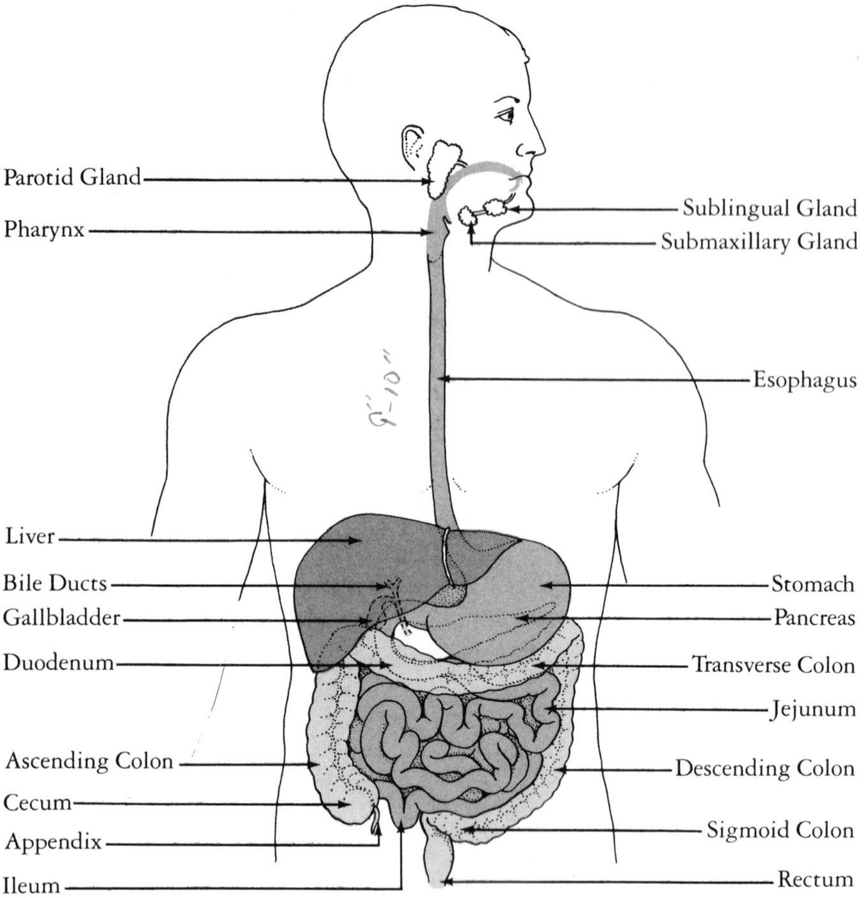

Figure 6–1 The digestive tract.

alveoloplasty (alveol/o/plast/y)—surgical process improving the shape and condition of tooth sockets in preparation for denture construction

6.2 **appen-** appendix

The appendix is a sac-like appendage extending from the large intestine, technically termed the vermiform appendix. The element *vermi-* means worm, so it is a worm-shaped appendage. A patient may have appendicealgia or appendicitis which is relieved by an appendectomy.

EXAMPLES:

appendicitis (appendic/itis)—inflammation of the appendix

appendiceal (appendic/e/al)—pertaining to an appendix; a synonym for appendicular

6.3 **bili-** bile; gall

Bile is a thick, sticky yellow or green fluid secreted by the liver into the gallbladder where it is stored and then sent to the intestines for mixture with gastric fluids as an aid to digestion, particularly the digestion of fats.

EXAMPLES:

biliary (bili/ary)—pertaining either to bile or collectively to bile, bile ducts, and gallbladder

biliary tract (bili/ary tract)—region that secretes and transmits bile; bile duct and gallbladder

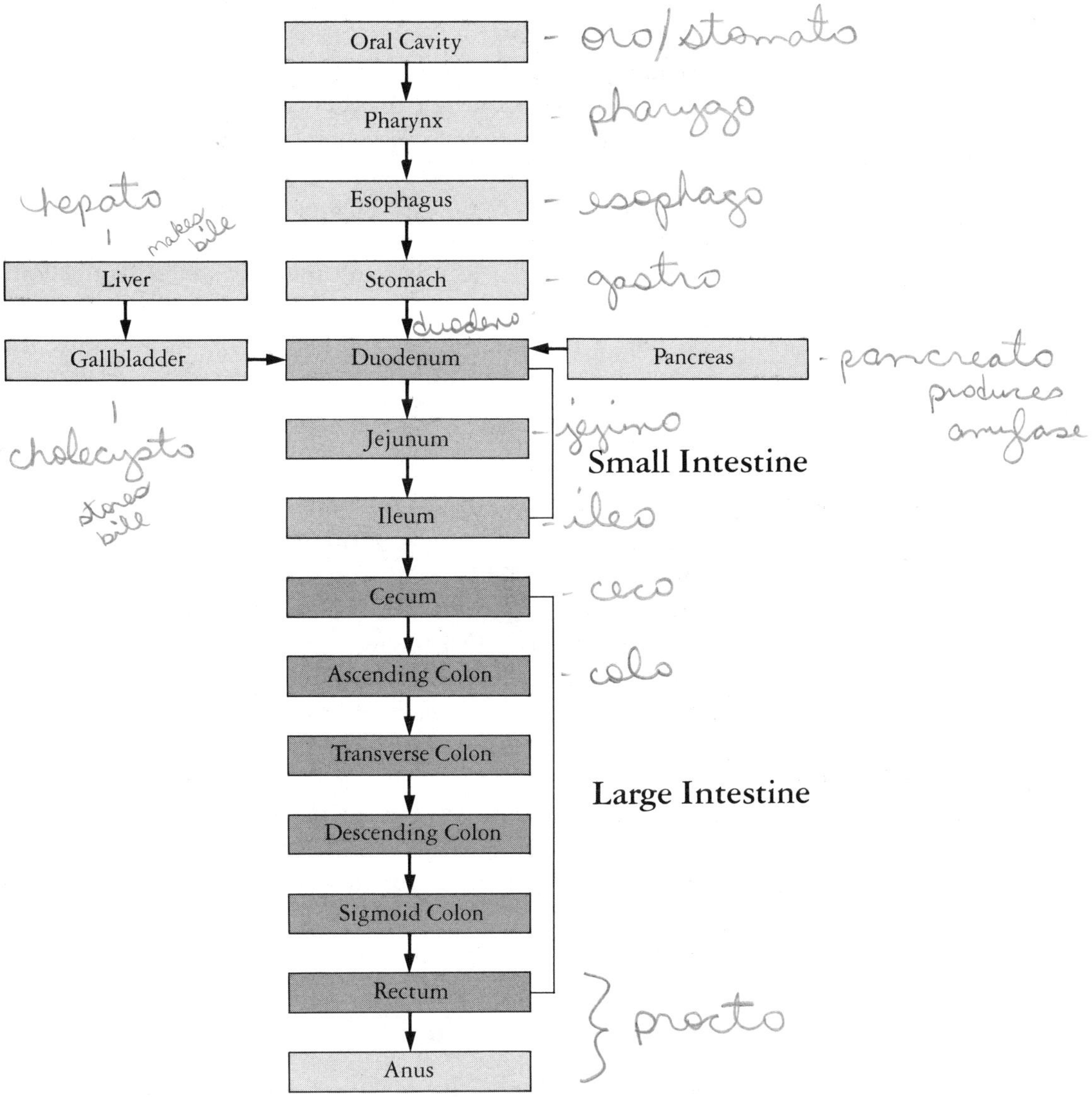

Figure 6–2 Flowchart of digestive pathway from entry to exit.

The root *chole-* is also associated with bile. A cholecyst, for example, is the sac or pouch in which bile is stored; the gallbladder. A choledocho is a common bile duct.

6.4 **bucca-** cheek; fleshy portion of the mouth

EXAMPLES:

buccal (bucc/al)—pertaining to cheek and mouth
buccinator (bucc/inator)—cheek muscle

6.5 **cec-** blind passage

A blind passage is a space having only one outlet so that smooth passage or flow through the space cannot occur. Even though the root may be used to refer to any such passage in the body, it usually denotes the cecum (cec/um), a pouch at the beginning of the large intestine having only one opening. Incidentally, the appendix hangs at the end of the cecum.

EXAMPLES:

cecotomy (cec/otomy)—incision into the cecum
cecectomy (cec/ectomy)—removal of the cecum
cecostomy (cec/ostomy)—provide the cecum with an artificial mouth or opening
cecorrhaphy (cec/o/rrhaphy)—suture of the cecum
cecopexy (cec/o/pexy)—fixation of the cecum to the abdominal wall

The actions named above may result from disease or injury affecting the cecum:

cecoptosis (cec/o/ptosis)—falling (downward displacement) of the cecum
cecorrhexis (cec/o/rrhexis)—rupture of the cecum; cecorrhexis may produce a hernia (cec/o/cele)
cecal (cec/al)—pertaining to the cecum

6.6 **cheil-** lip; therapeutics or conditions of the lip

The word root *labi-* also refers to lip; usually the lips of the vulva.

EXAMPLES:

cheilocarcinoma (cheil/o/carcin/oma)—cancer of the lip
cheilorrhaphy (cheil/o/rrhaphy)—suturing of the lips
cheiloplasty (cheil/o/plast/y)—fixation of the lip
cheilosis (cheil/osis)—condition of the lip

6.7 **chole-** bile; gall

Bile aids digestion of food, particularly fats. It is formed in and secreted by the liver (hepato-) and stored in the gallbladder (cholecyst) where it is discharged through the bile duct (cholangi-) into the intestines (enter-).

EXAMPLES:

choleic (chole/ic)—pertaining to or derived from the bile; of the bile; from the bile
cholangi- (chol/angi-)—bile vessel; bile duct, the tube through which bile passes
cholecyst (chole/cyst)—bile bladder; gallbladder

One of the bile ducts is the *choledoch-*. This is the common bile duct formed by the union of the common hepatic duct and the cystic duct.

6.8 **col-** colon

The colon is the large intestine. It is divided into the ascending, transverse, descending, and sigmoid (pelvic) sections. The colon is approximately fifty-nine inches long, extending from the ileum to the anus.

EXAMPLES:

colic (col/ic)—pertaining to the colon; also used to denote acute abdominal pain
colocentesis (col/o/centesis)—surgical perforation (puncture) of the colon; synonyms are colipuncture (col/i/puncture) and colopuncture (col/o/puncture)
colopexy (col/o/pexy)—fixation of a bend of the colon to the abdominal wall

6.9 **duodeno-** duodenum

The duodenum is the first section of the small intestine immediately following the stomach.

EXAMPLES:

duodenal (duoden/al)—of, pertaining to, or situated in the duodenum
duodenocholangitis (duoden/o/chol/ang/itis)—inflammation of the duodenum and common bile duct
duodenocholecystostomy (duoden/ochole/cyst/ostomy)—surgical creation of an opening (communication) between the gallbladder and duodenum

6.10 **enter-** intestines

EXAMPLES:

enteral (enter/al)—pertaining to the intestines
enteric (enter/ic)—pertaining to the intestines
gastroenter- (gastr/o/enter-)—pertaining to the stomach and intestines

6.11 **esophag-** esophagus

The esophagus is a tube through which food passes from the pharynx to the stomach. The word root *esophag-* is a combination of two elements, the prefix *eso-* meaning inner or inward and *phage-*, meaning to eat (swallowing). Just as the mouth and throat provide the outer swallowing of food for digestion in the stomach, the esophagus takes care of the inner swallowing, the final stage of food passage to the stomach.

EXAMPLES:

esophageal (esophag/e/al)—pertaining to or belonging to the esophagus
esophagoptosis (esophag/o/ptosis)—prolapse (falling down or downward displacement) of the esophagus
esophagocele (esophag/o/cele)—abnormal distention of the esophagus; hernia of the esophagus; protrusion of the mucous and submucous coats of the esophagus through a rupture in the muscular coat, producing a pouch or sac; diverticulum

6.12 **gastr-** stomach

EXAMPLES:

gastrointestinal (gastr/o/intestin/al) system—digestive system; combination of the stomach and intestines, responsible for digestion of food
gastroenteric (gastr/o/enter/ic)—pertaining to the stomach and intestines; pertaining to the digestive system
gastradenitis (gastr/aden/itis)—inflammation of the glands of the stomach

6.13 **gingiv-** gum; mouth gums forming collars around each tooth

EXAMPLES:

gingivitis (gingiv/itis)—inflammation of mouth gums
gingivectomy (gingiv/ectomy)—excision of mouth gums
gingivoplasty (gingiv/o/plast/y)—plastic repair or surgery of mouth gums

6.14 **glosso-** tongue

EXAMPLES:

hypoglossal (hypo/gloss/al)—underneath the tongue
glossorrhaphy (glosso/rrhaphy)—suture of the tongue
glossodynia, glossalgia (glosso/dyn/ia, gloss/algia)—pain in the tongue

A synonym for *glosso-* is *lingua-*.

6.15 **ile-** ileum

The ileum is the lowest part of the small intestine and opens into the large intestine.

EXAMPLES:

ileac (ile/ac)—pertaining to the ileum
ileitis (ile/itis)—inflammation of the ileum
ileus (ile/us)—intestinal obstruction

6.16 **labi-** lip; any lip-like structure, especially the lips of the face

The root *labi-* is the common form used to refer to a lip or lip-like structure; the root *cheil-,* however, is used to describe conditions of or therapy applied to the lip.

EXAMPLES:

labium (labi/um)—fleshy border or edge
labial (labi/al)—pertaining to a lip; pertaining to a labium
labiodental (labi/o/dental)—pertaining to the lips and teeth
labiology (labi/ology)—study of lip movements

6.17 **laryng-** larynx

The larynx is a structure composed of muscle and cartilage located below the pharynx, what is commonly termed the Adam's apple. It acts in three ways: (1) as a passageway for air into the lungs; (2) as an aid in swallowing; (3) as the voice box; that is, the container for the vocal cords that form sounds.

EXAMPLES:

otolaryngology (ot/o/laryng/ology)—the combination of otology (the study of the ear) and laryngology (the study of the throat), considered a single specialty area
rhinolaryngology (rhin/o/laryng/ology)—the combination of rhinology (the study of the nose) and laryngology, considered a single specialty area
otorhinolaryngology (ot/o/rhin/o/laryng/ology)—the combination of otology, rhinology, and laryngology, considered a single specialty area; also designated by the abbreviation E.N.T. (ear, nose, and throat)

6.18 **lingua-** tongue

EXAMPLES:

lingual (lingu/al)—pertaining to the tongue
lingula (ling/ula)—small tongue; generally a part of the body which is shaped like, and projects like, a tongue, especially part of the upper lobe of the left lung
lingually (lingu/al/ly)—toward the tongue

This word root carries the same meaning as the root *gloss-*. While both refer to the tongue in the mouth, they are used for different purposes. *Lingu-* is used to designate the tongue as a structure or point of reference (landmark), as in the term retrolingual, meaning behind the tongue. *Gloss-* is the word root used to denote diseases, injuries, and the therapeutic procedures used to alleviate diseases and injuries of the tongue.

6.19 **lith-** stone; mass composed of extremely hard material; calculus

EXAMPLES:

lithic (lith/ic)—pertaining to a stone or stones

-lithia, -lithiasis (-lith/iasis)—abnormal formation of stony material
Abnormal formations of stony material may occur throughout the body. Familiar terms may be gallstones (cholelith) and kidney stones (nephrolith). The condition *-lithia* or *-lithiasis* may occur in the joints (arthrolithiasis), the urinary bladder (cystolithiasis), or the appendix (appendicular lithiasis).

6.20 odont- tooth

EXAMPLES:

odontic, odontal (odont/ic, odont/al)—pertaining to a tooth or to the teeth
-odontia (-odont/ia)—form, condition, or treatment mode of the teeth
odontogenic (odont/o/gen/ic)—originating in the teeth

6.21 oment- covering of internal abdominal organs

EXAMPLES:

omentum (oment/um)—membraneous cover of the abdominal organs
omental (oment/al)—pertaining to the omentum
omentopexy (oment/o/pexy)—attachment of the omentum to another tissue or organ

6.22 or- mouth; structure bounded at the front by the lips, containing tongue and teeth

This word root is seen in the word oral, which means pertaining to the mouth.

EXAMPLES:

orad (or/ad)—toward the mouth
circumoral (circum/or/al)—area around the mouth (*circum-* means around, as in circumference—the distance around a circle)

The root *or-* is used to designate the mouth as an anatomical part; *stom-* or *stomat-* is used to designate diseases, injuries, and therapy of the mouth.

6.23 palat- soft structure separating nose from mouth

EXAMPLES:

palatine (palat/ine)—palate bones
palatitis (palat/itis)—inflammation of the palate
palatoplasty (palat/o/plast/y)—corrective surgery of the palate

6.24 peps-, pept- digest

EXAMPLES:

pepsin (peps/in)—substance secreted in the stomach that begins the digestive process
peptic (pept/ic)—pertaining to digestion, such as peptic ulcer which is an open sore on the lining of the stomach or duodenum
-pepsia (-peps/ia)—condition of digestion
dyspepsia (dys/peps/ia)—faulty digestion; indigestion
bradypepsia (brady/peps/ia)—slow digestion

6.25 phage- eat

EXAMPLES:

onychophagy (onych/o/phag/y)—nail biting
phagomania (phag/o/mani/a)—insatiable craving for food; literally, an eating mania

6.26 **pharyng-** pharynx

The pharynx is the muscular membranous cavity of the digestive tube leading from the mouth and nasal passages to the larynx and esophagus. It is about five inches long and serves as a common pathway for both air and food.

EXAMPLES:

pharyngocele (pharyng/o/cele)—hernial protrusion of part of the pharynx

pharyngalgia (pharyng/algia)—pain in the pharynx; a synonym is pharyngodynia

pharyngomycosis (pharyng/o/myc/osis)—any fungus disease of the pharynx

6.27 **plak-** plate

This word root appears as *-plakia* (-plak/ia) and indicates patches of eruption, usually on mucous membrane.

EXAMPLES:

leukoplakia (leuk/o/plak/ia)—disease marked by white thickened patches on the mucous membrane of the cheeks, gum, and tongue, due to irritation

malacoplakia (malac/o/plak/ia)—formation of soft patches on the mucous membrane of a hollow organ

This root may also appear as plaque:

plaque—any patch or flat area

dental plaque—deposit of material on the surface of a tooth

6.28 **proct-** anus; rectum

The anus is the last part of the digestive tube, measuring about seven inches in length, through which feces are expelled from the body. It consists of three parts: (1) the anus (an/us)—the opening through which feces are expelled; (2) the anal (an/al) canal—approximately one and one-half inches long, through which feces are conducted; and (3) the rectum (rect/um)—approximately five inches long, which serves as a storage pouch for feces. The root *proct-* usually is restricted to words that refer to the rectum. However, medical usage has broadened the application of the element to include the anus, the anal canal, and the rectum in its entirety.

EXAMPLES:

proctology (proct/ology)—branch of medicine dealing with the anus, the anal canal, and the rectum

proctologist (proct/ologist)—physician skilled in proctology

proctoplasty (proct/o/plast/y)—plastic surgery (surgical repair) of the anus, anal canal, or rectum

6.29 **stoma-** mouth; opening

The element *stoma-* is the word root of *-ostomy*, meaning a mouth-like opening. It may also appear as *stomat-*.

EXAMPLES:

stomatology (stomat/ology)—branch of medicine that treats the mouth and its diseases

stomal, stomatal (stom/al, stomat/al)—pertaining to a mouth

The relationship between the elements *stom-* and *-ostomy* is clarified by the meaning of *-ostomy*; to create a new opening is to create a new mouth or *stoma-*.

6.30 **uvula** grape-like projection hanging from soft palate

EXAMPLES:

uvular (uvul/ar)—pertaining to the uvula
uvulitis (uvul/itis)—inflammation of the uvula
uvulotomy (uvul/otomy)—excision of the uvula

Terminology Trivia

Tooth Decay

Generations of Americans have been raised on the advertising slogan: "A clean tooth never decays." Although most believe it, it is simply not true. Despite our vast scientific knowledge, we do not yet know the causes of tooth decay and we know no satisfactory way to prevent it. Yet, tooth decay is the most common affliction of the human race; at least ninety percent of people in the United States suffer from it.

Wild animals, even meat-eating animals, do not have cavities and because of this fact it used to be thought that cooked foods were people's undoing. Later, candy and soft drinks were held to be the chief causes, and it was further believed that cavities were a just punishment for children who did not brush their teeth twice a day and go to the dentist every six months. Yet, millions of people who brush their teeth every morning and evening every day of their lives and never miss a dental appointment have mouths full of fillings. On the other hand, we hear stories about people with perfect teeth who never brush them or go to the dentist. Are these stories true? Yes, there are many cases of people with good teeth who take little care of them, especially in Mediterranean countries.

We do know that acid is a primary cause of decay, produced by bacteria that live on the teeth. Bacteria generate decay from sugars that remain in the mouth. So, diet is a factor, but not the only factor. A clean mouth (from brushing the teeth) is certainly another factor. Heredity is still another factor. Diet, including the ingestion of fluoride, is also important. The composition of the saliva is a factor. The body's own metabolism may sometimes be a factor, for there are many cases of people working under great nervous strain whose teeth seem almost to disintegrate from within.

Obviously, there are many variables that can affect the condition of teeth. The sad fact is that a clean tooth can decay and it is even sadder that we do not know how to prevent it.

Orthodontia

Many people believe that teeth are straightened simply for cosmetic purposes. In point of fact, however, most orthodontic treatment is performed for functional reasons; both so the occlusion (fit) of the teeth is proper and so periodontal breakdown will not occur when people reach the ages of fifty, sixty, or seventy. At the same time, incidentally, appearance also improves.

Pronunciation and Meaning of New Terms

cheiloplasty (ki′ lo plas″ te) Surgical repair of a defect in the lip.

cheilosis (ki lo′ sis) Splitting and scaling of the lips and angles of the mouth, a characteristic of riboflavin deficiency.

colic (kol′ ik) Painful spasm of a hollow or tubular soft organ; pertaining to the large intestine.

colopexy (ko′ lo pek″ se) Surgical fixation of the large intestine to the abdominal wall.

duodenal (du″ o de′ nal) Pertaining to the duodenum.
d. carcinoma, cancer of the duodenum.

enteral (en′ ter al) Pertaining to the small intestine.

gingivectomy (jin″ jī vek′ to me) Cutting away part of the gums.

gingivitis (jin″ jī vi′ tis) Inflammation of the gums.

glossorrhaphy (glō sor′ ah fe) Suture of the tongue.

Self-test

1. For each set, match Column A with Column B.

Column A	*Column B*
___ bucca-	a. word root meaning tongue
___ cheil-	b. grape-like structure at the back of the mouth
___ glossa-, lingua-	c. inside of the cheek
___ labia	d. roof of the mouth
___ os-, ora-	e. opening into the mouth
___ palate	f. the lips
___ stoma-	g. word root meaning lip
___ tonsil	h. mouth
___ uvula	i. oval mass of tissue on each side of the throat

2.

Column A	*Column B*
___ alveol-	a. word root meaning gum
___ cementum	b. bony sockets for the teeth
___ plaque	c. tooth
___ denti-	d. narrow portion of the tooth
___ odont-	e. tissue holding tooth in place
___ gingiv-	f. deposit of hard material
___ gum	g. Firm, fleshy tissue covering the alveolar parts of the jaw
___ neck	h. word root meaning tooth
___ periodontal	i. fibrous connective tissues around the tooth

3.

Column A

___ duodenum
___ ileum
___ ileocecal foramen
___ appendix
___ cecum
___ descending colon
___ sigmoid colon
___ rectum
___ anus
___ procto-

Column B

a. opening between ileum and cecum
b. distal portion of small intestine
c. first section of small intestine
d. last section of colon
e. ring-like opening at the end of alimentary tract
f. word root meaning anus or rectum
g. section of bowel that moves downward
h. distal portion of the large intestine
i. part of colon with blind pouch
j. organ hanging down from the cecum

4.

Column A

___ chole-
___ gall
___ hepar-
___ cholecyst
___ hepatic duct
___ cystic duct
___ common bile duct
___ pancreatic duct
___ omentum

Column B

a. word root meaning bile
b. word root meaning liver
c. bile
d. gallbladder
e. membrane covering abdominal organs
f. tube from the liver
g. tube formed from joining of ducts
h. tube from the pancreas
i. tube from the gallbladder

5.

Column A

___ anorexia
___ appendicitis
___ colic
___ labiology
___ cholecystitis
___ cholelithiasis
___ cirrhosis
___ diarrhea
___ diverticulosis
___ duodenal ulcer
___ dyspepsia

Column B

a. inflammation of gallbladder
b. difficulty in digestion, indigestion
c. small tubular projections in the intestines
d. loss of appetite
e. flow through of undigested food
f. sore in the duodenum
g. inflammation of the appendix
h. study of lip movement
i. bile stones
j. disease in which liver becomes dark yellow
k. acute abdominal pain

6.

Column A

___ emesis
___ proctoplasty
___ gastritis
___ hemorrhoids
___ hepatitis
___ hyperacidity
___ intestinal obstruction
___ jaundice
___ malocclusion
___ peptic ulcer

Column B

a. protrusion of an organ from its normal place
b. blockage in the intestinal tract
c. surgical repair of the anus
d. erosion of stomach or duodenum
e. vomiting
f. inflammation of the stomach
g. dilated veins near the anus
h. inflammation of the liver
i. high acid content
j. disease in which skin becomes yellow
k. teeth not coming together when jaws are closed

7.

Column A

d abdominocentesis
h analplasty
b appendectomy
f cholecystectomy
g colectomy
a colostomy
c esophagectomy
i exodontia or extraction
e proctitis

Column B

a. formation of a permanent opening into the colon
b. removal of the appendix
c. removal of the esophagus
d. puncture of abdominal wall
e. inflammation of the rectum
f. removal of the gallbladder
g. removal of the colon
h. repair of the anal region
i. removal of teeth

8.

Column A

g gastrectomy
e gastroscopy
c gastrostomy
b glossectomy
a herniorrhaphy
f ileostomy
d intestinal anastomosis

Column B

a. repair of a hernia
b. removal of the tongue
c. making a somewhat permanent opening into the stomach
d. two ends of intestinal tract sewn together
e. visualizing the inside of the stomach
f. opening into the ileum
g. removal of the stomach

9.

Column A

c pancreatectomy
d pancreatic–ojejunostomy
e endoscopic papillotomy
b polypectomy
a proctoscopy
f sigmoidoscopy
i antacid
k antidiarrhetic
g antiemetic
j cathartic
h digestant

Column B

a. visualization of anal and rectal regions
b. removal of a polyp
c. removal of the pancreas
d. opening into jejunum for the pancreatic duct
e. viewing device passed inside body to enlarge the ampulla
f. visualization of sigmoid colon
g. drug used to control vomiting
h. drug used to aid digestion
i. drug used to control acid condition
j. substance used to cleanse bowel
k. drug used to control diarrhea

* See page 160

Seven
Genitourinary System

parenchymal - essential part of organ (does work)

The genitourinary system includes the urinary organs and the reproductive organs.

Functions of the Genitourinary System

The urinary organs consist of kidneys, ureters, bladder, and urethra. (See Figure 7–1.) These organs are found both in males and females, with essentially the same construction in both except that the male urethra is much longer than the female urethra and conveys secretions produced by reproductive glands.

Every twenty minutes the body's blood filters through the kidneys. A large branch of the aorta enters each kidney as the renal artery. It progressively divides to become arterioles with each afferent arteriole leading to a tuft of

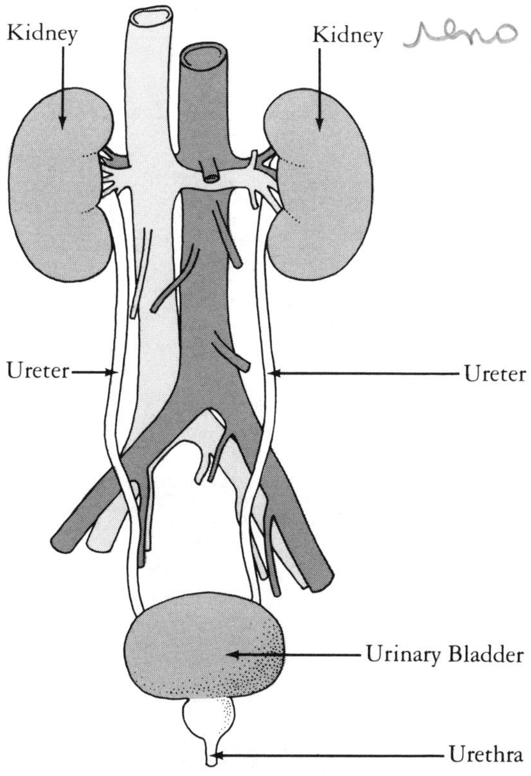

Figure 7–1 The urinary system.

Micturition - act of voiding or urination

coiled capillaries called a glomerulus. As the heart pressures blood into the renal arteries, fluid and salt pass through the glomerulus into a hollow tube. Each tubule, with its accompanying capillaries, is called a nephron. There are over two million nephrons in each kidney. Figure 7–2 presents a flowchart of the body's urinary pathway.

The essential organs of the male reproductive system are testes, or testicles (singular forms are testis and testicle), epididymides (singular form is epididymis), vas deferens, ejaculatory ducts, urethra, and penis. Accessory organs consist of seminal vesicles, prostate gland, and Cowper's glands. (See Figure 7–3.)

Sperm cells, or spermatozoa, are formed in the testes, stored in the epididymides, and travel through the vas deferens to the short ejaculatory ducts that end in the urethra. During sexual intercourse, sperm cells, together with fluid excreted by the prostate gland and the seminal vesicles, pass through the urethra and are deposited in the upper end of the vagina. The combination of sperm cells with fluid is called semen.

The female genital organs that constitute the pelvic group, as shown in Figure 7–4, are ovaries, fallopian (or uterine) tubes, uterus, and vagina. The external organs, termed the vulva, consist of mons pubis, labia majora bordering the pudendal cleft, labia minora, clitoris, vestibule, and greater vestibular glands. The urethra, through which urine is voided, is not considered a part of the female reproductive system.

Childbirth is referred to as parturition and occurs in three stages. It begins with uterine contractions that press the amniotic sac into the cervix, where it is ruptured. The fluid from the sac lubricates the cervical canal, facilitating passage of the fetus's head.

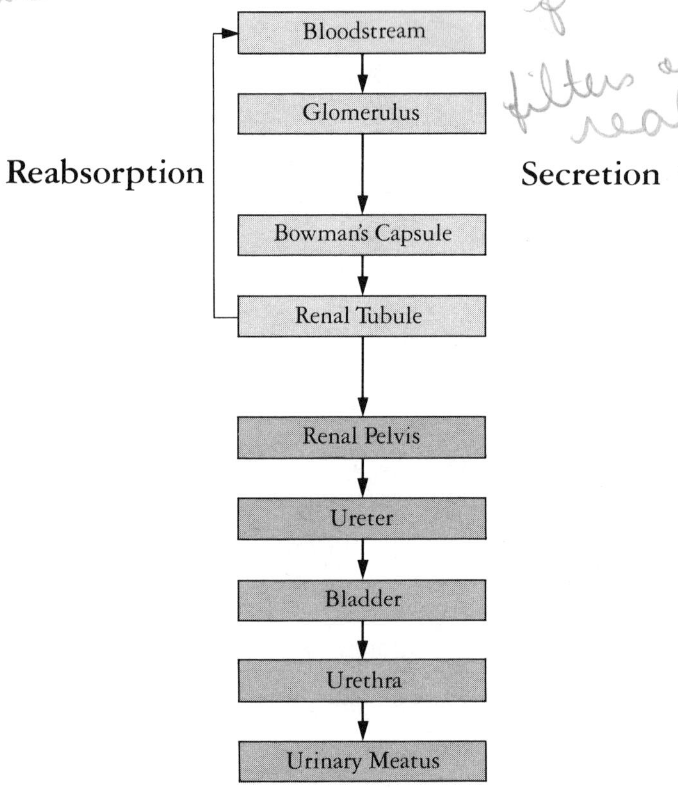

Figure 7–2 Flowchart of urinary pathway from bloodstream to exit.

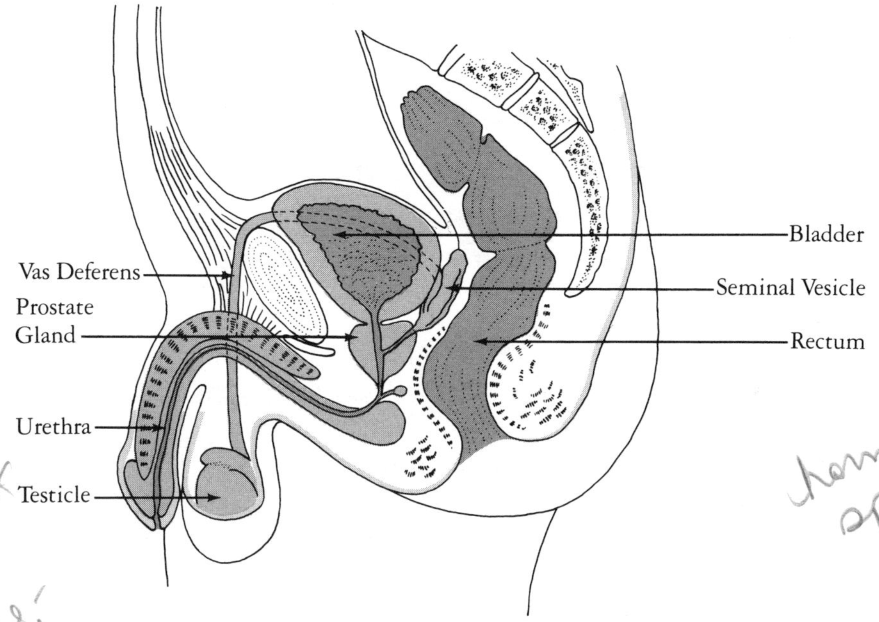

Figure 7–3 Male reproductive system.

Uterine contractions become more concentrated in the next stage and are aided by contractions of abdominal muscles moving the fetus through the vagina. During this stage, what remains of the amniotic fluid is expelled. When the child is delivered, the umbilical cord is immediately ligated (tied) and severed.

In the third stage, which occurs following birth, the placenta is expelled from the mother's body. The placenta is the organ contained within the uterus that maintains communication between mother and fetus. It consists of a fetal

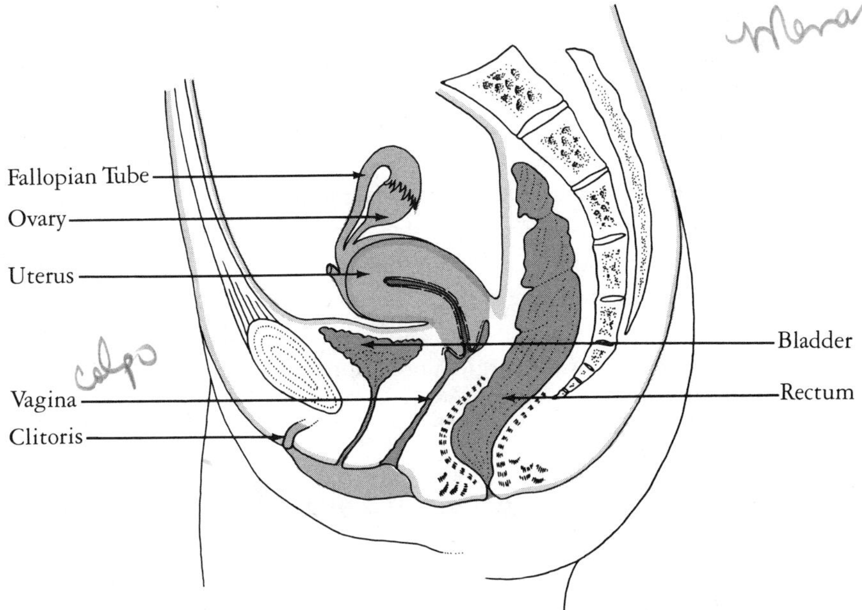

Figure 7–4 Female reproductive system.

portion—amnion, chorion, and villi—and a maternal portion divided in lobes or irregular outlines—the cotyledons.

Word Roots Relating to the Genitourinary System

7.1 **colpo-** hollow; vagina

The element *-colpos* (-colp/os) is a suffix used to denote a vaginal disorder of some specific type.

EXAMPLES:

pyocolpos (py/o/colp/os)—collection of pus within the vagina
hematocolpos (hemat/o/colp/os)—accumulation of menstrual blood in the vagina
colpitis (colp/itis)—inflammation of the vagina
colpotomy (colp/o/tomy)—incision into the wall of the vagina

The element *vagin-* is a word root used to denote relationships with any sheath-like structure, especially the vagina.

7.2 **gravid-** pregnant

EXAMPLES:

gravidic (gravid/ic)—occurring during pregnancy
gravidity (gravid/ity)—condition of being with child; pregnancy
gravidocardiac (gravid/o/cardi/ac)—pertaining to heart disease of pregnancy

7.3 **hyster-** womb; uterus

EXAMPLES:

hysteralgia (hyster/algia)—pain in the uterus
hysterectomy (hyster/ectomy)—surgical removal (excision) of the uterus
hysterology (hyster/ology)—study of the uterus

7.4 **metr-** womb; uterus

The word root *-metrium* (-metr/ium) refers to a part or layer of the uterus.

EXAMPLES:

myometrium (my/o/metr/ium)—smooth muscle coat of the uterus
endometrium (end/o/metr/ium)—mucous coat (lining) of the uterus

The form *-metra* (-metr/a) refers to a condition of the uterus. Although we are accustomed to using *-ia* as the word terminal denoting condition, the use of *-a* with *metr-* is an exception:

hematometra (hemat/o/metr/a)—accumulation of blood in the uterus

The roots *hyster-* and *metr-* are used interchangeably, with a tendency to use *hyster-* when denoting surgical procedures (operations) and *metr-* when denoting structural parts.

7.5 **nephr-** kidney

The kidneys consist of two bean-shaped glands found in the lower back.

EXAMPLES:

nephromegaly (nephr/o/megal/y)—enlargement of a kidney
nephritis (nephr/itis)—inflammation of a kidney
nephroma (nephr/oma)—tumor of the kidney

7.6 **oophor-** ovary; egg carrier

The elements *oophor-* and *ovar-* are synonyms; *ovar-* is more frequently used to designate the anatomical part, while *oophor-* is more frequently used to name diseases, abnormalities, and therapeutic procedures.

EXAMPLES:

oophoron (oophor/on)—ovary

oophoropexy (oophor/o/pexy)—surgical fixation or attachment of the ovary

hystero-oophorectomy (hyster/o/oophor/ectomy)—surgical removal of uterus and ovaries

7.7 **orchido-** testicle

EXAMPLES:

orchidoplasty (orchido/plasty)—surgical transfer of an undescended testicle to the scrotum

orchiectomy (orchi/ectomy)—excision of a testicle

orchiodynia (orchio/dynia)—testicular pain

7.8 **ovar-** egg; ovary

The ovary is the female reproductive organ that produces eggs and sex hormones; the root *ov-* means egg, with ovum the singular form and ova the plural form. The combination of elements in *ovar-* literally means a place for the ova.

EXAMPLES:

ovary (ov/ar/y)—female sexual gland in which ova are formed

ovariogenic (ovari/o/gen/ic)—produced in or arising from the ovary

ovariocentesis (ovari/o/centesis)—surgical puncture of an ovary

7.9 **para-** woman who has produced offspring

This word root should not be confused with the prefix *para-*, which means near, around, or beside.

EXAMPLES:

multipara (multi/para)—woman who has given birth more than once

nullipara (nulli/para)—woman who has never borne children

primipara (primi/para)—woman having her first child

7.10 **part-** labor; birth; delivery

This word root refers to the process whereby the mother is separated or parted from her offspring.

EXAMPLES:

parturition (part/ur/ition)—act or process of giving birth to a child

postpartum (post/part/um)—occurring after childbirth or after delivery

prepartal (pre/part/al)—occurring before or just prior to labor

7.11 **prostate-** gland of the male reproductive system

The prostate is a gland that surrounds the neck of the bladder and urethra in the male and contributes fluid to semen.

EXAMPLES:

prostatic (prostat/ic)—concerning the prostate gland

prostatitis (prostat/itis)—inflammation of the prostate gland
prostatorrhea (prostat/orrhea)—abnormal discharge of the prostate gland

7.12 ren- kidneys

EXAMPLES:

renal (ren/al)—pertaining to the kidney
supraren- (supra/ren-)—situated above the kidney; used especially when referring to the suprarenal gland (adrenal gland)

The word root *ren-* is used as a landmark or point of reference when locating other nearby structures. The word root *neph-* is used principally to name conditions affecting the kidneys and surgical procedures performed on the kidneys.

7.13 salpingo- tube, especially the uterine tube

EXAMPLES:

salpingostomy (salping/ostomy)—surgical opening made in the fallopian (uterine) tube because the natural opening has closed
endosalpinx (end/o/salpin/x)—mucus membrane lining the salpinx (fallopian or uterine tube)

7.14 semen- seed

Semen is the whitish fluid secreted by male reproductive organs that carries and transfers sperm for fertilization purposes. It may also appear in the form, *semin-*.

EXAMPLES:

semenology (semen/ology)—study of semen
seminal (semin/al)—pertaining to semen
semination (semin/ation)—introduction of semen into the female genital tract

7.15 ureter- urine-carrying tube

The ureter is a tube that carries urine from the kidney to the bladder. The word root *ur-* is found in the words ureter and urethra and means urine.

EXAMPLES:

ureteric, ureteral (ureter/ic, ureter/al)—pertaining to the ureter
ureterectasis (ureter/ectasis)—distention of the ureter

7.16 urethra- urethra

The urethra is the canal through which urine is discharged from the bladder to the outside; in males, semen is also discharged through the urethra.

EXAMPLES:

urethral (urethr/al)—pertaining to the urethra
urethrocele (urethr/o/cele)—prolapse (hernia) of the urethra
urethroplasty (urethr/o/plast/y)—plastic surgery of the urethra; operative repair of a wound or defect in the urethra

7.17 utero- uterus

The uterus is a muscular organ found in females that serves to protect and nourish the developing embryo and fetus during pregnancy. The roots *hyster-* and *metr-* also refer to the uterus. The baby being formed in the uterus is called an embryo during its first three months; thereafter, until birth, it is called a fetus.

EXAMPLES:

uterovesical (uter/o/vesic/al)—pertaining to the uterus and the bladder
uteropexy (uter/o/pexy)—fixation of a displaced uterus; a synonym is hysteropexy
uteritis (uter/itis)—inflammation of the uterus; a synonym is metritis

7.18 **vesic-** bladder; urinary bladder

EXAMPLES:

vesico- (vesic/o-)—word form relating either to a bladder or to the urinary bladder
vesical (vesic/al)—pertaining principally to the urinary bladder
vesicule (vesic/ule)—small bladder; blister

The elements *vesic-* and *cyst-* have the same meaning. *Vesic-* is the root generally used when naming various bladders or bladder-like structures in the body, while *cyst-* is the root generally used when naming diseases and therapeutic procedures that involve these structures.

Terminology Trivia

Obstetrics

The first obstetricians were women, known as midwives (obstetrix means midwife). In primitive times, women were assisted during delivery by midwives who tried to coax children out of their mothers' bodies with promises of food. During their last week of pregnancy, women were not given anything to eat in the belief that their children would emerge by themselves in search of milk. Labor was held to be a conscious act on the part of children, who desired escape. Pregnant women were often shaken, head down, or bounced on a blanket to facilitate delivery; some were even hung from trees with straps under their arms to allow gravity a chance to aid delivery.

During the sixteenth century Wertt, of Hamburg, dressed himself as a woman to attend an obstetrical case, but was recognized by a midwife and subsequently was burned to death. It was not until the seventeenth century that physicians in Europe began to attend obstetrical cases.

Semmelweis (1818–1865) was the first person to advocate a thorough washing of the hands before examination or delivery of pregnant women; he also advocated cleansing delivery rooms with calcium chloride to overcome high infant and maternal mortality rates. His views were prompted by his observation that death rates were highest in clinics in which medical students entered obstetric wards immediately after dissecting bodies. When Semmelweis introduced aseptic procedures in his wards, death rates dropped. Despite this proof, his colleagues believed fever could not possibly be introduced by the hands of physicians or nurses; they maintained blood poisoning was caused by certain diets or odors. Semmelweis became a victim of persecution and later died in a mental institution.

The Caesarean section, performed today in difficult births, was named for the law of the Roman Caesars that dictated every woman dying in advanced pregnancy undergo surgical operation to extract the fetus. There is a record from ancient times of a successful Caesarean operation performed by a pig farmer: His wife was in labor for a prolonged period of time, and since he had often operated on sows, he performed the same operation on his wife.

Gynecology

Until the fifteenth century, female ovaries were thought to be undescended testicles. The ovary was given its name by Farrari, a physician at Padua University. Until the ovum was identified in 1827 by Von Baer, the manner in which pregnancy occurred was unknown. In the seventeenth century, de Graaf discovered the ovarian follicles (Graafian follicles). It was William Harvey (1578–1657) who first theorized that life comes from eggs in the ovaries of females; the theory popular in his day held that minute human beings were preformed in the body. It is now known that there are about 200,000–400,000 ova in each human ovary, present from the moment of a woman's birth. Only some 400 of these mature, however, usually only one egg per menstrual cycle.

Modern gynecology probably originated in America in the early part of the nineteenth century when McDowell (1771–1830), of Danville, Kentucky, successfully removed an ovarian tumor without benefit of anesthesia or antisepsis. His patient rode a mule to his home, her large tumor resting on the saddle horn. She was accompanied by her two brothers, both carrying shotguns, who threatened to kill McDowell if their sister died. McDowell's patient sang hymns during the operation.

Breast cancer and uterine cancer are the two most common malignancies found in women. About fifty-seven percent of uterine cancer occurs in the cervix or endocervix. Widespread use of the Papanicolaou smear, which tests for the presence of precancerous cells, has resulted in a decline in mortality rates for cancer of the cervix.

Pronunciation and Meaning of New Terms

hysterectomy (his″ tĕ rek′ to me) Removal of the uterus.

nephromegaly (nef″ ro meg′ ah le) Enlargement of the kidney.

oophoropexy (o of′ o ro pek″ se) Surgical fixation of the ovary.

ovary (o′ vah re) The female gonad; either of the paired female organs in which eggs are formed.

parturition (par″ tu rish′ un) Childbirth.

postpartum (pōst par′ tum) After childbirth.

renal (re′ nal) Pertaining to the kidney.

r. dialysis, diffusion of blood across a semipermeable membrane to remove materials that the kidneys would normally remove if they were present and functioning properly.

r. failure, inadequate functioning of the kidneys, which leads to uremia.

*r. **pelvis,*** funnel-shaped cavity in the kidney that collects urine from many nephrons.
*r. **transplant,*** replacement of a diseased kidney with a healthy one from a donor.
*r. **tubule,*** that part of a nephron where formation of urine occurs.

salpingostomy (sal″ ping gos′ to me) Formation of an opening into a uterine tube for the purpose of drainage; surgical restoration of the patency of a uterine tube.

urethrocele (u re′ thro sēl) Herniation of the urethra.

Self-test

1. In each set, match Column A with Column B.

Column A

____ nephr-
____ Bowman's capsule
____ renal
____ ureter
____ glomerulus
____ nephron
____ bladder
____ urinary meatus
____ vesical
____ genitourinary
____ urethra

Column B

a. word root meaning kidney
b. pertaining to the kidney
c. collecting unit surrounding glomerulus
d. tubule plus capillaries—the functioning unit of the kidney
e. ball of capillaries in nephron
f. tube that transports urine from kidney to bladder
g. urinary bladder
h. reproductive and urinary organs
i. opening of tube from bladder to the outside
j. receptacle for urine
k. tube leaving the bladder

2.

Column A

____ urethrocele
____ dysuria
____ enuresis - bed wetting
____ glomerulonephritis
____ hematuria
____ nephrolithiasis
____ nephroptosis
____ nocturia
____ oliguria
____ pyelonephritis
____ polyuria
____ nephrectomy
____ renal calculi
____ uremia
____ ureteritis
____ vesical fistulas

Column B

a. ~~prolapse~~ of the urethra hernia
b. difficulty in urination
c. involuntary urination
d. blood in the urine
e. kidney stones
f. dropped kidney
g. inflammation of the renal glomeruli
h. frequent urination at night
i. opening between bladder and nearby organs
j. waste products remaining in the blood
k. inflammation of the kidney pelvis
l. inflammation of the ureter
m. scant or small amounts of urine
n. removal of a kidney
o. frequent urination
p. excessive urinary output

3.

Column A	*Column B*
_a_ anorchism	a. absent testes
_f_ cryptorchism	b. inflammation of epididymis and testes
_g_ epididymitis	c. collection of fluid around the testes
_b_ epididymoorchitis	d. removal of one or both testes
_c_ hydrocele	e. undersecretion of sex–related hormones
_e_ hypogonadism	f. undescended testicles
_l_ oligospermia	g. inflammation of epididymis
_j_ orchitis	h. removal of all or part of the prostate gland
_h_ prostatectomy	i. abnormal discharge from the prostate
_o_ prostatitis	j. inflammation of the testes
_n_ spermatocele	k. inflammation of the penis
_m_ vasectomy	l. small amount of sperm produced
_i_ prostatorrhea	m. removal of a section of the vas deferens
	n. cystic distention of the epididymis
	o. inflammation of prostate gland

4.

Column A	*Column B*
_c_ cervicitis	a. painful intercourse in women
_f_ vaginitis	b. white patches on external reproductive organs
_a_ dyspareunia	c. inflammation of the cervix
_g_ endocervicitis	d. endometrial tissue found in various locations of the pelvic cavity
_d_ endometriosis	e. inflammation of external female genitalia
_e_ vulvitis	f. inflammation of the vagina
_b_ leukoplakia of the vulva	g. inflammation of the lining of the cervix
_j_ amenorrhea	h. bleeding after menses have ceased
_i_ dysmenorrhea	i. painful menstruation
_k_ menorrhagia	j. lack of menstrual flow
_l_ metrorrhagia	k. excessive menstrual flow
_h_ postmenopausal bleeding	l. flow of blood from uterus at irregular intervals

5. Use the following terms to complete the statements below.

a. ~~birth control~~
b. colpectomy
c. colpocleisis
d. colporrhaphy
e. ~~dilation and curettage~~
f. ~~endometrial~~ biopsy
g. ~~pelvic examination~~

1. The action taken to prevent the birth of a child is called _birth control_.
2. _Dilation & curettage_ is a procedure to widen the opening of the cervix and scrape the lining of the uterus.
3. _d_ is the repair of the vaginal walls.
4. _f_ is an examination of tissue from the lining of the uterus.
5. The removal of the vagina is called _b_.
6. The procedure to close the vagina with sutures is called _c_.
7. The procedure in which the internal female reproductive organs are examined is called a _pelvic examination_

6. Match Column A with Column B.

Column A

- b hysterectomy
- f oophorectomy
- c salpingectomy
- e salpingo–oophorectomy
- d salpingorrhaphy
- a vulvectomy

Column B

- a. removal of the vulva
- b. removal of the uterus
- c. removal of uterine tubes
- d. repair of uterine tubes
- e. removal of uterine tubes and ovaries
- f. removal of ovaries

7. Use the following terms to complete the statements below.

- a. abruptio placenta
- b. ectopic
- c. spontaneous abortion
- d. hyperemesis gravidarum
- e. intrauterine death
- f. placenta previa
- g. premature

1. A pregnancy that develops in other than its normal place is called (a) an __b__ pregnancy.
2. Labor that starts before the full term of pregnancy is complete is __premature__ labor.
3. __d__ means excessive vomiting during pregnancy.
4. __a__ is a situation in which the placenta prematurely separates from the uterus.
5. __f__ means the placenta is nearer to the uterine outlet than is the baby.
6. The loss of the fetus from natural, unplanned causes is called a __spontaneous abortion__.
7. When a child dies before it is born, an __e__ has occurred.

8. Use the following terms to complete the statements below.

- a. amnionitis
- b. dystocia
- c. eclampsia
- d. stillborn
- e. toxemia

1. A difficult labor is called __dystocia__.
2. The condition in which harmful substances are existant in the blood of the mother is called __toxemia__.
3. A sudden development of convulsions in pregnancy is called __eclampsia__.
4. Inflammation of the amnion is called __amnionitis__.
5. A child who is born dead is called __stillborn__.

9. Match Column A with Column B.

Column A

- d gravida two, para one
- a multipara
- c nullipara
- b primipara

Column B

- a. woman who has given birth more than once
- b. woman giving birth to her first child
- c. woman who has never had children
- d. woman who has been pregnant twice and has one living child

Eight
Nervous System

Functions of the Nervous System

The central nervous system consists of the brain and the spinal cord, along with nerve trunks and fibers. The brain lies in the cranial cavity, while the spinal cord is continuous with the lower end of the brain, passing through the foramen magnum, a passage through the occipital bone of the head, and continuing down the vertebral canal. The brain and spinal cord are protected from injury by the bones of the skull and the arched vertebrae. (See Figure 8–1.)

The central nervous system has been compared to a computer: The brain acts as the central command unit and relays messages by way of the spinal cord through nerve fibers (part of the peripheral nervous system) reaching every structure in the body. Most of the body's physical actions are under the control of motor nerves. Sensory nerves, and special sense organs such as eyes and ears, are responsible for reactions of the body to its outside environment.

The nervous system is a combination of the central, peripheral, and autonomic nervous systems: the central nervous system includes the brain and spinal cord; the peripheral nervous system is composed of the nerves that enter (sensory nerves) and exit (motor nerves) the spine; and, the autonomic nervous system includes the sympathetic and parasympathetic systems that control and harmonize the work of vital organs. (See Figure 8–2.)

CNS- brain, spinal cord

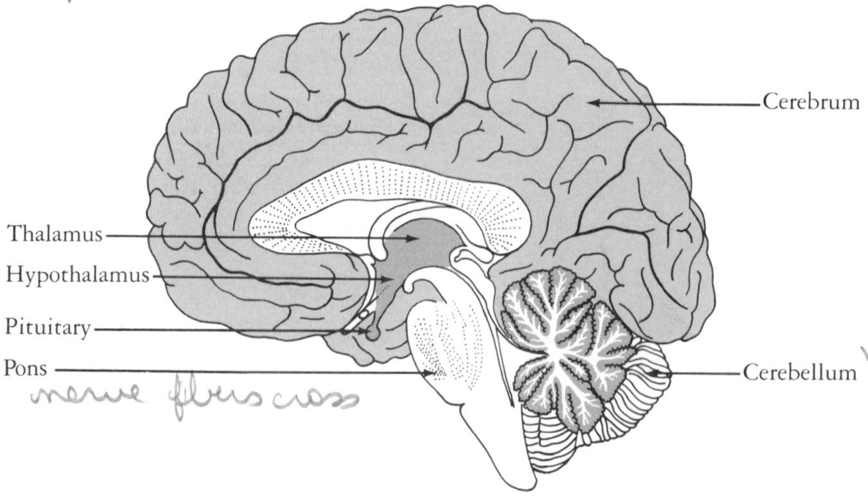

Figure 8–1 Sagittal section of the brain.

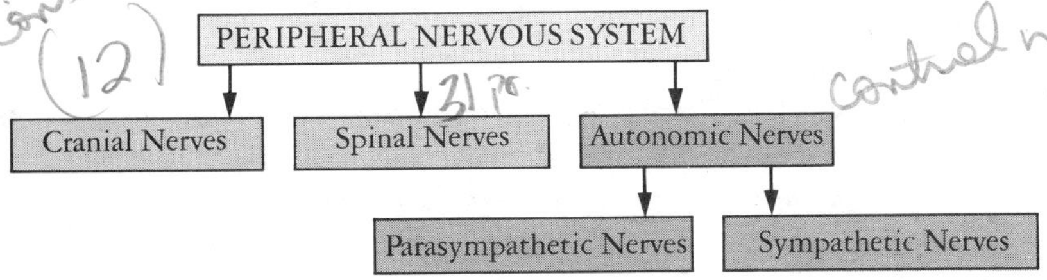

Figure 8–2 The peripheral nervous system components.

Word Roots Relating to the Nervous System

8.1 **cephal-** head

The word root *cephal-* refers to the head in its entirety, including cranium, brain, and organs of special sense (eyes, ears, and so on).

EXAMPLES:

cephalalgia (cephal/algia)—headache
cephalocele (cephal/o/cele)—protrusion of the brain through the cranial cavity
cephalopathy (cephal/o/pathy)—any disease of the head or brain

8.2 **cerebr-** brain

EXAMPLES:

cerebrospinal (cerebr/o/spin/al)—pertaining to the brain and spinal cord
cerebrosis (cerebr/osis)—any condition or disease of the brain
cerebromalacia (cerebr/o/malacia)—softening of the brain

The cerebrum is the main part of the brain in which the higher mental processes take place. It is sometimes used to denote either the entire brain or mental processes taking place in the brain.

8.3 **dendr-** tree; branching

This word root can be interpreted to mean a branching when describing body structures or parts that resemble the branching of a tree. It is most often used to describe nerve fibers that extend from a nerve cell.

EXAMPLES:

dendrite (dendr/ite)—name for nerve fibers that extend from a nerve cell
dendritic (dendr/it/ic)—resembling a dendrite; branching like a tree
dendroid (dendr/oid)—branching like a tree

8.4 **dura-** hard

The root *dura-* is a shortened form of dura mater; the outermost, toughest, and most fibrous of three membranes covering the brain and spinal cord.

EXAMPLES:

dura mater (or dura)—outermost of three membranes covering the brain and spinal cord
induration (in/dur/ation)—hardness; act or process of becoming hard
superdural (super/dur/al)—situated above or external to the dura mater

8.5 **encephal-** brain

EXAMPLES:

encephalic (en/cephal/ic)—pertaining to the brain; lying within the cranial cavity

encephalon (en/cephal/on)—name for the brain

encephalitis (en/cephal/itis)—inflammation of the brain; prolonged sleep, giving this condition the name sleeping sickness.

The root *encephal-* refers to the entire brain; the tissue structure that constitutes the organ of thought and neural coordination.

8.6 **ependym-** wrapping

The root *ependym-* refers to the membrane lining the cavities of the brain and the canal enclosing the spinal cord.

EXAMPLES:

ependyma (ependym/a)—membrane lining the cavities of the brain and the canal enclosing the spinal cord

ependymal (ependym/al)—pertaining to or composed of ependyma

ependymopathy (ependym/o/pathy)—any disease of the ependyma

8.7 **gangli-** swelling; knot-like mass

This word root denotes relationship to a ganglion; either a mass of nerve cells outside the brain and spinal column or an abnormal tumor or cyst consisting of tendon tissue that usually appears on wrists or ankle.

EXAMPLES:

gangliocytoma (gangli/o/cyt/oma)—tumor containing ganglion cells

ganglioplexus (gangli/o/plex/us)—network (plexus) of nerve fibers in a ganglion

ganglionectomy (gangli/on/ectomy)—excision of a ganglion

8.8 **lobo-** section of any organ, especially the brain and glands

EXAMPLES:

lobe (lob/e)—name for a well-defined portion of an organ; organs having such parts are the brain, the lungs, the liver, the glands, and the ears

lobectomy (lob/ectomy)—excision of a lobe

lobar (lob/ar)—of or pertaining to a lobe or section

8.9 **mening-** membranes covering brain and spinal cord

EXAMPLES:

meninges (mening/es)—name for the membranous sheath that envelops the brain and spinal cord

meningoencephal- (mening/o/encephal-)—word form for the meninges and the brain

meningitis (mening/itis)—inflammation of the meninges

8.10 **neuro-** nerve; nervous system

EXAMPLES:

neuron (neur/on)—nerve cell

psychoneurosis, neurosis (psych/o/neur/osis, neur/osis)—terms used to designate any of various psychic or mental disturbances

-neuria (-neur/ia)—suffix denoting condition of nerve function

dysneuria (dys/neur/ia)—impairment of nerve function
gastrohyperneuria (gastr/o/hyper/neur/ia)—excessive activity of stomach nerves
-neurium (-neur/ium)—suffix denoting nerve tissue
perineurium (peri/neur/ium)—connective tissue cover around nerve fibers

8.11 plexus- braid; network of nerves or vessels, such as veins or lymph

EXAMPLES:

plexal (plex/al)—pertaining to a plexus
plexiform (plex/i/form)—resembling a plexus or network
subplexal (sub/plex/al)—situated beneath a plexus

8.12 thalam- inner chamber

The root *thalam-* refers to the large gray mass that is part of the brain.

EXAMPLES:

thalamus (thalam/us)—name for the large gray mass in the brain
thalamic (thalam/ic)—pertaining to the thalamus

It is in the thalamus that sensations of pain, smell, and touch are integrated and relayed to specific topographic parts of the surface (cortex) of the brain. The word root is used as a landmark. The thalamus, epithalamus, hypothalamus, and subthalamus are terms used to name chambers of a large brain cavity called the diencephalon.

Terminology Trivia

Psychotherapy

The terms psychiatrist and psychoanalyst are often confused. Psychiatrists, always medical doctors, do not use the couch as an invariable accessory in treatment, usually preferring instead to see their patients face–to–face across a desk. Psychoanalysts, on the other hand, who may or may not be medical doctors, do use the couch if they practice the classic psychoanalysis associated with Freud. Psychoanalysts themselves undergo psychoanalysis in addition to studying its principles.

Psychiatrists may also be psychoanalysts if they have undergone psychoanalysis. Psychiatrists, analysts or not, use various treatment techniques with their patients: medication, behavior modification, supportive therapy, and electric shock, to name a few. Although Freud was a physician, he trained nonmedical persons as analysts, postulating that a medical background might actually hinder the practice of psychoanalysis.

A prevalent misconception concerns the idea that psychiatry and psychoanalysis deal with intellectual problems; indeed, intellectuals themselves tend to believe this. The truth is, however, that psychotherapy deals not with the mind, but with the emotions. If mere intellect could solve our problems, they surely would long since have vanished. For example, as far back as one can go in history, logical arguments against war have been common; war simply has no intellectual defense. So, why do we still have wars?

During ancient and medieval times, persons who were mentally ill often were chained in cells or otherwise isolated from society. Many believed to be possessed by evil spirits were even killed. For centuries, the plight of the insane was ignored, and no steps were taken even to study the condition. Between the years 1500–1700, almost 750,000 people were accused and convicted of witchcraft. According to clinical information contained in trial records, many of these people were psychotic. By the year 1564, the witch craze had spread to England from many parts of Europe, finally reaching a peak in 1592. Various sources estimate that by the end of the seventeenth century, somewhere between 300,000 and nine million people in Europe were burned to death. This witch-hunting mania spread to the New World and was centered in Massachusetts, Connecticut, and Virginia.

Shakespeare was born during the witch craze in England and his plays indicate a great interest in the problems of the mentally ill. The play, *King Lear*, presents a good example of senile psychosis. Shakespeare advocates entertainment as a therapeutic approach to mental illness in his work, *Love's Labour's Lost*. *A Comedy of Errors*, *King Henry VI*, *The Taming of the Shrew*, *Hamlet*, and *Macbeth* are all plays that contain mentally ill characters.

Freud (1856–1939) pioneered the field of psychoanalysis. He was acquainted with Shakespeare's plays and often referred to them in his writings. Freud collaborated with Breuer on the use of hypnosis in the treatment of hysteria, later abandoning it for free-association theory. He was joined in this by Adler and Jung, but later they rejected his theories on infantile sexuality and the Oedipus complex. Adler maintained that personality disorders are based on people's overcompensation for personal deficiencies, environmental repressions, and inferiority feelings. Jung introduced the terms extroversion and introversion; used to describe personality types. Later, psychoanalysts branched out and were joined in the study of psychiatric problems by other members of the medical mainstream.

Psychologist is a more inclusive term than either psychiatrist or psychoanalyst. Psychologists engage in a variety of activities: marriage counseling, testing, therapy, research, consultation, teaching. Like the term social worker, the term psychologist is sometimes used by lay persons with less precision than professionals employ. Clinical psychologists customarily hold the Ph.D. and are more likely to engage in psychotherapy than are psychologists who hold the Ed.D., or Doctor of Education degree. Unlike psychiatrists and most psychoanalysts, psychologists are not doctors of medicine.

Pronunciation and Meaning of New Terms

dura mater (du′ rah ma′ ter) The outermost and toughest of the three membranes of the brain and spinal cord.

lobectomy (lo bek′ to me) Excision of a lobe, as removal of a lobe of the lung, brain, or liver.

meninges (mē nin′ jēz) The three membranes covering the brain and spinal cord: dura mater, arachnoid, and pia mater.

meningitis (men″ in ji′ tis) Inflammation of the meninges, the membranes that cover the brain and spinal cord. Meningitis is caused by a variety of infectious microorganisms.

cerebral m., inflammation of the membranes of the brain.
spinal m., inflammation of the membranes of the spinal cord.

neuron (nu′ ron) A nerve cell.

thalamus (thal′ ah mus) The largest subdivision of the diencephalon.

Self-test

1. In each set, match Column A with Column B.

Column A

___ cerebrum
___ mesencephalon
___ cerebellum
___ pons
___ spinal cord

Column B

a. small, round mass located in posterior section of cranium
b. largest portion of the brain
c. column of nervous tissue running down center of vertebrae
d. bridge-like structure
e. the midbrain

2.

Column A

___ cordotomy
___ cephalalgia
___ subdural
___ neuron
___ electroencephalogram
___ lobotomy
___ encephalitis
___ neurolysis
___ neurotripsy
___ dura mater
___ sympathectomy

Column B

a. recording of electrical activity of the brain
b. headache
c. cutting into a lobe of the brain
d. cutting into the spinal cord
e. inflammation of the brain
f. nerve cell
g. external to the dura mater
h. removal of a piece of a sympathetic nerve
i. cutting of nerve tissue
j. outermost covering of the central nervous system
k. crushing a nerve tissue

Nervous impulse - the result of physiochemical changes occurring in the membrane of nerve fiber

arteries - away from heart
arterioles
capillaries
venule
vein - blood to ♡

Nine

Cardiovascular and Lymphatic Systems

The cardiovascular system (also known as the circulatory system) includes the heart, arteries, veins, capillaries, and blood. (See Figure 9–1.) The lymphatic system is a separate, but closely associated, system. It is included with the cardiovascular system because of its physiological relationship.

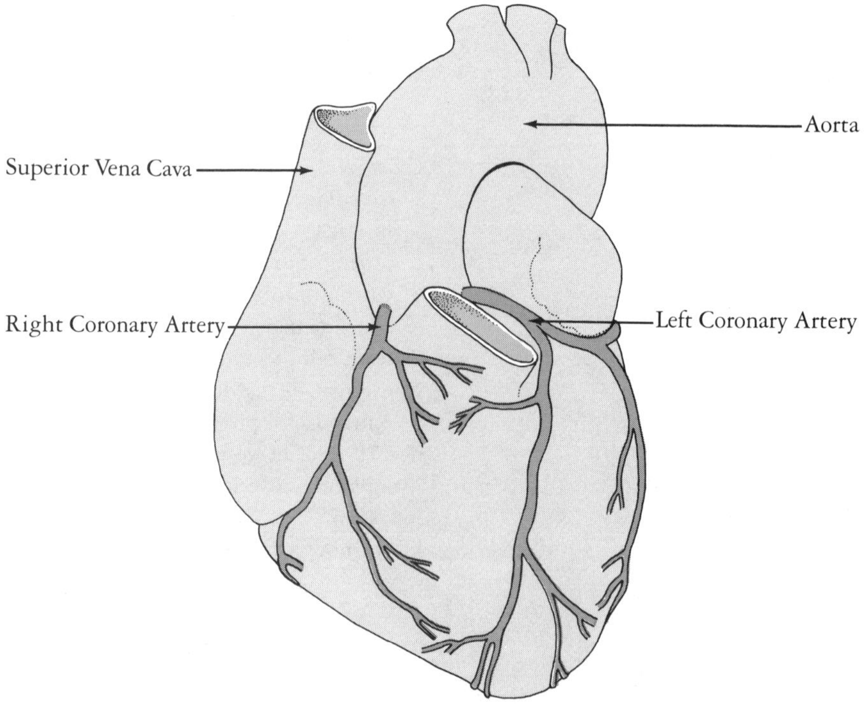

Figure 9–1 The heart/coronary arteries.

Functions of the Cardiovascular System

One of the functions of the cardiovascular system is the regulation of blood pressure. Blood pressure is the force the heart exerts on the walls of the arteries in pushing blood through the body. It is actually a measure of two types of blood pressure: systolic and diastolic. Systolic pressure is the higher of the two since it results from contractions of the heart's ventricles, or systole. Diastolic pressure is the lower pressure count because it occurs during relaxation of the heart's ventricles, or diastole. (See Figure 9–2.) Normal blood pressure

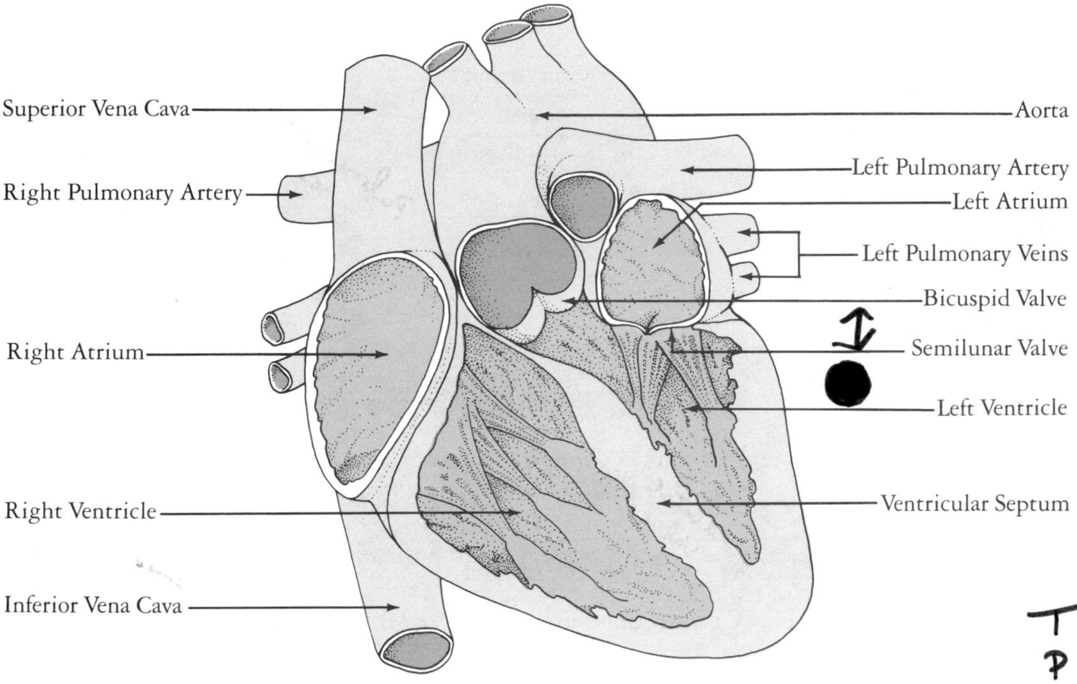

Figure 9–2 Internal view of the heart.

(measured by a sphygmomanometer) in a twenty–year–old adult is about 115 to 120 millimeters of mercury (*mm Hg*) at the systolic and 70 to 80 *mm Hg* at the diastolic. These readings are usually expressed as a fraction—120/80. A person's normal blood pressure can vary a great deal. For days, even weeks, many individuals can have an elevated blood pressure that causes them no harm. Exercise, tension, and excitement can raise blood pressure, as can age. At age sixty-five, a blood pressure reading of 135/85 would hardly be considered abnormal. Only when blood pressure is unduly high, over a prolonged period of time, is disease likely. A consistent systolic pressure of 150 is considered questionable, and a diastolic reading over 90 is considered high. The diastolic identifies the lowest constant arterial blood pressure in the body; it is, therefore, the more significant of the two pressure readings. Some factors that affect blood pressure include:

1. volume or amount of blood.
2. force or strength of the heartbeat.
3. condition of the arteries.
4. thickness or viscosity of the blood.

The condition in which blood pressure is elevated is called hypertension; abnormally low pressure is called hypotension. A flowchart of the body's circulatory pathway is shown in Figure 9–3.

Blood consists of plasma, white cells (leukocytes), red cells (erythrocytes), and platelets. Lymph is a virtually colorless fluid, rich in white blood cells and similar to blood plasma in appearance. It is circulated by lymph vessels located in every part of the body except the brain, spinal cord, eyeball, internal ear, nails, and hair. Part of the fluid discharged by blood capillaries to bathe tissues is reabsorbed by lymph capillaries; lymph capillaries also absorb particles

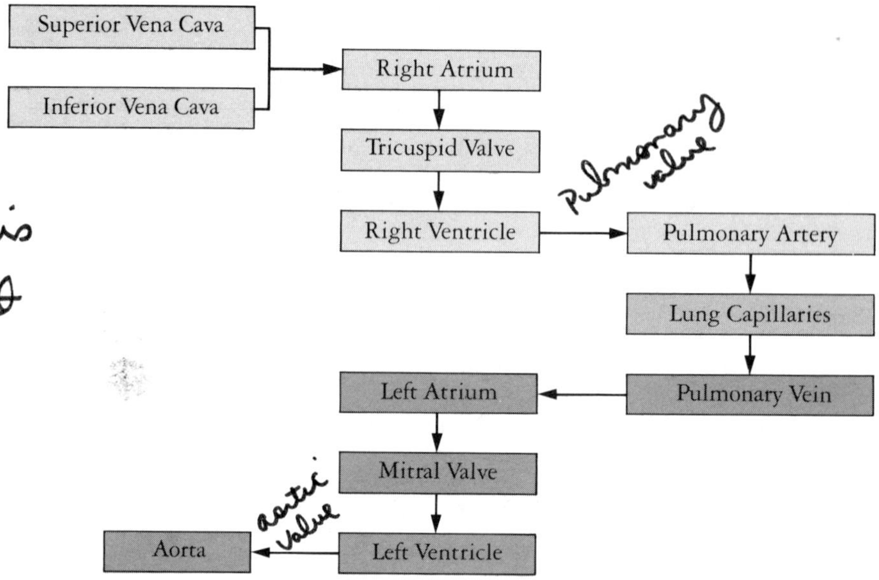

Figure 9–3 Flowchart of circulatory pathway from entry to exit of the heart.

of larger molecular size that cannot be absorbed by blood capillaries. (See Figure 9–4.)

Lymph vessels and lymph glands form a vast network throughout the body. They collect lymph and carry it toward the heart, eventually opening into the thoracic duct and right lymphatic duct which in turn empty into the left and right subclavian veins, respectively.

The lymphatic system is very important in defense against infection. For example, an acute infection of the hand will cause swelling, edema, and tenderness in the arm. This is called lymphangitis, commonly referred to as blood poisoning, because the lymph channels become inflamed. The redness

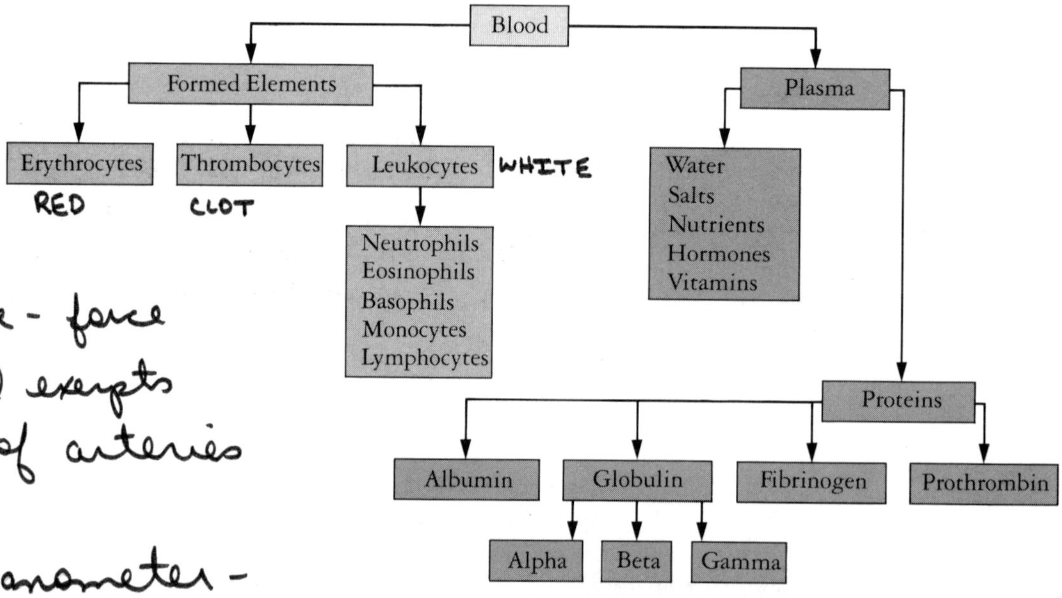

Figure 9–4 Blood cells and fluid components.

appears as streaking up the arm and, since blood is not really involved, the term blood poisoning is a misnomer. The inflammation may be arrested by lymph nodes (in this case, axillary nodes in the armpit that serve the lymph system from the arm) that become palpable and tender. This second condition is called lymphadenitis. Infections and cancer may also spread through the lymph vessels.

Word Roots Relating to the Cardiovascular and Lymphatic Systems

9.1 **angi-** blood vessel

This word root means vessel and so may be used to designate any of the tubes, ducts, or canals that convey body fluids. Its usual reference, however, is to the blood vessels.

EXAMPLES:

angiitis (angi/itis)—inflammation of a vessel, usually a blood vessel
angiectomy (angi/ectomy)—surgical removal of a vessel
angiomegaly (angi/o/megal/y)—enlargement of vessels

9.2 **arteri-** artery

An artery is any one of the system of large, thick-walled tubes that carry blood directly from the heart to the principal parts of the body. A vein, on the other hand, carries blood back to the heart.

EXAMPLES:

arteriectasis (arteri/ectasis)—dilation of an artery
arteriectopy (arteri/ec/top/y)—displacement of an artery from its normal location
arteriosclerosis (arteri/o/scler/osis)—hardening (sclerosis) and thickening of the arteries

9.3 **cardi-** heart

EXAMPLES:

cardiopathy (cardi/o/path/y)—any disease of the heart
carditis (card/itis)—inflammation of the heart
cardiology (cardi/ology)—study of the heart
tachycardia - fast heart beat

Bradycardia - slow heart beat

9.4 **cor-, coron-** heart

These elements are word roots used to designate the heart. They are introduced to mark their distinction from the element *cardi-*, used to name conditions and therapeutic procedures relating to the heart. The word roots *cord-* and *card-* are also used in reference to the heart.

EXAMPLES:

coronary (coron/ary)—arteries supplying blood to the heart muscle
cordate (cord/ate)—heart shaped
cordial (cord/ial)—stimulating the heart

9.5 **glom-** rounded mass; cluster

EXAMPLES:

glomus (glom/us)—small, round anatomical (normal) swelling composed of tiny blood vessels
glomic (glom/ic)—pertaining to a glomus
glomerulus (glomer/ul/us)—tufted structure or cluster generally

Diastolic - pressure when ventricles are relaxed

/80 90 ↑ - is too high

composed of blood vessels or nerve fibers; used principally to designate coils of blood vessels in the kidney

glomerul- (glomer/ul-)—word form for a glomerulus

glomerular (glomer/ul/ar)—pertaining to or of the nature of a glomerulus

This term is also used in conjunction with the renal system, where glomeruli are found.

9.6 **glyco-, gluco-** sweet; sugary

This word root is used chiefly to indicate the presence of sugar in the blood.

EXAMPLES:

glycemia (glyc/em/ia)—presence of sugar in the blood

hyperglycemia (hyper/glyc/em/ia)—abnormally high sugar content in the blood

glycolysis (glyc/o/lysis)—breaking down of sugar into simpler compounds

glycopenia (glyc/o/penia)—deficiency of sugar in body tissues

9.7 **hem(at)-** blood

EXAMPLES:

hematologist (hemat/ologist)—specialist in the study of blood

hematoma (hemat/oma)—tumor containing blood

hemorrhoid (hem/o/rrhoid)—dilated anal vein containing blood

If a word root begins with the letter *h*, it will retain the *h* if it begins a word. However, if the root is preceded by some other element, the *h* usually will be dropped. For example, the term anhemia becomes anemia when the *h* is dropped.

9.8 **hepat-** liver

EXAMPLES:

hepatitis (hepat/itis)—inflammation of the liver

hepatology (hepat/ology)—study of the liver

hepatomegaly (hepat/o/megal/y)—enlargement of the liver

9.9 **lien-** spleen

EXAMPLES:

lienal (lien/al)—pertaining to the spleen

gastrolienal (gastr/o/lien/al)—pertaining to stomach and spleen

lienorenal (lien/o/ren/al)—pertaining to spleen and kidney

9.10 **myel-** marrow; soft inner part of bones; cable-like tissue enclosed in canal formed by vertebrae

EXAMPLES:

osteomyel- (oste/o/myel-)—word form for bone marrow; relating to bone and its marrow

osteomyelitis (oste/o/myel/itis)—inflammation of bone and marrow

encephalomyel- (en/cephal/o/myel-)—word form for brain and spinal cord; synonym for myeloencephal-

Bone marrow and the spinal cord have structural similarities—both are surrounded by bone.

9.11 **phleb-** vein

EXAMPLES:

phlebectasis (phleb/ectasis)—enlargement (dilation) of a vein; a synonym is phlebectasia

phlebophlebostomy (phleb/o/phleb/ostomy)—surgical openings made to provide communication between two veins

phlebitis (phleb/itis)—inflammation of a vein

9.12 **pyle-, pyloro-** gate; opening; passage

The word root *pyle-* is used to express a relationship to the portal vein, a large important vein that carries blood from the digestive organs and spleen to the liver. For example, the term pylic (pyl/ic) means pertaining to the portal vein. The word root *pylor-* means gate keeper and is used to express a relationship to the pylorus, the opening from the stomach into the intestines through which stomach contents pass.

EXAMPLES:

pyloric (pylor/ic)—pertaining to the pylorus

gastropylor- (gastr/o/pylor-)—word form for the stomach and pylorus

gastropyloric (gastr/o/pylor/ic)—pertaining to the stomach and pylorus

gastropylorectomy (gastr/o/pylor/ectomy)—excision of the pyloric portion of the stomach

9.13 **splen-** spleen

EXAMPLES:

splenohepatomegaly (splen/o/hepat/o/megal/y)—enlargement of both the spleen and the liver

splenogenous (splen/o/gen/ous)—produced in or formed by the spleen

splenokeratosis (splen/o/kerat/osis)—hardening of the spleen

9.14 **thromb-** lump; clot

This word root is used to specify clotting properties and problems of the blood.

EXAMPLES:

thrombus (thromb/us)—clot in a blood vessel or one of the cavities of the heart, formed by coagulation of the blood

thrombosis (thromb/osis)—formation of a blood clot in a blood vessel or organ

thrombocyte (thromb/o/cyt/e)—clotting cell; small cell in the body that plays an important part in platelet clotting

9.15 **vas-** vessel; duct

The word roots *vas-* and *angi-* both mean vessel, especially blood vessel. Although their usage in medical terminology may overlap, *vas-* is generally used to name various ailments that affect vessels and therapies used to correct such ailments.

EXAMPLES:

cerebrovascular (cerebr/o/vas/cul/ar)—pertaining to the blood vessels of the brain's cerebrum

myovascular (my/o/vas/cul/ar)—pertaining to muscles and their blood vessels

vasectomy (vas/ectomy)—surgical excision of all or part of the duct through which sperm is secreted

9.16 **vena-** vein

Veins are vessels that carry blood toward the heart. This word root is used with descriptive words to name the many veins of the body. Diseases, abnormalities, and therapeutic procedures pertaining to veins are named using the root *phleb-*.

EXAMPLES:

venation (vena/tion)—distribution of veins to an organ

venae comitantes (venae co/mit/antes)—two or more veins accompanying an artery

venule (venule)—small vein continuous with a capillary

Terminology Trivia

Cardiology

Although human beings are dependent on the circulatory system for their very existence, it was not until the seventeenth century that much was known about it. Prior to that time, the Hippocratic doctrine had taught that the heart was the source of body heat, and that blood, collected in the liver, carried this heat to the left side of the heart. Galen thought the liver was the source of blood formation, with all veins originating from that organ. Credit for our current beliefs go to William Harvey (1578–1657), who performed experiments with animals and used mathematical proofs to uncover the true nature of blood circulation.

The important roles blood transfusions play in prolonging and saving lives today make it almost inconceivable that at one time blood-letting with leeches was the predominant treatment for disease. The idea behind blood-letting was that it would relieve pain, the aim being the cure or prevention of gastroenteritis, then believed to be the basis of all ailments.

Pronunciation and Meaning of New Terms

cardiology (kar de ol′ o je) The study of the heart and its functions.

cerebrovascular (ser″ ē bro vas′ ku lar) Pertaining to the blood vessels of the cerebrum.

c. accident, condition involving the blood vessels of the brain, generally associated with ischemic or hemorrhagic lesions.

gastrointestinal (gas″ tro in tes′ tī nal) Pertaining to the stomach and the intestines.

glycolysis (gli kol′ ī sis) The breaking down of glycogen or glucose.

hepatitis (hep″ ah ti′ tis) Inflammation of the liver.

hepatomegaly (hep″ ah to meg′ ah le) Enlargement of the liver.

osteomyelitis (os″ te o mi″ ē li′ tis) Inflammation of the bone and bone marrow.

thrombosis (throm bo′ sis) The presence of a blood clot.

thrombus (throm′ bus) A blood clot formed in the heart or a blood vessel.

phlebitis (flē bi′ tis) Inflammation of a vein.

Self-test

1. For each set, match Column A with Column B.

Column A

___ superior vena cava
___ pulmonary artery
___ right pulmonary vein
___ aorta
___ [redacted] tricuspid valve
___ glycemia
___ angi-
___ capillary
___ phleb-
___ venule

Column B

a. main artery of the body
b. blood vessel carrying blood to the lungs
c. sugar in the blood
d. valve on the right side of the heart between the atrium and ventricle
e. drains blood from upper part of the body to the heart
f. returns blood from right lung
g. hair-thin blood vessel
h. word root meaning vein
i. vessel
j. small vein

2.

Column A

___ angina pectoris
___ angiogram
___ vasodilation
___ arteriography
___ arteritis
___ bradycardia
___ cardiomyopathy
___ cardiomegaly
___ bacterial endocarditis
___ electrocardiogram
___ edema
___ neutrophils

Column B

a. pain in the chest
b. slow heart rate
c. x-ray of blood vessels, including arteries and veins
d. x-ray of arteries
e. inflammation of an artery
f. widening the diameter of blood vessels
g. disease of the heart muscle
h. record of electrical activity of the heart
i. inflammation inside the heart
j. swelling of parts of the body
k. enlarged heart
l. a type of leukocyte

Pg. 157

3.

Column A	*Column B*
___ thrombus	a. inadequate heart muscle action
___ hemangioma	b. inflammation of a vein
___ hematoma	c. dilated vein containing blood in anal area
___ hemorrhoid	d. low blood pressure
___ hypertension	e. swelling containing blood
___ hypotension	f. high blood pressure
___ phlebitis	g. clot of blood obstructing blood vessels
___ myocardial insufficiency	h. tumor consisting of blood vessels
___ phlebotomy	i. incision of a vein

4.

Column A	*ColumnB*
___ erythrocytes	a. blood fluid
___ leukocytes	b. red blood cells
___ plasma	c. white blood cells
___ hemoglobin	d. red coloring in red blood cells
___ albumin	e. protein substance that becomes spherical in solution
___ globulin	f. protein that produces fiber
___ fibrinogen	g. protein substance that coagulates like an egg white when heated
___ prothrombin	h. protein that is involved in blood clot production

5.

Column A	*Column B*
___ agranulocytosis	a. unequal size of red blood cells
___ anemia	b. blood more acid than normal
___ anisocytosis	c. blood more alkaline than normal
___ anoxia	d. deficiency of oxygen in blood
___ acidosis	e. reduced erythrocytes, hemoglobin, or packed red cells
___ alkalosis	f. lack of granulocytes

6.

Column A	*Column B*
___ hemostasis	a. disease of lymph glands
___ lymphadenitis	b. neoplasm of lymphatic tissues
___ lympadenopathy	c. inflammation of lymph glands
___ lymphatic metastasis	d. elevated blood sugar
___ lymphoma	e. stopping of blood
___ splenomegaly	f. enlargement of the spleen
___ hyperglycemia	g. the spread of disease through the lymphatic system

Ten
Respiratory System

The term respiration refers to the interchange of oxygen (O_2) and carbon dioxide (CO_2). This process involves the inhalation, or inspiration, of oxygen and the exhalation, or elimination, of carbon dioxide and other waste gases.

Functions of the Respiratory System

Before birth, the alveoli of the lungs contain only a small amount of fluid. The thorax is unexpanded and filled by airless lungs; only a small portion of the blood from the right ventricle passes through the lungs. The remainder of the blood passes to the aorta through the ductus arteriosus, a temporary channel from the pulmonary artery to the aorta. At the moment of birth, the diaphragm descends and the thorax expands. Simultaneously, a large portion of venous blood is conveyed through the lungs and the interior of the lungs comes in direct communication with the atmosphere through air passages. As the thorax expands, the lungs are filled both by the intake of air and by negative pressure. (See Figure 10–1.)

The act of respiration consists of three cycles: inspiration, which is the breathing of air into the lungs; expiration which is the exhalation of air out from the lungs; and, the interval between expiration and inspiration. The respiratory system in relation to the heart is shown in Figure 10–2.

Oxygen is one air element breathed into the lungs during inspiration. It is absorbed by the lungs, passed into the bloodstream (where it loosely combines with hemoglobin to form oxyhemoglobin), and is carried by the red blood cells to all tissues and cells of the body. The amount of oxygen retained by tissues and cells depends on their needs; tissues will not retain more oxygen than is needed. Increased activity on the part of tissues requires increased use of oxygen. During strenuous exercise, for example, oxygen utilization by muscles of the body may more than double and be accompanied by a marked increase in the amount of supplied blood.

Carbon dioxide is formed in the body and is carried by the venous bloodstream to the lungs for expiration. The amount of carbon dioxide produced by respiration varies with the health, size, and activity level of the individual.

Root Words Relating to the Respiratory System

10.1 **aer-** air

This element is an old spelling of air that persists in medical terminology.

EXAMPLES:

aerial (aer/i/al)—pertaining to air

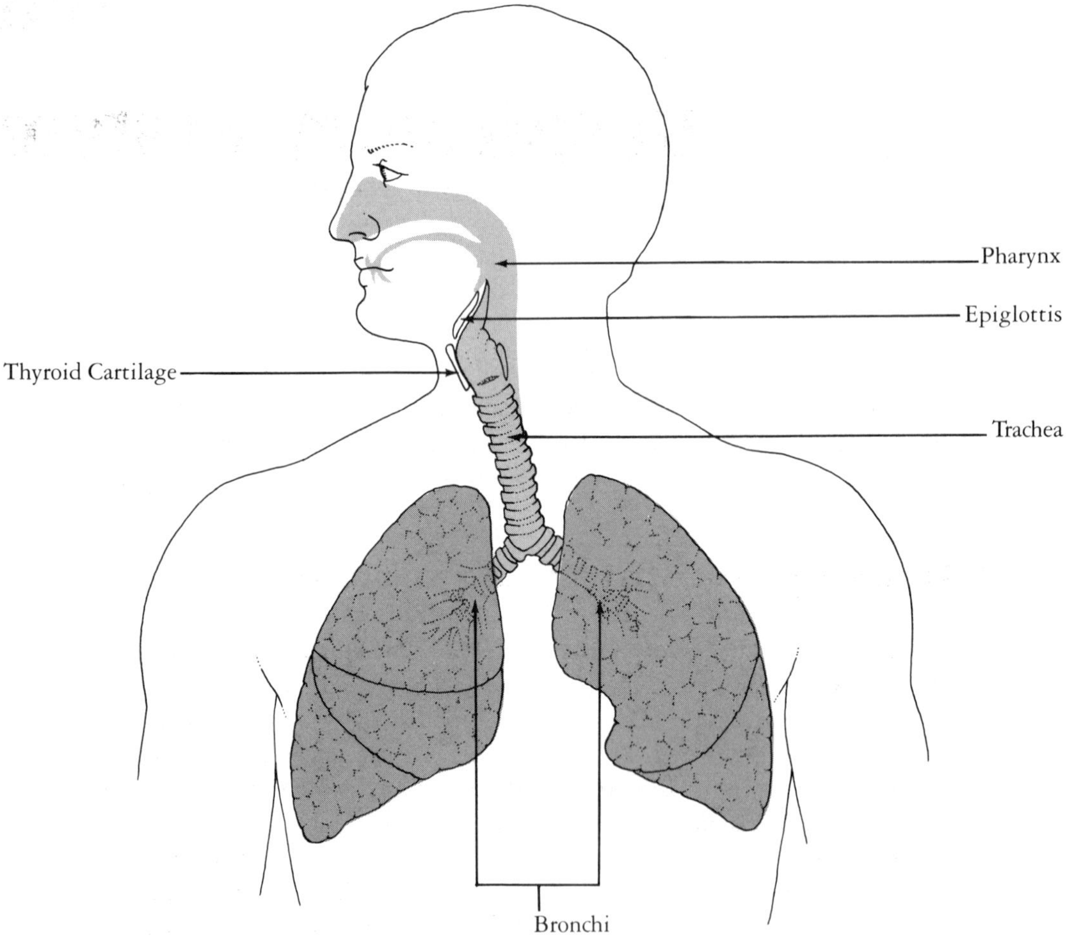

Figure 10–1 The respiratory system.

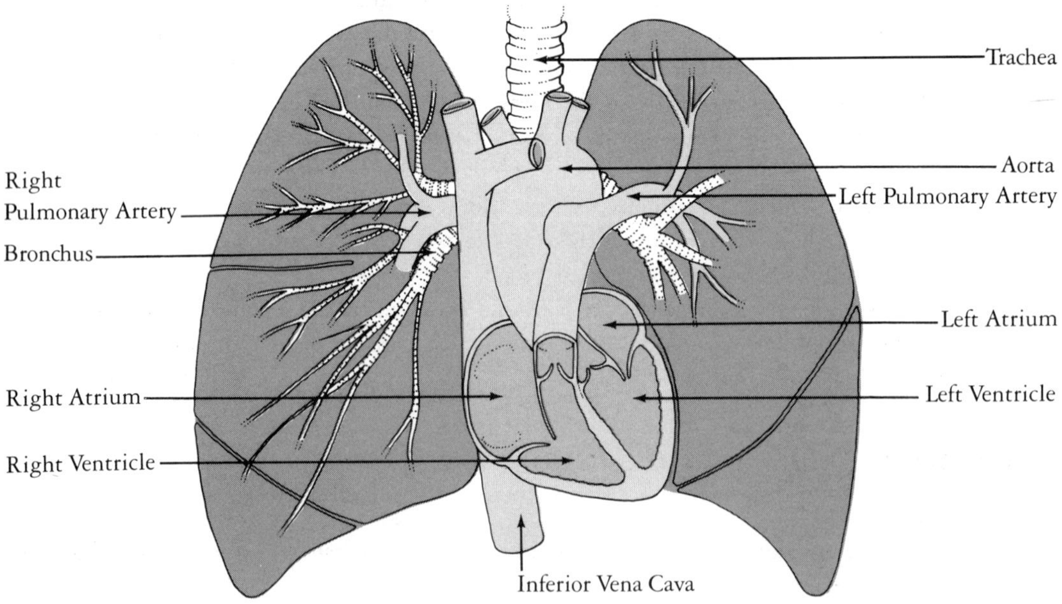

Figure 10–2 Respiratory system in relation to the heart.

aerosis (aer/osis)—production of gas in tissues or organs of the body
aeropathy (aer/o/path/y)—any disease due to a change in atmospheric pressure, such as the bends

10.2 **bronch-** bronchus

A bronchus is one of two main branches from the trachea or windpipe that carry air into the lungs. The plural of bronchus is bronchi. The point at which the bronchi branch from the trachea is named the tracheal bifurcation.

EXAMPLES:

bronchitis (bronch/itis)—inflammation of the bronchial tubes
bronchopneumonia (bronch/o/pneumon/ia)—name given to an inflammation of the lungs, that usually begins in the end of the bronchi
bronchopleuropneumonia (bronch/o/pleur/o/pneumon/ia)—pneumonia complicated by bronchitis and pleurisy

10.3 **phren-** mind; diaphragm; phrenic nerve

The diaphragm is the muscular wall or partition separating the chest cavity from the abdominal cavity

EXAMPLES:

phrenic (phren/ic)—pertaining to the mind; pertaining to the diaphragm
phrenic- (phren/ic-)—word form denoting relationship to the phrenic nerve

The suffix *-phrenia* is used to form words having to do with mental disorders:

bradyphrenia (brady/phren/ia)—slowness in mental activities such as initiative, interest, and speech; frequently accompanying encephalitis

The Greeks believed the diaphragm was the location of the mind. It would have been just as commonplace for the Greeks to describe a person as having a good diaphragm as it is for us to describe a person as having a good head; both indicate a good mind.

10.4 **pne-** lungs; air

The importance of air for the maintainence of life is reflected by the fact of its many word forms. The presence of the word root *pne-*, for example, indicates a relationship to breathing.

EXAMPLES:

hyperpnea (hyper/pne/a)—abnormal increase in the speed and depth of breathing
hypopnea (hypo/pne/a)—abnormal decrease in the speed and depth of breathing
bradypnea (brady/pne/a)—abnormal slowness of breathing
apnea (a/pne/a)—no breathing; absence of breathing

The forms *pneum-* and *pneumat-* indicate a relationship to respiration:

pneumal (pneum/al)—pertaining to the lungs
pneumatic (pneumat/ic)—of or pertaining to air or respiration
pneumatocele (pneumat/o/cele)—swelling anywhere in the body containing air; protrusion of the lung through a weak place in the wall of the chest

The form *pneumon-* is used to indicate a relationship to the lungs:

pneumonia (pneumon/ia)—inflamation of the lungs usually accompanied by chills, increase in temperature, pain, and coughing
pneumonitis (pneumon/itis)—condition of localized, acute inflammation of the lungs without the range of complications and symptoms accompanying pneumonia; benign pneumonia
pneumonic (pneumon/ic)—peretaining to the lung or to pneumonia

10.5 **pulmon-** lung

EXAMPLES:

pulmo (pulm/o)—lung; organ of respiration
pulmonic, pulmonary (pulmon/ic, pulmon/ary)—pertaining to the lungs
renopulmonary (ren/o/pulmon/ary)—pertaining to the kidneys and lungs

The forms *pulmo-* and *pulmono-* are generally used to indicate the lung as a landmark, while *pneumono-* is used principally to name conditions and therapeutic procedures relating to the lungs.

10.6 **spiro-** coil; wind; twist; breathe

EXAMPLES:

spiroid (spir/oid)—resembling a spiral or coil
spiradeno- (spir/aden/o-)—word form used interchangeably with *hidradeno-* (hidr/aden/o) to denote a sweat gland; so called because of the sweat gland's spiral shape
spirometer (spir/o/meter)—apparatus for measuring respiration
spirophore (spir/o/phore)—device used for artificial respiration

The root *spir-* also appears in words such as perspire, perspiration, aspiration, and respiration. In these words the element means breath or breathing.

10.7 **trachel-** neck; neck-like structure

The root *trachel-* relates to a neck or neck-like structure and is most frequently used with reference to the neck of the body or the neck (cervix) of the uterus.

EXAMPLES:

trachelitis (trachel/itis)—inflammation of the cervix
trachelopexy (trachel/o/pexy)—surgical fixation of the cervix to an adjacent part

A word root closely resembling *trachel-* is *trache-*, which refers to the windpipe; the main trunk of the system of tubes through which air passes to and from the lungs:

trachea (trache/a)—name for the windpipe
tracheal (trache/al)—pertaining to the windpipe
tracheotomy (trache/otomy)—incision into the trachea for insertion of a tube to overcome an obstruction

Terminology Trivia

Pulmonary Disease

The invention of the stethoscope by Laennec in the seventeenth century was a major contribution to diagnosis of respiratory diseases. Laennec (1781–1826) noticed children using hollow tubes to listen to sounds made by tappings on hollow logs. From this, he proposed that hollow cylinders of paper, and later hollow wooden tubes, would be useful for examining the human chest. His descriptions of breathing sounds, such as cavernous respiration, and crepitant, mucous, sonorous, or bubbling rales, have been useful to this present day. Laennec also described such illnesses as phthisis (tuberculosis), bronchiectasis, emphysema, pneumothorax, and cancer of the lungs. His invention of the stethoscope as an instrument for diagnosis permitted physical diagnosis far beyond anything previously used. His description of a chronic pleurisy found in alcoholics led to the discovery of an accompanying change in the liver, named cirrhosis because of its yellowish color. This condition is now known as Laennec's cirrhosis.

Leprosy

Counter to the impression so often given in Hollywood versions of biblical stories, lepers do not simply rot away, nor do their fingers and toes fall off. Nor is leprosy, as portrayed, a highly contagious disease characterized by open, running sores. No one really knows whether the leprosy mentioned in the Bible is the same disease as the one known today. Around a hundred years ago it was discovered that leprosy is caused by a bacteria similar to the type responsible for tuberculosis.

Leprosy can take either of two forms: a relatively mild tuberculoid infection whose victims are invariably discharged from hospitals after relatively short stays, and a lepromatous type, which can persist for life. Much remains to be learned about leprosy, but one thing is certain: it is not, counter to almost universal belief, easily acquired by contact with sufferers. None of the nurses, nuns, or doctors at the United States Public Health Service Hospital for Lepers at Carville, Louisiana, has ever contracted it; even where the disease is most prevalent, in parts of India, only five percent of the population is affected. None of the many attempts by courageous doctors—or less courageous doctors who used volunteers—to deliberately infect themselves or others with leprosy has succeeded.

Only one common belief about leprosy appears to have any basis in fact. It is true that one of the effects of the disease is to desensitize the skin. Thus, when the movie camera shot a close-up picture of the forgotten cigarette burning the fingers holding it (an actual scene from a movie set in the tropics, years ago), it at least had some foundation in fact. It seems doubtful, however, that the disease could have progressed so far as this without some previous indication.

Pronunciation and Meaning of New Terms

bronchitis (brong ki′ tis) Inflammation of the bronchi.

bronchopneumonia (brong″ ko nu mo′ ne ah) Inflammation of the lungs as well as the bronchi.

pulmonary (pul′ mo ner″ e) Pertaining to the lungs.

spirometer (spi rom′ ē ter) The instrument used in spirometry.

Self-test

1. Match Column A with Column B.

Column A

c apnea
f dyspnea
a hyperventilation
e laryngotracheobronchitis
b orthopnea
i pneumoconiosis
g pneumothorax
j pulmonary edema
k tracheotomy
h tachypnea

Column B

a. excessive breathing
b. condition in which breathing is easier in upright position
c. absence of breathing
d. inflammation of the pleura
e. inflammation of larynx, trachea, and bronchi
f. difficulty breathing
g. air in thoracic cavity outside lungs between two pleura
h. fast rate of breathing
i. lung condition caused by inhalation of dust particles
j. excessive fluid in lungs
k. cutting into the trachea

pg. 159–160

protects organs
aids in movement
gives shape

Eleven
Skeletal System

The skeleton is the jointed framework, composed of over 200 bones and cartilages, that supports and gives shape to the body. (See Figure 11–1.)

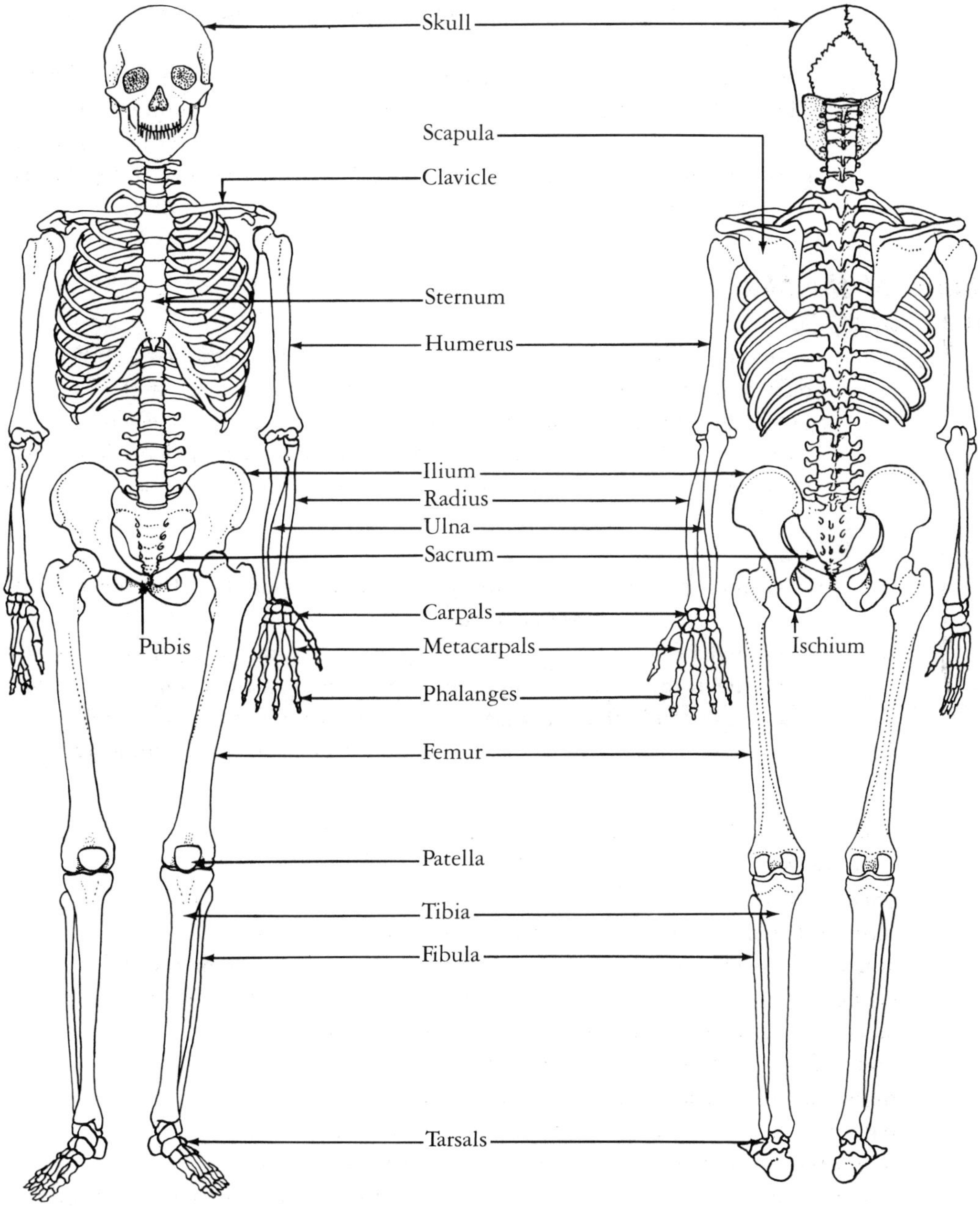

Figure 11–1 Anterior and posterior view of the skeleton.

Classification of Bones

Bones are classified according to their shape—either long, flat, short, or irregular. The femur (bone between the hip joint and the knee) is an example of a long bone, as is the humerus (bone between the shoulder and elbow). The short bones are those of the wrists, ankles, toes, and fingers (carpals, tarsals, and phalanges, respectively). The flat bones are those of the skull, sternum, shoulder blades (scapulae), and pelvis. The vertebrae are examples of irregular bones.

11.1 **ost-** bone; bone tissue

This element may appear in the forms *ost-*, *oste-*, *oss-*, *ossi-*, and *osse-*.

EXAMPLES:

osseous (osse/ous)—of the nature or quality of bone or bone tissue; bony

osteal (oste/al)—of the nature or quality of bone or bone tissue; bony

The roots *oss-*, *ossi-* and *osse-* are most often used when naming anatomical parts involving bone or when naming normal biological processes involving bone or bone tissue. The roots *ost-* and *oste-* are used when naming disease conditions and the therapeutic procedures used to correct them.

Bones of the Skull

11.2 **crani-** skull; cranium

Cranium is used in three different ways to refer to bones of the head: to refer to all the bones of the head; to refer to all the bones of the head except the jaw (mandible); and to refer to the brain case or enclosure—that is, all the bones surrounding the brain (eight bones). This last usage includes all the bones of the head except the jaw and other bones forming the face.

EXAMPLES:

cranial (crani/al)—pertaining to the skull or cranium; directional term for a body part nearer to the head

cranial bones (crani/al bones)—eight bones forming the brain case

craniectomy (crani/ectomy)—excision of part of the skull

craniomalacia (crani/o/malacia)—abnormal softening of the skull

The skull, as shown in Figures 11–2 to 11–4, is divided into the following areas:

frontal (front/al)—bone located in the front of the skull
occipital (occipit/al)—bone located in the back of the skull
parietal (pariet/al)—bones that compose the sides and roof of the skull
temporal (tempor/al)—bones found on the sides of the temples
sphenoid (sphen/oid)—wedge-shaped bone located at the base of the skull
ethmoid (ethm/oid)—sieve-like bone situated at the base of the skull
lacrimal (lacr/i/mal)—bone found under the tear duct
facial (faci/al)—bones that compose the face
nasal (nas/al)—bones that compose the nose
palatine (palat/ine)—bones of the roof of the mouth or palate
mandible (mand/ible)—lower jawbone that permits chewing
maxilla (maxill/a)—upper jawbone. There are two such bones, the left maxilla and the right maxilla, joined at the center of the face
zygomatic (zyg/o/matic)—cheek bones situated below the eyes

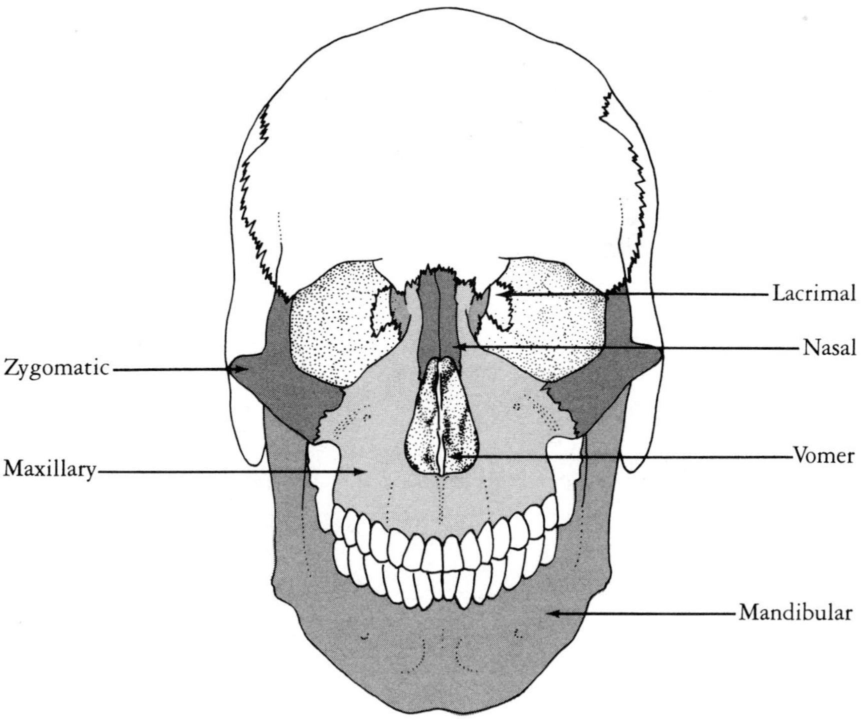

Figure 11–2 Facial bones.

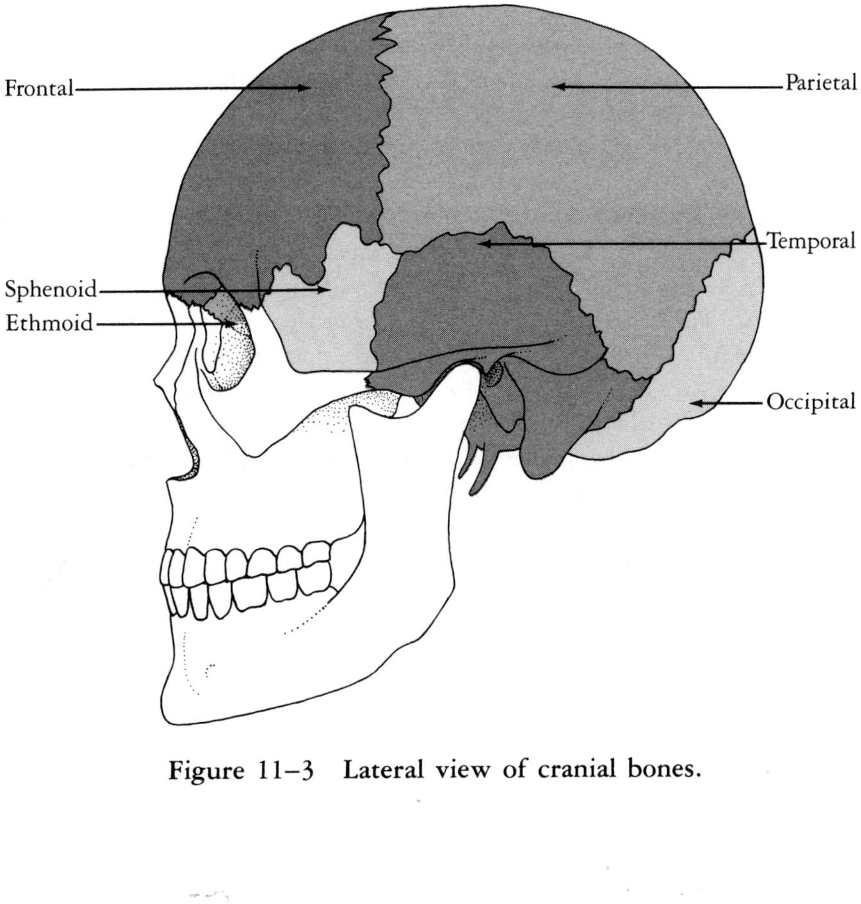

Figure 11–3 Lateral view of cranial bones.

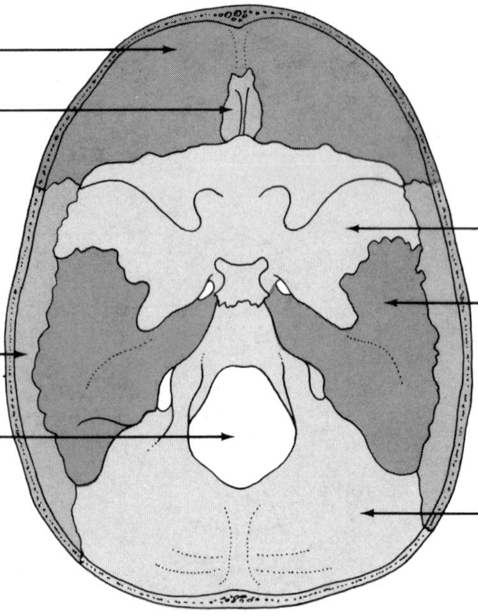

Figure 11–4 Bones of the skull cap viewed from the inside.

Bones of the Trunk and Extremities

The vertebral or spinal column is composed of twenty-four vertebrae (singular form is vertebra), the sacrum (five pieces), and the coccyx (nine pieces). The coccyx is the rudimentary tail. The vertebral column shelters the spinal cord, supports the skull and thorax, stiffens the trunk, and anchors the pelvic girdle. It is composed of: cervical (neck) vertebrae; thoracic (chest) vertebrae, which also serve as a place of attachment for ribs; lumbar (lower back) vertebrae, which support the lower trunk; sacral vertebrae for attachment of the pelvic girdle; and the coccyx. (See Figure 11-5.)

Each vertebra has a body (anterior portion) and an arch (posterior portion). The body bears weight, while the arch helps to form the canal that houses the spinal cord. Between the vertebrae are intervertebral disks, which consist of cartilage and serve as cushions. There are seven cervical vertebrae located in the neck. The first is called the atlas; its function is to support the skull. Rotation of the skull on the neck is the function of the joint, (called the axis), between the first and second cervical vertebrae. The axis has a broad base on which the atlas turns. The rest of the cervical vertebrae have no names and are known only by number. There are twelve thoracic vertebrae that support the chest and serve for articulation of the ribs. Five lumbar vertebrae located in the small of the back carry most of the weight of the trunk. The sacrum is composed of five sacral vertebrae that are fused into a single bone to which the pelvic girdle is anchored. The rudimentary tail, or coccyx, of the vertebral column is composed of four, or sometimes fewer, fused vertebrae.

11.1 **calc-** heel; stone

This element may appear as *calc-* when referring to the element calcium.

EXAMPLES:

calcic (calc/ic)—of or pertaining to calcium

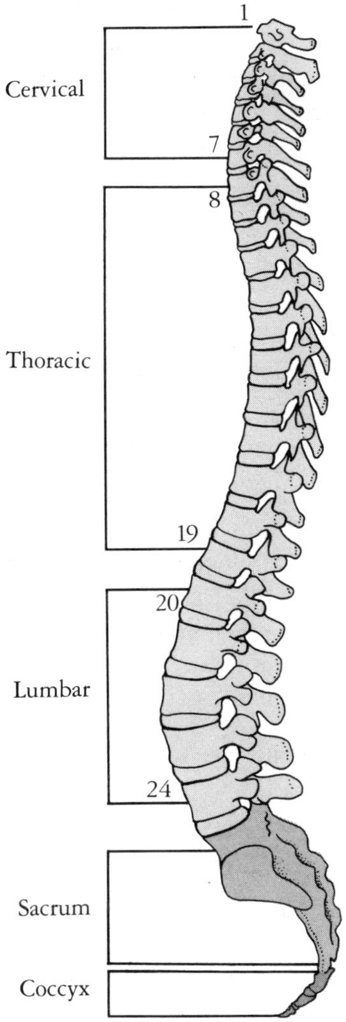

Figure 11–5 Vertebral column.

calcemia (calc/em/ia)—presence of an abnormally large amount of calcium in the blood

It may also appear as *calcan-* when referring to the heel bone:

calcaneus (calcane/us)—name for the heel bone, the large tarsal (ankle) bone that forms the heel

It may also appear as *calcare-* when referring to the various chemical compounds containing calcium; lime and chalky substances are chemical forms containing calcium:

calcareous (calcare/ous)—pertaining to or containing lime or calcium; chalky

11.2 carpo- wrist; eight bones of the wrist

EXAMPLES:

carpal (carp/al)—pertaining to the wrist
carpectomy (carp/ectomy)—excision of all or part of the wrist
carpoptosis (carp/optosis)—dropping of the wrist

11.3 cauda- tail; rear end; tail-like appendage (something hanging on a main structure)

EXAMPLES:

caudal (caud/al)—pertaining to the tail or tail-like appendage

cauda (caud/a)—name for a tail-like appendage
caudad (caud/ad)—directed toward a cauda or tail
caudalward (caud/al/ward)—toward the caudal, tail, or back end
caudal anesthesia (caud/al an/esthesia)—loss of sensation produced by an injection of an anesthetic into the lower (caudal) portion of the spinal cord

11.4 cost- rib

EXAMPLES:

costal (cost/al)—pertaining to a rib; related to or situated near ribs
chondrocostal (chondr/o/cost/al)—of or pertaining to rib cartilage
epicostal (epi/cost/al)—situated on a rib
costa (cost/a)—rib

11.5 dactyl-, digit- finger or toe

EXAMPLES:

dactylion (dactyl/ion)—union of fingers or toes
dactylomegaly (dactyl/o/megaly)—abnormally large fingers or toes
dactylospasm (dactyl/o/spasm)—cramp of a finger or toe
digital (digit/al)—pertaining to the digits (fingers or toes)

11.6 hallux great toe; big toe

EXAMPLES:

hallux flexus (hallux flex/us)—hammertoe
hallux valgus (hallux valg/us)—displacement of the great toe toward other toes
hallux varus (hallux var/us)—displacement of the great toe away from other toes

11.7 ili- ilium

The ilium is the flat, uppermost portion of the three hipbone sections.

EXAMPLES:

iliac (ili/ac)—pertaining to the ilium
iliocostal (ili/o/cost/al)—pertaining to ilium and ribs
iliolumbocosto-abdominal (ili/o/lumb/o/cost/o-abdomin/al)—pertaining to iliac, lumbar, costal, and abdominal regions

11.8 pelvi- pelvis

The pelvis refers to any basin-like or funnel-shaped structure; specifically, it refers to the bones in the hip or pelvic girdle (formed by the ilium, ischium, and pubis) that support the spinal column.

EXAMPLES:

pelvic (pelv/ic)—pertaining to the pelvis
pelvitherm (pelv/i/therm)—apparatus for heat application to the pelvic organs through the vagina
pelvospondylitis (pelv/o/spondyl/itis)—inflammation of the pelvic portion of the spine

11.9 rachi- vertebral column

EXAMPLES:

rachis (rachi/s)—name for the spinal column
rachidial, rachidian (rachidi/al, rachidi/an)—pertaining to the spinal column
rachitis (rach/itis)—inflammation of the spine; disease commonly known

as rickets—failure to form bones properly or a softening of bones in children due to lack of vitamin D

11.10 sacro- sacrum

The sacrum is a thick, triangular bone of the vertebral column, located above the tailbone. It joins with the hip bones to form the back of the pelvis.

EXAMPLES:

sacral (sacr/al)—pertaining to the sacrum; region around the sacrum
sacrad (sacr/ad)—toward the sacrum or sacral region
sacroplex (sacr/o/plex)—plexus (network of nerves) stemming from the sacrum

11.11 spondyl- spinal column; vertebra

EXAMPLES:

spondylous (spondyl/ous)—pertaining to a vertebra or to the spinal column
spondylic (spondyl/ic)—pertaining to a vertebra or to the spinal column

11.12 tarso- ankle region; instep

EXAMPLES:

tarsus (tars/us)—ankle region
tarsal (tars/al)—pertaining to the instep or to ankle bones (tarsal bones)
metatarsus (meta/tars/us)—part of the foot between the ankle (tarsus) and toes

The bones of the foot may be seen in Figures 11–6 and 11–7.

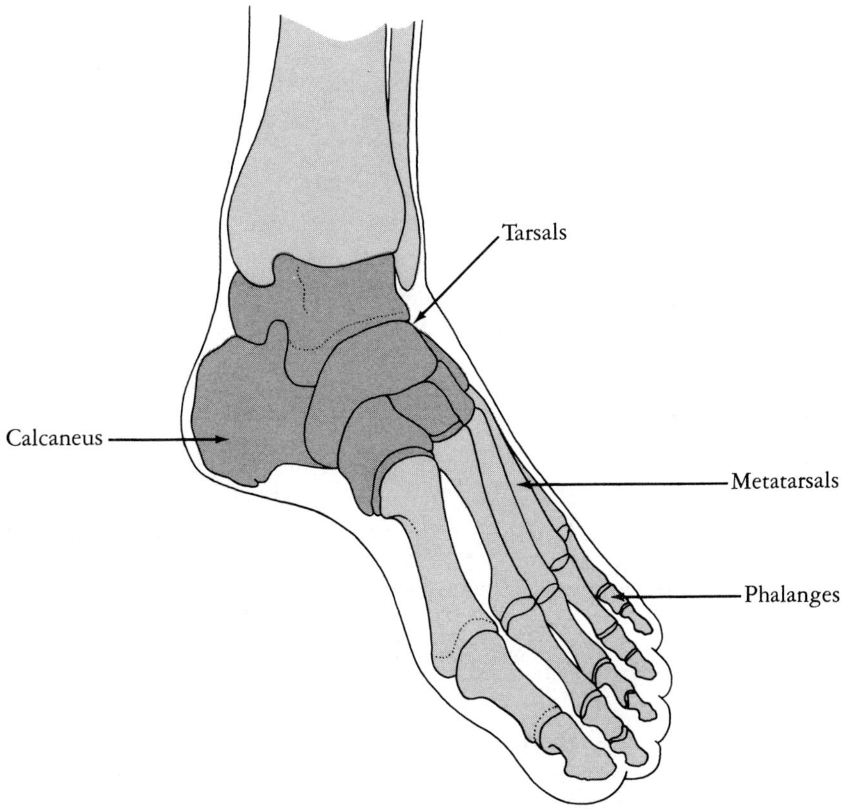

Figure 11–6 The left foot and ankle.

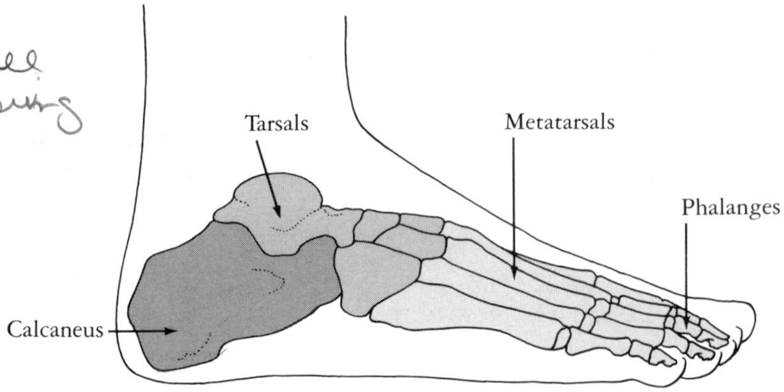

Figure 11–7 Lateral view of right foot.

Joints and Supporting Structures

The term used to refer to the study of joints is arthrology (arthro means joints). The joint is a structure that holds bones together in such a manner as to permit or prohibit motion. Bones are capable of different degrees of motion, depending on the mechanical construction and functions of their connecting joints. Most bones are capable of moving over one another, but at the same time they are held in place by ligaments of connective tissue. The term joint, or articulation, is applied to any union of bones, whether or not there is movement.

Joints are described according to their tissue formation. There are three types of joints—fibrous, cartilaginous, and synovial; synovial joints are the most important. Joints are classified as being either freely movable (diarthrosis), slightly movable (amphiarthrosis), or immovable (synarthrosis).

Word Roots Relating to Joints

11.13 **arthr-** joint; body joint; point where two bones come together

EXAMPLES:

arthral (arthr/al)—pertaining to a joint
arthritis (arthr/itis)—inflammation of a joint
arthrotomy (arthr/otomy)—cutting into or incision of a joint

11.14 **burso-** sac; any bag-like cavity; sac containing lubricating fluid

The bursae are closed sacs containing fluid that lie between surfaces that glide over each other. They lie between tendons and surfaces on which tendons glide to reduce friction.

EXAMPLES:

bursitis (burs/itis)—inflammation of a bursa
bursopathy (burso/path/y)—any disease of a bursa

11.15 **chondr-** cartilage; firm elastic tissue connecting body parts

Important formations of cartilage are found in joints, in connections between ribs and breastbone (sternum), and in bone development.

EXAMPLES:

chondral (chondr/al)—pertaining to cartilage
chondroma (chondr/oma)—tumor composed of cartilage
chondropathology (chondr/o/path/ology)—study of diseases of the cartilage

11.16 lig- ligament

The element *lig-* means tie or bind. A ligament is a band of tough tissue connecting (tying) bones or holding (binding) organs in place.

EXAMPLES:

ligate (lig/ate)—bind or tie with a ligature
ligature (lig/at/ure)—thread or wire for surgical tying
ligation (lig/at/ion)—application of a ligature

11.17 tens- stretch

The word root *ten-* means stretch and conveys the idea of stretcher (a thing that stretches) or stretching (the act, or action, of extending or reaching out). The root appears in several forms: *teno-*, *tenono-*, or *tenonto-* (ten/o-, tenon/o-, tenont/o-).

EXAMPLES:

tendon (tend/on)—any cords of tough, fibrous connective tissue that attach muscles to bones or other body parts
tenotomy (ten/otomy)—cutting of a tendon
tendonitis, tenontitis (tendon/itis, tenont/itis)—inflammation of a tendon
tensor (tens/or)—any muscle that stretches or tenses some body part
tension (tens/ion)—act or condition of being stretched or strained
neurotension (neur/o/tens/ion)—surgical stretching of a nerve

Terminology Trivia

Siamese Twins

The use of the term, Siamese twins, is something of a misnomer. It was first used to refer to Chang and Eng who, though born in Siam in 1811, were actually three-fourths Chinese; their father was fully Chinese, and their mother was one-half Chinese. Their story is indeed a fascinating one. In time, they became American citizens, taking the name Bunker, and were slave holders in North Carolina before the start of the Civil War.

Many who know Mark Twain's account of a siamese pair, "Those Extraordinary Twins," assume that he made up the tale of Luigi and Angelo and added that typically Twainian literary touch of ensuring that one brother (Luigi) was a heavy drinker, while the other brother (Angelo) was a teetotaler. The fact is, though, the real Chang actually was a heavy drinker and the real Eng actually was a teetotaler.

One would assume there must be descendants of Chang and Eng, and there are. Chang had seven daughters and three sons; Eng, seven sons and five daughters. Speculations as to methodology are left to the reader.

Pronunciation and Meaning of New Terms

arthritis (ar thri′ tis) Inflammation of the joints.

bursa (ber′ sah) A sac or pouch of fluid situated in places in tissues where friction would otherwise occur, especially about joints.

chondrocostal (kon″ dro kos′ tal) Pertaining to the cartilage and ribs.

frontal (frun′ tal) Pertaining to the forehead; a plane.

iliac (il′ e ak) Pertaining to the ilium, a bone of the pelvis.

pelvic (pel′ vik) Pertaining to the pelvis.

sacral (sa′ kral) Pertaining to the sacrum, the triangular bone below the lumbar vertebrae.

tarsus (tahr′ sus) The seven bones composing the articulation between the foot and the leg; also the cartilaginous plates of the eyelids.

nasal (na′ zal) Pertaining to the nose.

palatine (pal′ ah tīn) Pertaining to the palate.

Self-test

1. For each set, match Column A with Column B.

Column A

b myelo-
c osteoblasts
e osteal
a osteocytes
d ossification

Column B

a. bone cell
b. marrow
c. cells that form bone
d. process of bone-cell production
e. bony

2.

Column A

f osteoarthritis
a osteochondritis
i osteochondroma
k osteochondrosis
d osteoclasia
b osteodystrophies
e osteoma
h osteomalacia
g osteomyelitis
c osteopenia
j osteoporosis

Column B

a. inflammation of bone and cartilage
b. group of diseases in which there are growth disturbances
c. decrease in bone mass
d. condition in which bone is destroyed
e. bone tumor
f. inflammation of bone joint
g. inflammation of bone and marrow
h. softened bones
i. tumor of bone and cartilage covering the bone
j. porous bones
k. group of diseases affecting growth centers of bone and articular cartilage

3.

Column A	*Column B*
____ cranium	a. back of skull
____ frontal	b. pertaining to the face
____ occipital	c. sieve-like bone
____ temporal	d. upper jaw
____ sphenoid	e. sides and roof of skull
____ ethmoid	f. bone in front of skull
____ facial	g. wedge-shaped bone
____ nasal	h. cheekbones
____ zygomatic	i. enclosing the brain
____ parietal	j. pertaining to the nose
____ palatine	k. bones at the temples
____ maxilla	l. lower jaw
____ mandible	m. roof of the mouth

4.

Column A	*Column B*
____ spondylous	a. five vertebrae of the loin
____ cervical vertebrae	b. vertebra that allows head to turn
____ axis	c. toward the lower portion of the spinal column
____ thoracic vertebrae	d. twelve vertebrae of back and chest
____ lumbar vertebrae	e. breastbone
____ sacral vertebrae	f. seven bones of the neck
____ coccygeal vertebrae	g. cervical vertebrae that may be felt
____ sternum	h. spinal column
____ rachis	i. five fused vertebrae
____ caudal	j. pertaining to vertebrae or spinal column
	k. four fused vertebrae of the tailbone

5. Match Column A with Column B. There are two answers for some items in Column A.

Column A	*Column B*
____ clavicle	a. single bone of upper arm
____ scapula	b. bones in fingers and thumb
____ humerus	c. small bone in forearm on the thumb side
____ ulna	d. larger bone in forearm
____ radius	e. bones of the wrist
____ carpal bones	f. collarbone
____ metacarpal bones	g. shoulder blade
____ phalanges	h. bones in the hand

6. Match Column A with Column B.

Column A	*Column B*
____ pelvis	a. place where pubic bones grow together
____ ilium	b. shaped like a basin
____ symphysis pubis	c. superior portion of hip
____ femur	d. kneecap
____ patella	e. anklebone
____ tibia	f. thighbone
____ fibula	g. outer, thinner bone of the lower leg
____ tarsal bones	h. bones of the foot
____ metatarsal bones	i. inner, larger bone of the lower leg

7. Match Column A with Column B.

Column A

___ carpectomy
___ hallux valgus
___ diskectomy
___ osteoclasis
___ osteoplasty
___ osteotomy
___ dactylion
___ spinal fusion
___ chrondroma
___ arthrotomy
___ tenotomy

Column B

a. removal of wrist bones
b. great toe displaced toward other toes
c. removal of intervertebral cartilage
d. joint taken apart and limb removed
e. reconstruction or repair of bone
f. surgical breaking of bone
g. cutting into bone
h. two or more vertebrae joined together
i. union of fingers
j. incision of a joint
k. tumor of cartilage
l. incision of a tendon

Twelve

Muscular System

The study of muscles is called myology. The term muscle is derived from the Latin word, *mus*, or the Greek word, *mys*, both meaning mouse, because muscle movements were thought by the ancients to resemble mice crawling under cloth.

Components of the Muscular System

The muscular system is composed of the following important elements:

tendons—the strong, fibrous white bands that attach muscles to bones. They enable muscles to apply force at some distance from contracting parts. A good example of this is the leg; tendons control movements of ankles and toes from muscles in the calf. If movement of the ankle depended on its own muscles, the ankle would have to be many times its normal size.

fascia—muscle fibers are held together in muscle bundles by fibrous connective tissue. Groups of bundles are held together by sheaths, or fascia. These sheaths keep muscles in place during movement and allow them to slide freely over one another.

ligaments—the strong bands of tissue that hold bones together and keep organs in place.

origins—the immovable attachment of a muscle, at the point where it is anchored by a tendon, to bone that is stationary during action.

insertions—the more movable attachment of a muscle to bone that moves.

motor nerves—the nerve that causes muscle to move. Nerves leading to a muscle contain both sensory and motor fibers. Bundles of these fibers divide continuously until each motor nerve axon supplies a definite group of muscle fibers, sending a branch to each; the branch terminates in a motor endplate on the surface of the muscle cell. The combination of nerve cell, axon, and muscle-cell group is called a neuromotor unit.

tone—tonus, or tone, of muscles refers to their state of tension.

The muscles of the body are identified in the following four ways:

1. Muscles *identified by their function.* These will usually have a word root, end in a suffix (*-or* or *-ens*), and be followed by the name of the affected structure. Examples: extensor carpi (extension of wrist); flexor hallicus (flexing of great toe); levator scapulae (raising of shoulders); constrictor pharynges (constricting of the pharnyx); and opponens pollicus (flexing and opposing of thumb).
2. Muscles *identified by joining the names for points of origin and attachment* with a word terminal (*-eus* or *-is*). Examples: brachioradialis (upper arm and radius);

sternoclavicularis (sternum and clavicle); palatopharyngeus (palate and pharnyx); and occipitofrontalis (back and front of head).

3. Muscles *identified by their form or position*. These usually contain a descriptive adjective followed by the name for the location of the muscles. Examples: obliquus abdominis externus (oblique abdominal external muscle); teres major (large muscle in scapular region); tibialis anterior (anterior tibial muscle); longissimus thoracis (long muscle in the thorax); pectoralis minor (small chest muscle).
4. Muscles *identified by figurative names* (named for resemblance to some object, shape, or the way they are used). Examples: buccinator (trumpeter—cheek muscle used in blowing of a trumpet); cremaster (hanger—muscles suspending the testes); gastrocnemius (muscle on back of lower leg, shaped something like the stomach); gemmellus (twin muscles); platysma (flat); piriformis (pear-shaped); pyramidalis (shaped like a pyramid); risorius (laughter—facial muscle used in laughing); splenius (bandage or compression); trapezius (flat surface); sartorius (tailors muscle—muscle on top of the leg that allows it to cross in the fashion of a tailor).

There are over 400 skeletal muscles in the body. There are only about 200 names for them because there are similar muscles on the right and left sides of the body. For example, the deltoid muscle is the triangular muscle of the shoulder; there is both a right deltoid muscle and a left deltoid muscle. Figures 12–1 and 12–2 present posterior and anterior views of the body's muscular system.

Most muscles also exist as pairs. If there is a muscle that extends a body part, there is also a muscle that flexes that part. For example, flexor carpi ulnaris flexes the wrist and extensor carpi ulnaris extends the wrist. The flexor is called an agonist and the muscle that works against the contraction is an antagonist. One that works along with other muscles is a synergist.

Terms Used to Name Muscles

Quality	Word Root	Meaning
Size	maximus	largest
	minimus	smallest
	major	larger
	minor	smaller
	longus	long
	brevis	short
	vastus	great, large, vast
	gracilis	slender, delicate
Shape	cuneiform	wedge-shaped
	deltoid	triangular
	fusiform	spindle-shaped
	latus	broad
	lumbrical	worm-like
	penniform	feather-like, pennate
	platy-	flat
	pyramidal	cone-shaped
	quadrilateral	four-sided
	rhomboid	four-sided, with opposite sides parallel
	serratus	saw-like edge
	teres	long and round
	trapezoid	four-sided with two parallel sides

Fiber Arrangement	bipennate	muscle fibers joining a central tendon from both sides in a feather-like fashion
	unipennate	muscle fibers joining a central tendon from one side
	curved	fibers in a bent arrangement
	oblique	a somewhat slanted or angled arrangement
	parallel	fibers that extend in the same direction and do not cross or separate
	rectus	straight
	transversus	lying across
Action	adductor	moving a part toward midline
	abductor	moving a part away from midline
	flexor	bends a part
	extensor	straightens a part
	levator	raises a part
	depressor	lowers a part
	tensor	tightens a part
Number of Muscle Divisions	triceps	three (tri) heads (ceps)
	biceps	two (bi) heads (ceps)
	quadriceps	four (quadri) heads (ceps)
	digastric	two (di) bellies (gastric)
Points of Attachment (selected examples)	sternocleidomastoid	attached to the sternum, the collar bone (cleido), and the mastoid process of the temporal bone
	peroneus longus	long muscle attached to the fibula (peroneus)
Location (selected examples)	intercostal	between (inter) the ribs (costal)
	tibialis posterior	behind the tibia
	epicranial	upon (epi) the skull (cranium)
	medial pterygoid	muscle toward midline attached to a wing-shaped bone
	subclavius	under (sub) the clavicle (clavius)
	extensor digitorum profundus	deeply (profundus) situated muscle that extends (extensor) the finger (digitorum)

Word Roots Relating to the Muscular System

12.1 **kines-** motion

EXAMPLES:

kinesalgia (kines/algia)—muscle pain with movement
kinesia (kines/ia)—motion sickness
kinesiology (kines/i/ology)—study of muscles and muscle movement

12.2 **leio-** smooth (involuntary) muscles

This root may be used when referring to any smooth surface; it is used in the description of tumors to identify smooth muscles generally found in the walls of the stomach, intestines, vessels, and glands. They are also in the very small muscles of the skin and, when contracted, produce what is called goose flesh.

EXAMPLES:

leiomyoma (lei/my/oma)—tumor composed of smooth muscle fibers
leiodermia (leio/derm/ia)—abnormal glossiness or smoothness of the skin

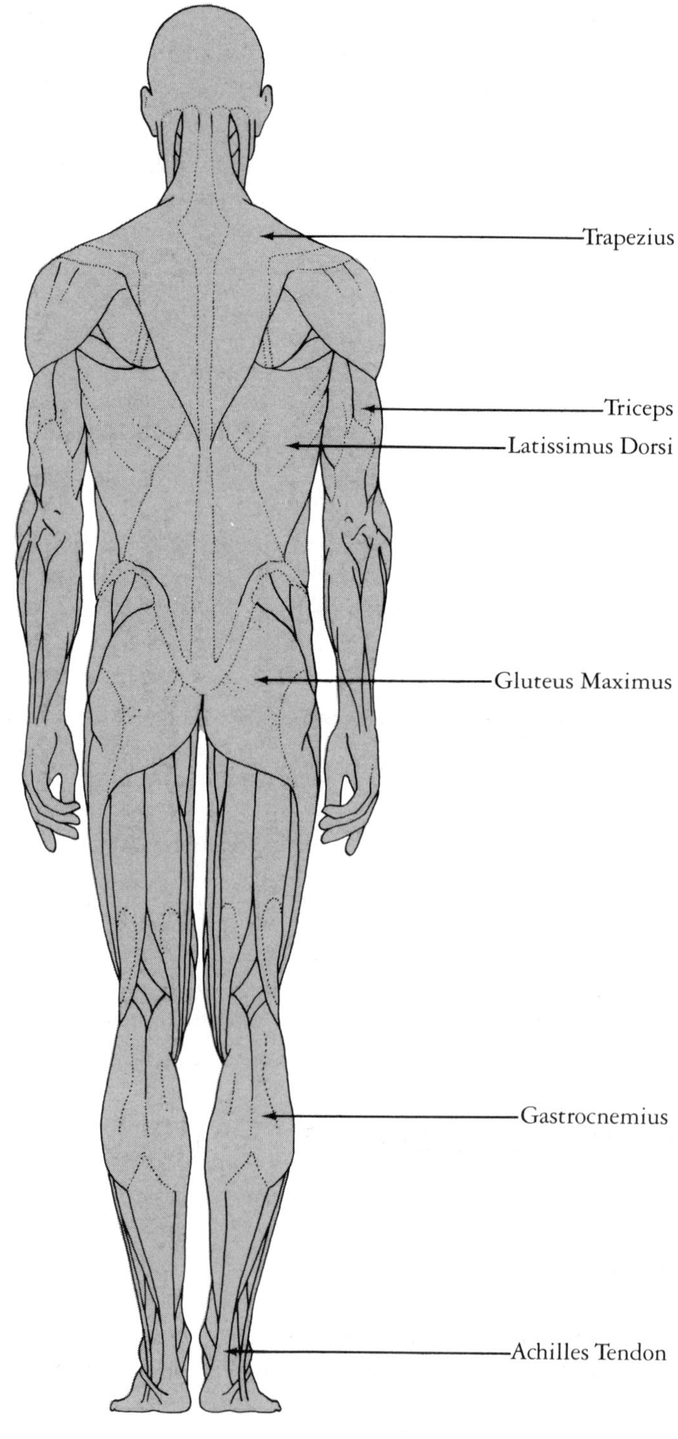

Figure 12–1 Muscles visible immediately beneath the skin (common ones labeled).

12.3 lumbo- loin; lower back

EXAMPLES:

lumbar (lumb/ar)—pertaining to the loins

lumbago, lumbodynia (lumb/ago, lumb/o/dyn/ia)—pain in the lumbar region; lower back pain

dorsolumbar (dors/o/lumb/ar)—pertaining to the back and loins

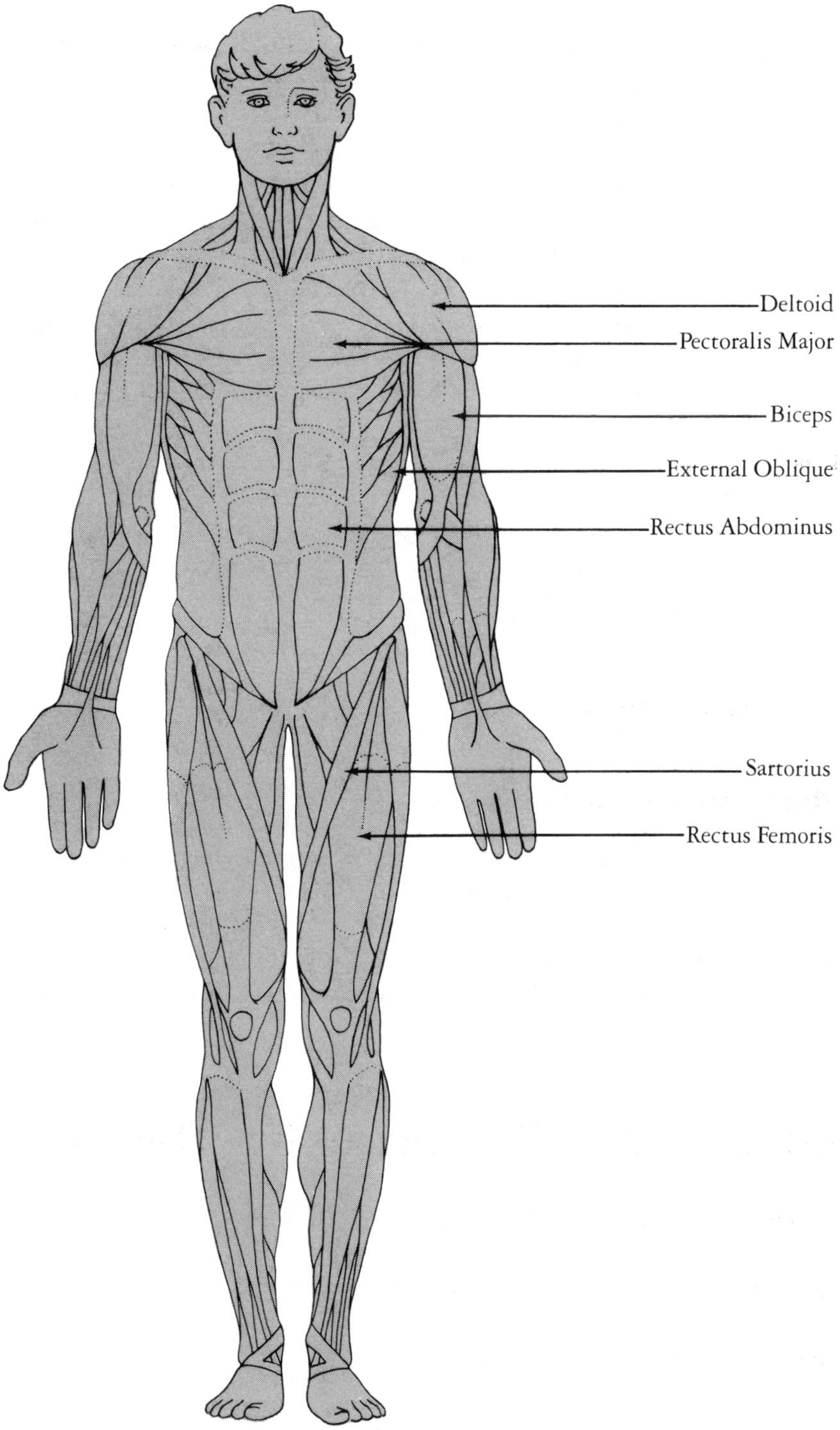

Figure 12–2 Muscles visible immediately beneath the skin.

12.4 my- muscle

EXAMPLES:

myoma, -myoma (my/oma, -my/oma)—tumor consisting of muscular elements

angiomyoma (angi/o/my/oma)—tumor consisting of blood vessels and muscle elements

12.5 spas- pull; draw

A form of this root, *-spasm*, means involuntary contraction. The root *spas-* indicates any involuntary muscular movement, ranging from mild muscle twitches to severe cramps.

EXAMPLES:

-spasia (-spas/ia)—condition of muscular contraction
myospasia (my/o/spas/ia)—spasmodic condition in which rigidity of the muscles is followed immediately by relaxation
-spasmia (-spasm/ia)—disease characterized by spasms
myospasmia (my/o/spasm/ia)—disease characterized by uncontrollable muscle spasms
spastic (spast/ic)—of the nature of or characterized by spasms

12.6 sthen- strength

EXAMPLES:

sthenia (sthen/ia)—normal strength, as opposed to asthenia
sthenic (sthen/ic)—active or strong
sthenometer (sthen/o/meter)—device for measuring muscular strength

Terminology Trivia

Copper Bracelets and Arthritis

There is no scientific evidence that copper, or any such metal, worn on the wrists or ankles has an effect on arthritis. However, even the great seventeenth–century physician, Paracelsus, said that a ring made of electrum would protect the wearer from epilepsy, apoplexy, palsy, and pain. More recently, in Canada, there spread the false belief that a copper wire bound tightly around the waist would ward off rheumatism.

Pronunciation and Meaning of New Terms

buccinator (buk′ in ā tor) The muscle of the cheek.

cuneiform (kune′ ī form) A wedge-shaped muscle.

deltoid (dell′ toy d) Triangular muscle.

fascia (fash′ ah) Sheath of connective muscle.

gastrocnemius (gas trōk′ nemi us) Calf muscle shaped like a stomach (*gastr-*).

gracilius (gras′ il ē us) A slender, delicate (gracious) muscle.

kinesalgia (kin ēs al gee ah) Muscle movement accompanied by pain.

leimyoma (lie′ my ō mah) Tumor composed of smooth muscle tissue.

medial pterygoid (me′ de al tery′ goy d) A muscle toward the midline attached to a wing-shaped bone.

myospasia (my ō spaz ah) Rigid muscles followed by relaxation.

obliquus (ō bleek us) A Latin word for oblique, used to denote the angle of a muscle.

sternocleidomastoid (stern′ ō klyd ō mast oyd) A muscle attached to the sternum, clavicle (*cleido-*), and the mastoid process of the temporal bone.

synergist (sinner jist) A muscle that functions in cooperation with another.

trapezius (trap ē zee us) A flat triangular muscle covering the posterior surface of the neck and shoulder.

Self-test

1. For each set, match Column A with Column B.

Column A

___ origin
___ belly
___ insertion
___ fascia
___ tendon
___ agonist
___ antagonist
___ kine-
___ sthen-
___ synergist

Column B

a. end of a muscle attached to bone that moves
b. fibrous cord by which a muscle is attached
c. end of muscle attached to bone that does not move
d. layer of thin fibrous tissue between muscles and enclosing muscles
e. long extension of a muscle
f. muscle that works against a contracting muscle
g. word root meaning motion
h. contracting muscle; the prime mover
i. word root meaning strength
j. muscle that works with other muscles

2.

Column A

___ maximus
___ minimus
___ major
___ minor
___ longus
___ brevis
___ cuneiform
___ deltoid
___ fusiform
___ penniform
___ platy-
___ quadrilateral
___ rhomboid
___ serratus
___ trapezoid

Column B

a. smallest
b. largest
c. larger
d. long
e. short
f. smaller
g. feather-like, pennate
h. four-sided
i. wedge-shaped
j. four-sided with opposite sides parallel
k. flat
l. saw-like edge
m. spindle-shaped
n. four-sided with two parallel and two nonparallel sides
o. triangular
p. kite-shaped

3.

Column A

___ bipennate
___ curved
___ oblique
___ parallel
___ rectus
___ adductor
___ flexor
___ extensor
___ depressor
___ tensor

Column B

a. joining a tendon from both sides
b. slanted or angled arrangement
c. extends in same direction and does not cross
d. bent arrangement
e. straight
f. muscle that straightens
g. muscle that tightens a part
h. muscle that moves a part away from midline
i. muscle that lowers a part
j. muscle that moves a part toward midline
k. muscle that bends a part

4.

Column A

___ smooth muscles
___ myasthenia gravis
___ muscle hypertrophy
___ muscular dystrophy
___ myospasmia
___ skeletal muscles
___ kinesia
___ polymyositis

Column B

a. muscle weakness
b. abnormal development of muscles
c. inflammation of many muscles
d. excessive growth; muscle enlargement
e. motion sickness
f. breakdown of striated muscle
g. involuntary muscles
h. lack of growth; muscle shrinkage
i. muscle rigidity
j. voluntary muscles

flexion/extension
dorsiflexion/plantar flexion
abduction/adduction
rotation
supination/

154

Thirteen
Integumentary System

Components of the Integumentary System

The study of skin is called dermatology. The Greek term for skin is derma; the Latin term is cutis. The integumentary system includes not only skin but also hair, nails, mammary glands, sweat glands, and sebaceous glands.

The skin is composed of two layers: the epidermis, or epithelium, which is the outer skin layer visible to the naked eye, and the dermis, or corium, which is the internal skin layer. The layers of the epidermis, from the dermis outward, are the stratum germinativum or germinal layer, the stratum granulosum, the stratum lucidum, and the stratum corneum. These strata, or layers, are differentiated by means of their cell types. As these cells move outward from the stratum germinativum to the stratum corneum, they become keratanized (hardened).

Among the deeper cells in the basal layer of the epidermis are those that contain pigment. Through its color and quantity, pigment is the chief factor determining complexion color. This pigmentation of the skin results mainly from the presence of granules of melanin. The quantity of melanin pigment varies in persons of different races. Pigmentation of the skin is protection from injurious light rays, and for this reason white people cannot withstand the sun of the tropics as well as blacks, unless their skin has become deeply tanned from exposure to the sun's rays.

The epidermis is firmly adherent or interlocked to the inner layer, the dermis. The shafts of the sweat glands and hair follicles that traverse the epidermis also help to keep it firmly anchored to the inner layer.

The corium, or dermis, is a dense network of fibrous and elastic tissue that contains blood vessels and nerves. The deep surface of this layer merges with the fat-containing subcutaneous connective tissue. In the dermis lie the hair shafts, sebaceous glands, and sweat glands. They are actually part of the epidermis, but are located in little depressions found in the dermis. The dermis is attached to the epidermis by papillae. The sensation of pain cannot be elicited from the outer, or epidermal layer of the skin, but only from the inner layers, which have nerve endings that produce sensations of pain, touch, heat, and cold.

The structure of the skin on the palms of the hands and soles of the feet is different from that on the rest of the body. It is composed of papillary ridges that are formed during intrauterine life and are permanent. These are numerous and capable of forming their own unique patterns. Each person's fingerprints are different from those of every other person. In many hospitals, it is routine practice to make prints of newborns' feet for identification purposes.

The skin varies in thickness; it is thick on the palms of the hands and soles of the feet, but thin on the eyelids. Skin also varies in moistness and smoothness, in accord with the presence of sebaceous (oil-producing) glands and sweat glands. It is firmly elastic in youth and wrinkles with age. The inner layer of skin is resistant to the penetration of water. However, watery solutions made up of phenols (cleaning agents) can penetrate the skin. Also, alcoholic solutions and suspensions in fats, ointments, and liniments can pass through skin layers and be absorbed. The papillae in gooseflesh are produced by the contraction of small bundles of muscles in the skin, called the arrector pili (arrector means raise and pili refers to the hair), which also cause compression of the sebaceous glands near these papillae. These small muscle bundles are attached at one end to the hair follicles; it is these muscles that cause the hair to stand on end.

The nails, like hair, are a modified form of epidermis. The Latin term for nail is unguis; the Greek term is onyx or onycho. The nails are hardened, flat, resilient plates of epidermis from the stratum lucidum layer. They derive their translucent, pale, or delicate pink appearance from underlying capillaries and grow from their roots. The soft, uncornified, whitish portion at the base of the nail is partly covered and forms the lunula. This moon-shaped lunula at the base of the nail may be partially or completely concealed by the overlapping cuticle.

The breasts, or mammae, in the pectoral region (pectus means breast) are rudimentary in the males, but form hemispherical structures in females (see Figure 13–1.) They contain the milk-secreting mammary glands. The soft hemispherical form of the mamma is due to the superficial fascia that are heavily laden with adipose tissue (fat) that surrounds the mammary gland. Cooper's ligaments support the breast. In the center of the breast is the nipple with its encircling halo, called the areola. Lactation is the process by which milk is produced. Milk is formed in the lactiferous sinus and flows down the lactiferous duct to the nipple.

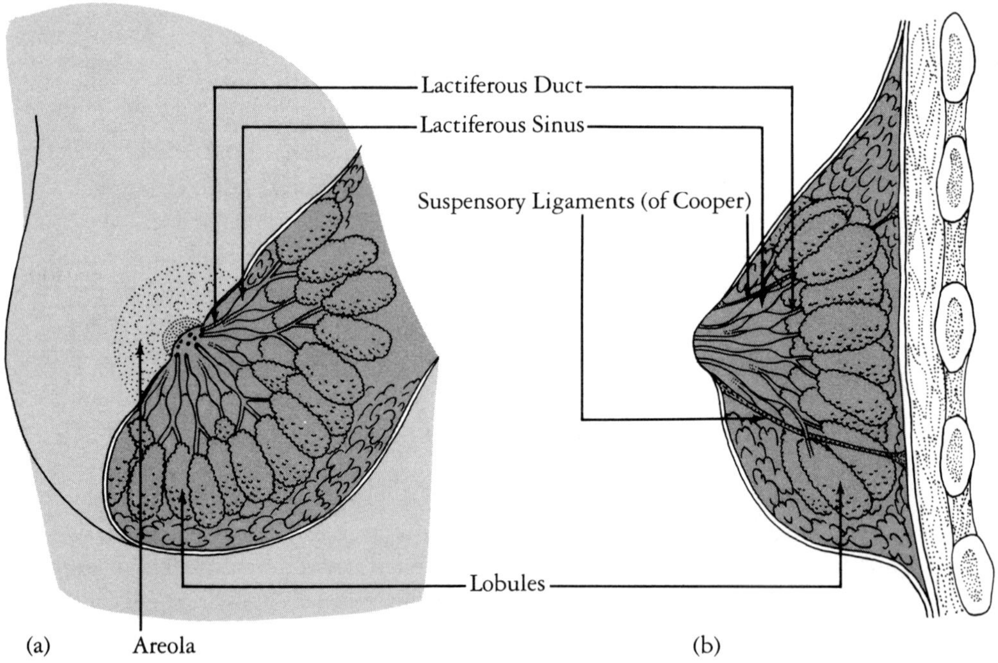

Figure 13–1 Female breast.

Word Roots Relating to the Integumentary System

13.1 **cut-** skin

EXAMPLES:

cutis (cut/is)—skin; protective outer covering of the body
cuticle (cut/icle)—outer layer of the skin; a synonym is eponychium
cutaneous (cutan/eous)—pertaining to skin
-cutaneous (-cutan/eous)—suffix denoting relationship to skin
subcutaneous (sub/cutan/eous)—situated or occurring beneath skin
transcutaneous (trans/cutan/eous)—through skin
cutitis (cut/itis)—inflammation of the skin

13.2 **dermat-, derm-** skin

EXAMPLES:

dermal (derm/al)—pertaining to skin
dermis (derm/is)—skin
dermatitis (dermat/itis)—inflammation of the skin

13.3 **hidr-** perspiration; sweat

EXAMPLES:

hidradenoma (hidr/aden/oma)—tumor of the sweat glands
hidropoiesis (hidr/o/poiesis)—formation of sweat
hidrorrhea (hidr/o/rrhea)—abnormal sweating

13.4 **macul-** spot, stain, blotch on the skin

EXAMPLES:

macula (macul/a)—spot or blotch
macule (macul/e)—macula
maculation (macul/ation)—spotted condition; formation of spots or macules

Tumors (*-oma* or *onc-*) are usually discolored but are always characterized by swelling. A macule is a discolored spot or patch that is flat; neither swollen nor depressed. Birthmarks and freckles are examples of macules that are not signs of disease. Macula indicative of disease are spots that accompany some infectious diseases.

13.5 **mamm-** breast

EXAMPLES:

mammi-, mammo- (mamm/i-, mamm/o-)—forms denoting relationship to the breast or to the milk-secreting gland in the breast of the female
mamma (mamm/a)—name for the breast
mammary (mamm/ary)—pertaining to the breast
mamilla (mamill/a)—name for the nipple or any nipple-like structure

The root *mamm-* is generally used to designate the breast as a structure or landmark:

mammose (mamm/ose)—having large breasts
mammoplasty (mamm/o/plast/y)—surgical reconstruction of the breast

The root *mast-* is used to designate the female breast and mammary gland and the diseases and corrective procedures relating to them:

mastalgia (mast/algia)—pain in the mammary gland

mastectomy (mast/ectomy)—excision of the breast

There is a small bony projection behind the ear called the mastoid (mast/oid) process, so named because its shape resembles that of a breast; *masto-* may be encountered in reference to the mastoid process, but usually is accompanied by a word element that limits its meaning.

13.6 onych- nail; claw

EXAMPLES:

onychomycosis (onych/o/myc/osis)—fungal infection of the nails
-onychium (-onych/ium)—region of the fingernail or toenail
eponychium (ep/onych/ium)—cuticle; narrow band of skin (epidermis) that extends from the nail wall to the nail surface

The word roots *unguo-* and *onyx-* also refer to nails.

13.7 pilo- hair

EXAMPLES:

pilus (pil/us)—a hair
pilomotor (pil/o/motor)—movement of hair, as in gooseflesh
pilocystic (pil/o/cyst/ic)—cyst-like mass containing hair; describes certain skin tumors
depilation (de/pil/ation)—process of hair removal (the agent for hair removal is called a depilatory)

13.8 tegument skin; covering

The word tegument is a shortened form of integument, meaning a covering, used to denote the skin.

EXAMPLES:

integumentary (integument/ary)—pertaining to or composed of skin; serving as a covering, like the skin
integumentary system (integument/ary system)—used to designate the entire covering of the body, including skin, hair, nails, skin glands, breasts, and mammary glands
tegumental (tegument/al)—concerning the skin

13.9 theli- nipple; thin layer of tissue

EXAMPLES:

thelium (thel/ium)—nipple
thelitis (thel/itis)—inflammation of the nipple
epithelium (epi/thel/ium)—tissue covering surfaces, forming glands, and lining most cavities of the body
endothelium (end/o/thel/ium)—layer of cells (tissue) lining the inside of blood and lymph vessels, the heart, and other closed cavities

13.10 trich- hair

EXAMPLES:

-trichia, -trichosis (-trich/ia, -trich/osis)—condition of the hair
leukotrichia (leuk/o/trich/ia)—whiteness of the hair
sclerotrichia (scler/o/trich/ia)—hard, dry state of the hair
atrichosis (a/trich/osis)—absence of hair; baldness
trichoesthesia (trich/o/esthesia)—sense by which one perceives skin hair being touched

trichogenous (trich/o/gen/ous)—promoting the growth of hair
atrichosis (a/trich/osis)—without hair; preferred term is alopecia

Terminology Trivia

The Invention of the Bra

A man invented the bra! Actually, it was two men acting independently in two different countries who accomplished this task.

Otto Titzling not only contributed this ingenious device (or garment) to the world, but also unwillingly contributed his name to form a euphemism for the female breast. Otto was born in 1884 in Hamburg, where he worked through his teenage years for his uncle in the garment trade. In 1910, he moved to New York where he met and fell in love with a budding opera singer, Swanhilda Olafson.

Swanhilda had overwhelming upper proportions that were bound by the full-length undergarments of the time. This put her at a disadvantage when she had to produce vocal sounds from deep within her abdomen. Otto recognized her problem and designed the "chest halter" to replace the restrictive corset Swanhilda formerly had to wear. The initial design was a crude massive undertaking that he completed in 1912.

The outbreak of World War I interrupted Otto's research and development of women's support garments. Otto's uncle came to Washington during this time and obtained a contract to produce woolen military uniforms. He thought the speculative chest halter could only be marketed to a limited number of women, and so the idea lay dormant for several years until a Frenchman, Philippe de Brassiere, unveiled his creation.

Although the war stifled Otto's efforts, it ultimately contributed to the new garment's development. Women were now in the workforce and the old corsets they wore hampered their productivity. Then, in 1913, a by-product of wartime research came in the form of elasticized material. It was just what Otto needed to rekindle his interest in the chest halter. At the same time, women were becoming more fashion conscious and they looked to Europe to set the standards; de Brassiere, by this time, had covered the European market. A demand was created to which Otto and his wife Swanhilda responded. They produced bras for American women and to this day, they are wrongfully dubbed as copiers of Brassiere's invention.

Pronunciation and Meaning of New Terms

corium (kor′ e um) Internal layer of skin.

dermal, dermatologic (derm′ ȧl, der″ mah to loj′ ik) Pertaining to the skin.

dermatitis (der″ mah ti′ tis) Inflammation of the skin.

epidermus (epi′ der mis) External layer of skin.

lunula (loon u la) The whitish portion at the base of nails.

onychomycosis (on′ ik o my ko sis) A fungus infection of nails.

pilus (peel′ us) Hair.

thelium (theel′ e um) Nipple.

trichoesthesia (trick′ es thes ē ah) Sense by which one perceives skin hair is being touched.

trichogeneous (trick′ ō gen ē us) Promoting hair growth.

Self-test

1. Match Column A with Column B.

Column A

___ sebaceous glands
___ sebum
___ lunula
___ cuticle
___ paronychial

Column B

a. moon shaped
b. oily, glandular secretion
c. small area of dead skin around base of nail
d. glands that open into hair follicles or directly onto surface of skin
e. area around the nail

2. Use the following terms to fill in the blanks.

a. areola
b. galact or lacto
c. mammary gland
d. mast- or mamm-
e. theli-
f. lactation

1. The word root for tip or point of the breast is ________.
2. The small area of color around the nipple is called the ________.
3. The breast of the female is sometimes called the ________.
4. The process of producing milk is called ________.
5. The word root for milk is ________.
6. The word root for breast is ________.

3. Use the following terms to fill in the blanks.

a. hyperhidrosis
b. hypertrichosis
c. hypomastia
d. laceration
e. macula
f. melanoma
g. epithelioma
h. mottled skin
i. depilation

1. The process for removing hair is ________.
2. Another name for a spot or blotch is ________.
3. A wound in which there is an irregular tear is called a ________.
4. An excessive amount of sweating is called ________.
5. A term meaning very small, underdeveloped breasts is ________.
6. A tumor of the skin is ________.
7. A condition in which there is an excessive amount of hair is called ________.
8. A condition in which there is variation in the color of skin produced by underlying blood vessels is called ________.
9. A tumor of the melanocyte cells is called a ________.

4. Match Column A with Column B.

Column A

___ scleroderma
___ dermabrasion
___ depilatory
___ sebaceous cyst
___ emollient
___ keratolytic lotion
___ thelitis
___ mammography
___ mammoplasty
___ mastectomy

Column B

a. scraping skin to remove acne scars
b. preparation used to soften skin
c. chemical preparation for removal of hair
d. inflammation of a nipple
e. liquid preparation used to break down a hard layer of skin
f. a sac-like structure filled with sebum
g. hardening of the skin
h. x-ray examination of breasts
i. plastic surgery on breasts
j. removal of a breast

Fourteen
Special Senses

The Components of Special Senses

The special senses include smell, taste, sight, hearing, and touch. The peripheral organ of smell is the nose (*naso-* and *rhino-* are terms that refer to nose), along with external parts and nasal cavities. Odor is perceived by the olfactory membrane of the nose through stimulation of its cells. The olfactory (*olfact-* refers to smell) receptors are confined to the nasal mucosa over a relatively small area; either side of the nose interior on the walls of a narrow niche formed by the superior nasal concha (concha means shell-shaped), the upper part of the septum, and the roof of the nasal cavity.

Infections in the mucous membrane lining the nose are easily spread. The nasopharynx, the auditory canal, the middle-ear cavity, the sphenoidal, ethmoidal, frontal, and maxillary sinuses, the palatine bones, and the tear ducts are all continuous with the mucous membrane of the nose.

The organs of taste are the taste buds, located mainly on the surface of the tongue. They are also found in the mucous membrane that covers the soft palate, the pharynx, and the epiglottis.

The sense of taste is limited to four simple, primary, or fundamental tastes—sweet, sour (acid), salt, and bitter. Various other tastes are blends of these four. A substance will arouse a sensation of taste only if it is dissolved either in solution or by saliva, which accounts for the location of the taste buds on a moist surface. Many substances we imagine are tasted are actually only smelled; their "taste" depends on their aroma.

The organ of sight is the eye, along with extrinsic muscles, eyelids, and tear apparatus. (See Figure 14–1.) The eye includes the bulb of the eye, or eyeball, and an optic nerve that connects the eye to the brain. This system

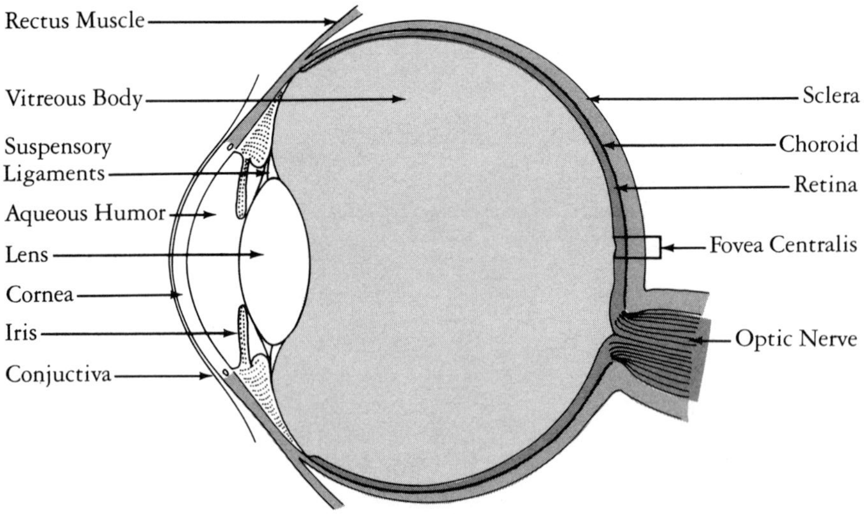

Figure 14–1 Transverse section of the eye.

constitutes the essential part of the organ of sight. The terms orbit and optic refer to the eye. A flowchart of the eye's visual pathway is shown in Figure 14–2.

Eyes are the most important sense organs in the body. It is with them that we receive most of our information, not only from what we see around us, but also from what we learn through the printed word. The eyeballs lie to the right and left of the nose root and are shaped almost like spheres. Attached to each eyeball and contained in their orbital cavities are the optic nerves, ocular muscles, and various other nerves and vessels. A soft mucous membrane, called the conjunctiva, covers the exposed one third of each eyeball. The eyes are protected by eyelids (referred to as palpebrae) that are fringed with rows of eyelashes (called cilia).

Eyeballs may be likened to hollow spheres whose walls are comprised of three concentric coats and are filled with three transparent refracting media. The external, fibrous coat is composed of the sclera located behind the eye and the cornea located in front of the eye. The intermediate, or vascular, pigmented coat is composed of three layers named, from the back of the eye forward: the choroid, the ciliary body, and the iris. The internal, nerve-filled coat contains the retina and is continuous with the optic nerve. (See Figures 14–3 and 14–4.)

The eyes each have an opening in front, called the pupil, that allows in light and a lens behind this opening that focuses the rays of transmitted light

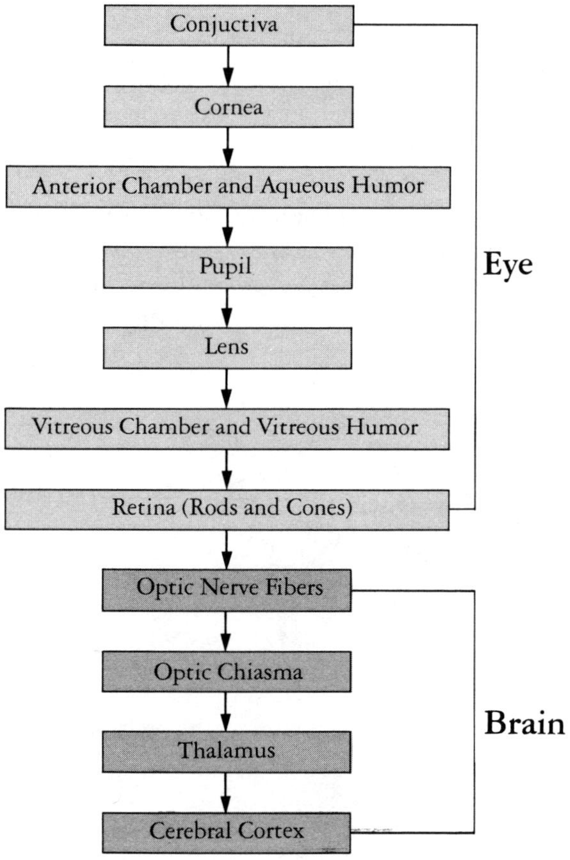

Figure 14–2 Flowchart of visual pathway from image to neurological interpretation.

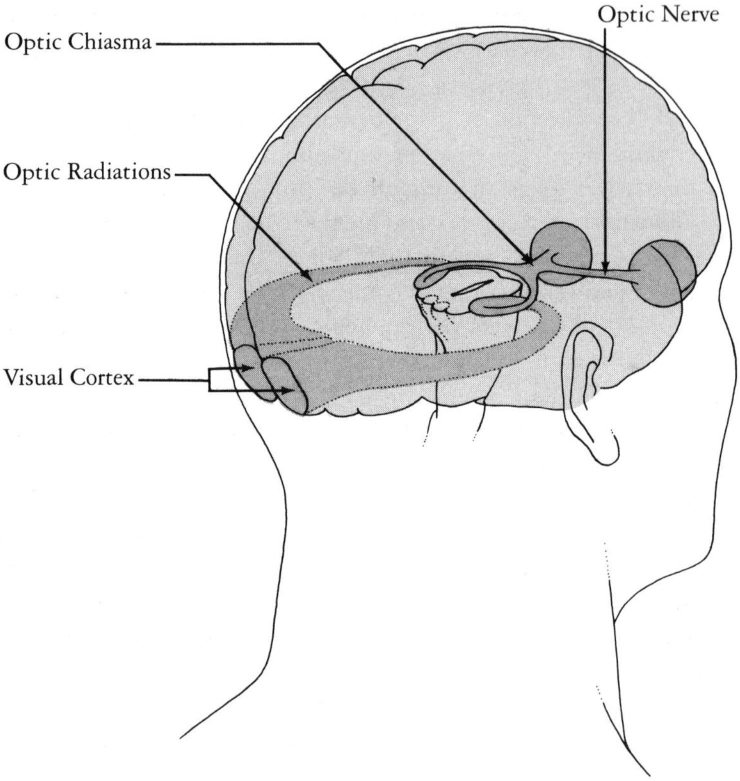

Figure 14–3 Visual pathways.

to form images on the retina. The retina is the inner coat of the eyes and contains light receptors—rods and cones. Optic nerves carry impulses from the retinas to the visual areas and are, therefore, the sensory pathway for impulses received in the retinas by rods and cones.

The ears are not simply organs of hearing, but are actually compound organs that are sensitive both to sound waves and to the effects of gravity. (See Figure 14–5.) They contain structures that are responsible for the body's equilibrium. A flowchart of the ear's auditory pathway is presented in Figure 14–6.

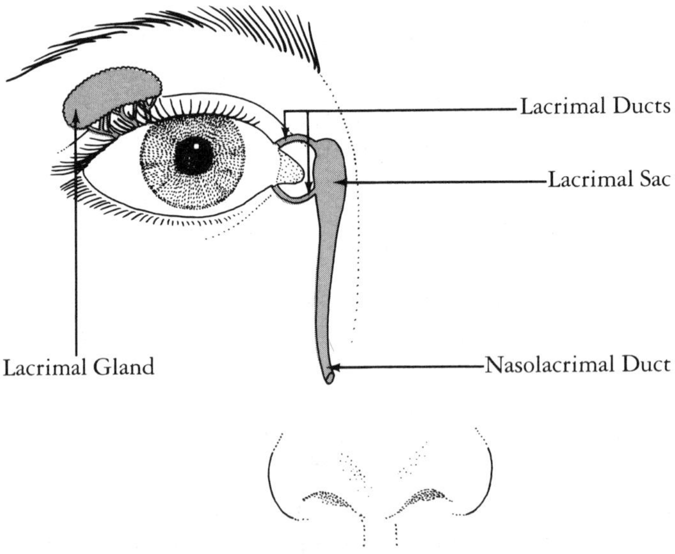

Figure 14–4 The tear apparatus.

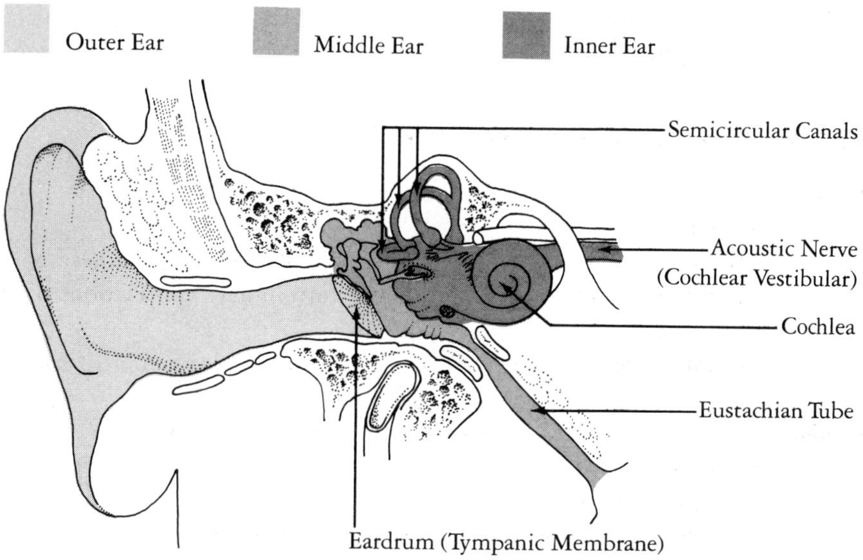

Figure 14–5 The ear.

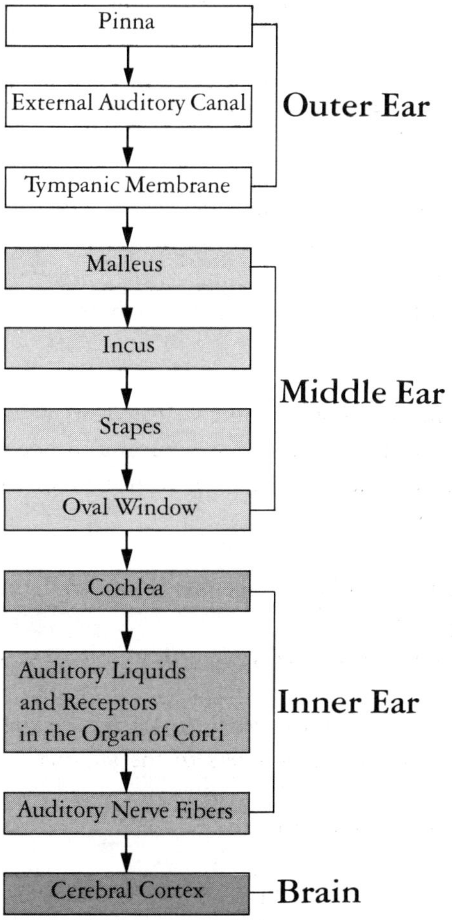

Figure 14–6 Flowchart of auditory pathway from sound to neurological interpretation.

The skin is a receptor for the sensation of touch, as well as being sensitive to heat, cold, pressure, and pain. It is an organ of the integumentary system.

Word Roots Relating to the Eyes and Vision

14.1 **blephar-** eyelid

EXAMPLES:

blepharoplasty (blephar/o/plast/y)—plastic repair or surgery of an eyelid
blepharospasm (blephar/o/spasm)—involuntary contractions of the eyelid
blepharadenoma (blephar/aden/oma)—glandular tumor of the eyelid

14.2 **cantho-** angle found at the end of the eyelid; corner of the eye

EXAMPLES:

canthal (canth/al)—pertaining to a corner of the eye
canthus (canth/us)—name for the corner of the eye

14.3 **cili-** eyelash

EXAMPLES:

cilium (cili/um)—eyelashes; eyelid or outer edge of eyelid; edge of eyelid from which eyelashes extend
supercilia (super/cilia)—eyebrows; above the eyelashes
ciliogenesis (cili/o/gen/esis)—formation or development of cilia

14.4 **corne-** horny; cornea

The cornea is the transparent part of the eyeball that covers the iris and pupil.

EXAMPLE:

corn (corn)—name for a build-up of thick, horny skin tissue, produced by friction and pressure
corneal (corne/al)—pertaining to the cornea of the eye
corneous (corne/ous)—horn-like or horny

14.5 **dacyr-** tear

This element is a root meaning tear or tears of the eye. The root *lacrim-* is used to denote body parts or structures associated with the production of tears. Medical conditions relating to tear production are generally denoted by the use of the root *dacry-*.

EXAMPLES:

dacryoadenitis (dacry/o/aden/itis)—inflammation of a lacrimal gland (a tear gland)
dacryocystectomy (dacry/o/cyst/ectomy)—excision of the wall of the lacrimal sac

Note that the word form *dacryadeno-* refers to the lacrimal (tear) gland, while the form *dacrycysto-* refers to the lacrimal (tear) sac.

14.6 **iris** rainbow; colored membrane of the eye

EXAMPLES:

iris (iris)—name for the colored membrane of the eye
iridic (irid/ic)—pertaining to the iris
iridization (irid/iz/ation)—patient's perception of colored halos around lights, occurring in glaucoma

14.7 kerat- horny; horny tissue; cornea of the eye

EXAMPLES:

keratoderma (kerat/o/derma)—horny skin or covering

hyperkeratosis (hyper/kerat/osis)—overgrowth (excessive growth) of the horny layer of the skin

keratomalacia (kerat/o/malacia)—softening of the cornea

The word root *corne-* identifies the cornea of the eye as a structure or landmark, while the root *kerato-* identifies horny tissues, conditions, and therapeutic procedures relating to the cornea.

14.8 lacrim- tear

EXAMPLES:

lacrimal glands (lacrim/al)—glands that secrete tears

lacrimal ducts (lacrim/al)—ducts (canals, or tubes) that convey secretions (tears) of the lacrimal glands to the corners of the eyes (canthus)

lacrimotomy (lacrim/otomy)—incision of the lacrimal duct

14.9 ocul- eye

EXAMPLES:

ocular (ocul/ar)—pertaining to the eye

oculus (ocul/us)—name for the eye

The word roots *ocul-*, *opt-*, *-opia*, and *ophthalm-* all relate to the eye. The root *ocul-* is generally used as a landmark, while *opt-* denotes relationship to vision or sight. The suffix *-opia* denotes a condition of vision or sight, while the root *ophthalm-* is generally used to designate conditions and therapies relating to the eye:

oculonasal (ocul/o/nas/al)—pertaining to the eye and the nose

oculopathy (ocul/o/path/y)—any disease or disorder of the eye

ophthalmolith (ophthalm/o/lith)—stone-like substance in the eye

ophthalmalacia (ophthal/malacia)—abnormal softening of the eye (note that the *m* in *ophthalm-* has been dropped because of the presence of the *m* in -malacia)

optic, optical (opt/ic, opt/ic/al)—pertaining to the eye; pertaining to vision or sight; pertaining to light

anopia (an/opia)—no vision

An ophthalmologist (ophthalm/ologist) is a doctor of medicine who specializes in the eyes. In addition to prescribing corrective lenses (eyeglasses), he or she is licensed to diagnose and prescribe drugs. An optometrist (opt/o/metr/ist) is one who is licensed to correct vision defects by measuring vision impairments and prescribing corrective lenses. The root *metr-* means measure. An optician (opt/ic/ian) is one who prepares lenses and supplies eyeglasses in accordance with the prescriptions of the ophthalmologist or the optometrist.

14.10 palpebr- eyelid

EXAMPLES:

palpebra (palpe/bra)—eyelid

palpebrate (palpebr/ate)—wink

palpebration (palpebr/ation)—abnormally frequent winking

This word root also refers to the eyelid; it is used for naming or referring to the eyelid as an anatomical part. The root *blephar-* is used principally for naming conditions and therapeutic procedures involving the eyelid.

14.11 phak- crystalline lens of the eye

EXAMPLES:

phakitis, phacitis (phak/itis, phac/itis)—inflammation of the crystalline lens of the eye
phacocele (phac/o/cele)—displacement or hernia of the eye lens
phacocyst- (phac/o/cyst-)—denotes relationship to the sac enclosing the crystalline lens of the eye

14.12 scler- hardness; white part of the eye

EXAMPLES:

sclerous (scler/ous)—hard; a synonym is indurated (in/dur/ated)
sclerosis (scler/osis)—a hardening; hardening of a body part, caused by inflammation

The word root *scler-* may be used in the form of the word ending *-sclerosis*. Another frequent use of the element *scler-* is in reference to the sclera, the white cover of the eyeball that surrounds the back five-sixths of the eyeball:

sclera (scler/a)—tough, white supporting cover of the eyeball
sclerotic (sclerot/ic)—pertaining to the sclera

14.13 tropia- deviation of eyes away from visual axis

EXAMPLES:

ametropia (a/metr/opia)—refractive disorder
tropometer (trop/o/meter)—device for measuring rotation of eyes
anisometropia (an/iso/me/tropia)—unequal focusing ability

Word Roots Relating to the Ear and Hearing

14.14 acousti- hearing; sound

EXAMPLES:

acoustic (acoust/ic)—pertaining to hearing
acoustogram (acoust/o/gram)—graphic tracings of sound measures such as decibel levels and frequencies per second

The basic word root meaning sound is *acous-* or *acus-*:

-acusis (-acu/sis)—word form used to denote a condition of hearing; a synonym is -acusia
anacusis (an/acu/sis)—condition of not hearing; total deafness (*an-* means not)
hemianacusia (hemi/an/acus/ia)—loss of hearing in one ear only

14.15 aur- ear

EXAMPLES:

auricle (aur/i/cle)—projecting part of the ear lying outside the head
auricul- (aur/i/cul-)—word form denoting relationship to the ear or to an ear-shaped appendage on a chamber of the heart
auriculocranial (aur/i/cul/o/crani/al)—pertaining to an ear and the cranium

14.16 ot- ear

The word root *ot-* also means ear and is used for identifying conditions of the ear and the therapeutic procedures used to correct them.

EXAMPLES:

otitis (ot/itis)—ear infection

parotid (par/ot/id)—situated near the ear; such as the parotid gland, a salivary gland located near the ear

epiotic (epi/ot/ic)—situated on or above the ear

entotic, endotic (ent/ot/ic, end/ot/ic)—situated in or arising in the ear

14.17 myring- eardrum

EXAMPLES:

myringa (myring/a)—eardrum

myringoscopy (myring/o/scop/y)—inspection of the eardrum using a myringoscope

myringoplasty (myring/o/plast/y)—surgical repair of eardrum defects

14.18 phon- voice; sound

This descriptive word root is generally used to denote speech or body sounds; the body sounds may be those arising within the body (heart beats) or created by such means as percussion (tapping).

EXAMPLES:

phonocardiogram (phon/o/cardi/o/gram)—record made of heart sounds

phonogram (phon/o/gram)—record made of any sound

phonomyogram (phon/o/my/o/gram)—record made of sound produced by muscle action

14.19 tympan- eardrum; eardrum enclosure

EXAMPLES:

tympanum (tympan/um)—name for enclosure or chamber in which eardrum is located; also called tympanic cavity

tympanic membrane (tympan/ic)—eardrum

tympanal (tympan/al)—pertaining to the tympanum or to the tympanic cavity

Word Roots Relating to Other Special Senses

14.20 lal- speech; babbling

EXAMPLES:

lalopathy (lal/o/path/y)—any speech disorder

lalophobia (lal/o/phob/ia)—fear or intense dislike of speaking (stage fright), often associated with stuttering

-lalia (-lal/ia)—speech disorder

14.21 odyn- pain

This word root has the same meaning as the element *-algia*.

EXAMPLES:

arthrodynia (arthr/odyn/ia)—pain in a joint; arthralgia

myodynia (my/odyn/ia)—pain in a muscle; myalgia

glossodynia (gloss/odyn/ia)—pain in the tongue; glossalgia

14.22 osmo- odor; sense of smell

EXAMPLES:

osmics (osm/ics)—science that deals with the sense of smell; study of odors
osmatic, -osmatic (osmat/ic, -osmat/ic)—pertaining to the sense of smell
anosmatic (an/osmat/ic)—having no sense of or only an imperfect sense of smell
anosmia (an/osm/ia)—absence of the sense of smell
hyposmia (hyp/osm/ia)—abnormally decreased sensitivity to odor

14.23 sinus hollow; recess

There are many cavities in the body designated as sinuses. The most familiar ones are the paranasal sinuses; air cavities in the cranial bones that communicate with the nasal cavity.

EXAMPLES:

sinusoid (sinus/oid)—resembling a sinus
sinusotomy (sinus/otomy)—surgical incision of a sinus
sinusology (sinus/ology)—branch of medicine that relates to the sinuses

14.24 somni- sleep

EXAMPLES:

somniferous (somni/fer/ous)—inducing or causing sleep (-ferous is a word ending that means producing)
insomnia (in/somn/ia)—inability to sleep; also called hyposomnia
hypersomnia (hyper/somn/ia)—excessive sleep; uncontrollable drowsiness

Terminology Trivia

Medical Instruments

Knowledge concerning diseases of the larynx and other respiratory passages was greatly advanced with the invention of the laryngoscope in 1855 by Garcia. Garcia was a gifted singer who invented this instrument so that he could observe the position of his vocal cords while singing. The ophthalmoscope was invented in 1850 by von Helmholtz, who made examination of the live retina possible for future generations.

Pronunciation and Meaning of New Terms

corneal (korn′ eel) Pertaining to the cornea of the eye.

dacryoadenitis (da′ kre ad en itis) Inflammation of the tear gland.

lacrimal (lak′ rĭ mal) Pertaining to the tears.

ocular (ok′ u lar) Pertaining to the eye.

phacocele (pha ko′ seal) Hernia of eyelid.

sclera (skler′ ah) White supporting cover of the eyeball.

auricle (or′ ik le) The external ear.

Self-test

1. For each set, match Column A with Column B.

Column A

___ blepharoptosis
___ canthus
___ caruncle
___ dacryopyrrhea
___ lacrimal gland
___ lacrimal duct
___ lacrimal sac
___ nasolacrimal duct

Column B

a. drooping upper eyelid
b. discharge of pus from lacrimal gland
c. corner of the eyelid
d. eyelashes
e. tissue that secretes tears
f. small canals that transport tears from eyes to nose
g. tube that carries tears down the nose
h. pouch-like area at beginning of duct in the nose
i. small, fleshy eminence

2.

Column A

___ amblyopia
___ ametropia
___ anisometropia
___ anopia
___ iridoplegia
___ blepharitis
___ blepharoptosis
___ iridomalacia

Column B

a. no vision, usually in one eye
b. paralysis of the iris sphincter
c. dull vision; lazy eye
d. softening of the iris
e. general term meaning a refractive disorder
f. drooping eyelid
g. inflammation of the eyelid
h. different focusing ability in each eye

3.

Column A

___ conjunctivitis
___ dacryoadenitis
___ dacryocystitis
___ detached retina
___ diplopia
___ enophthalmia
___ epicanthus
___ esotropia
___ exophthalmia
___ exotropia
___ plakatis
___ hyperopia
___ keratitis
___ keratoconjunctivitis

Column B

a. inflammation of tear gland
b. inside lining of eye pulled away
c. fold of skin over corner of the eye
d. inflammation of tear sac
e. eye appearing to be sunken into the orbit
f. inflammation of the outer lining of the eye
g. double vision
h. farsightedness
i. turning out of the eyes
j. protruding eyes
k. turning in of the eyes; cross-eyed
l. inflammation of the eye lens
m. inflammation of cornea and conjunctiva
n. inflammation of the cornea

4.

Column A

___ leukoma
___ nyctalopia
___ optic neuritis
___ ophthalmoplegia
___ proptosis
___ retinitis
___ retinopathy
___ scleritis
___ subconjunctival hemorrhage
___ sympathetic ophthalmia
___ trichiasis

Column B

a. dense, white opacity of cornea
b. paralysis of eye muscles
c. inflammation of optic nerve
d. night blindness
e. bulging eye
f. noninjured eye suffering with the injured eye
g. hairs of eyelid growing inward
h. bleeding under conjunctiva
i. inflammation of the retina
j. inflammation of the sclera
k. general term meaning disease of the retina

5.

Column A

___ bilateral otitis media
___ eustachian salpingitis
___ external otitis
___ myringa
___ mastoiditis
___ malleus
___ myringitis
___ otosclerosis
___ otalgia
___ otorrhagia
___ otorrhea
___ stapes

Column B

a. inflammation of auditory tube
b. tympanic membrane
c. injury to the ear due to a change in air pressure
d. middle ear inflammation in both ears
e. inflammation of the bony process of the temporal bone
f. inflammation of the external ear
g. last bone of the middle ear
h. bleeding from the ear
i. first bone of the middle ear
j. inflammation of tympanic membrane
k. pain in the ear
l. spongy bone replacing the hard bone of the labyrinth
m. discharge from the ear

Fifteen
Endocrine System

Functions of the Endocrine System

The complex communication among cells of the body is accomplished jointly by the endocrine (*endo* means within and *krinein* means to separate) system and the central nervous system. The central nervous system acts instantaneously. Actions of the endocrine glands are more delayed; glands slowly discharge their secretions into the bloodstream.

The endocrine system is composed of the ductless glands of internal secretion; called ductless glands because they have no ducts with which to carry away their secretions. The substances secreted by these glands are called hormones; hormone is a Greek word meaning to excite. Although most hormones are excitatory, some are inhibitory. Endocrine glands that secrete hormones are the thyroid, parathyroids, pituitary, adrenals, gonads, pineal body, thymus, pancreas, and intestinal glands.

Word Roots Relating to the Endocrine System

15.1 **adeno-** gland

A gland is a body part that separates and secretes certain elements.

Examples of Glands

Gland	Secretion
kidney	urine
mammary	milk
salivary	saliva

EXAMPLES:

adenosis (aden/osis)—any condition of a gland, especially finding a gland where it is not supposed to be

adenotomy (aden/otomy)—cutting into a gland

adenoma (aden/oma)—a tumor with a gland-like structure (a glandular tumor)

The term adenoma does not mean tumor of a gland, but rather a tumor with a gland-like texture or structure:

fibroadenoma (fibro/aden/oma)—adenoma with fibrous tissue

blepharadenoma (blephar/aden/oma)—glandular tumor of the eyelid (adenoma of the eyelid)

nephradenoma (nephr/aden/oma)—glandular tumor of the kidney (adenoma of the kidney)

15.2 **adreno-** adrenal gland

EXAMPLES:

adrenal (adren/al)—situated near the kidney; adrenal gland
adrenogenous (adren/o/gen/ous)—produced or arising in the adrenals
adrenalopathy (adren/al/o/path/y)—any disease of the adrenal glands; also called adrenopathy

15.3 **hormone** to excite

A hormone is a substance formed in an organ of the body, carried by a body fluid where it has a specific effect.

EXAMPLES:

hormonotherapy (hormon/o/therap/y)—treatment through use of hormones
hyperhormonal (hyper/hormon/al)—pertaining to hormone excess
hypohormonal (hypo/hormon/al)—pertaining to hormone deficiency

15.4 **thyro-** thyroid

The term thyroid may be used to indicate a body part, such as a cartilage, artery, nerve, and so on, in the region of the thyroid gland. The thyroid gland (*thyr/o/aden-*) is a large endocrine gland lying in front of and on either side of the trachea. It secretes a hormone that regulates body growth and metabolism.

EXAMPLES:

hypothyroidism (hypo/thyroid/ism)—deficiency of thyroid activity or the condition resulting therefrom; also called hypothyroidosis
hyperthyroidism (hyper/thyroid/ism)—hyperactivity (excess activity) of the thyroid gland; also called hyperthyroidosis
thyrochondrotomy (thyro/chondr/otomy)—surgical incision of the thyroid cartilage

An enlarged thyroid gland is called a goiter. It is a condition caused by a lack of iodine in the diet. Exophthalmic goiter is characterized by bulging eyeballs and enlarged thyroid, as well as by other minor symptoms. The cause of this condition is unknown, but dietary iodine is thought to be involved.

Terminology Trivia

Endocrinology

Graves (1796–1853) of Ireland was the first person to describe hyperthyroidism and one variety even bears his name: Graves' disease. From the days of Hippocrates, goiter, a chronic enlargement of the thyroid gland, has been treated with burnt seaweed, which is rich in iodine. In coastal areas, simple goiter is infrequent, due to the common dietary intake of sea life (plants and animals). In 1918, Marine found goiters present in ninety percent of the dogs tested in Cleveland, Ohio. He and his associates identified the value of iodine in prevention of goiter. The disease took its toll on sheep and had a major economic impact on the sheep and hog industries. Prophylactic (preventative) measures became a major activity with the help of dietary supplements of iodine.

Functions of the parathyroid glands were a mystery until 1892 when Gley, a French physiologist, found that if they were removed during goiter surgery, tetanic seizures resulted. The parathyroid glands regulate the level of serum calcium, necessary for proper functioning of heart, nerves, and muscle.

Pronunciation and Meaning of New Terms

adenoma (ah den ō mah) A tumor with a gland-like structure.

adrenal (ah dre′ nal) A flattened body above each kidney that secretes steroid hormones, epinephrine, and norepinephrine.

hyperthyroidism (hi″ per thi′ roi dizm) Increased activity of the thyroid gland.

hypothyroidism (hi″ po thi′ roi dizm) Decreased activity of the thyroid gland.

thyroid (thi′ roy d) A large endocrine gland in front of and on either side of the trachea.

Self-test

1. Match Column A with Column B.

Column A

b acromegaly
c adrenogenital syndrome
d exophthalmic goiter
a goiter
e hyperadrenocorticism
j hyperthyroidism
g hypothyroidism
f parathyroid tetany
h thyroiditis
k thyrotoxicosis

Column B

a. enlargement of the thyroid gland
b. enlarged extremities
c. hyperformation of adrenal cortex; includes symptom of early development of the reproductive organs
d. condition characterized by eyes protruding from their sockets
e. oversecretion of hormones from adrenal cortex
f. severe muscle contractions due to hormone deficiency
g. undersecretion of thyroid hormones
h. inflammation of thyroid gland
i. abnormal mucus deposits under the skin
j. oversecretion of thyroid hormones
k. toxicity caused by oversecretion of the thyroid gland

2501 How Endocrine System works
* # 2502 Miracle Months Hormone + development
# 2503 mind + Hormones

Roulette ISL

Filmstrip

Sign up on log book

Sixteen
Diagnosis and Disease

Diagnosis

Diagnosis is an early step in medical care. It is usually made after a medical history is taken and a physical examination is given. The medical history consists of information that is collected concerning past events that might relate to the patient's illness. A medical history includes the following:

Medical History	
Chief complaint	CC
History of present illness	HPI
Past medical history	PMH
Family medical history	FMH
Social history	SH
Review of systems	ROS

The purpose of a medical history is to help evaluate symptoms of a disease by gathering information that might be related to these symptoms. The information gathered from both the physical examination and the medical history is recorded in one place: the medical record.

The physical examination is a systematic evaluation of the body that includes the following:

inspection: looking into or at (inspecting) the patient with various instruments. For example, an ophthalmoscope is an instrument for viewing the inside of the eye (*ophthalmo*).

palpation: touching (palpating) or feeling specific areas of the patient's body. The body is palpated for irregularities in size, firmness, lumps, or other physical findings.

auscultation: listening to (ausculting) the sounds produced by or made in response to electronic devices. For example, a stethoscope is an instrument for listening to the sounds in the chest (*steth*).

percussion: striking (percussing) various parts of the body to determine the quality of sounds produced; the reflexes or reactions of nerves; and the existence of tenderness.

vital signs: measurements taken of temperature, pulse, respiratory rate, and blood pressure. These are commonly abbreviated as *T, P, RR,* and *BP.*

Diagnosis of disease condition involves the following terms:

acute: condition that is sudden.

ambulatory: able to walk. The sick person is not confined to a sickbed or clinic but is capable (*ory*) of walking (*ambulat*).

anomaly: irregularity; deviation from normal.
atrophy: wasting away of the body or an organ or a part, due to irritation or disease.
benign: mild disease.
chronic: condition that lasts a long time.
clinical: related to examination; first-hand observation of a disease resulting in diagnosis.
diagnosis: identification of a disease through (*dia*) knowledge (*gnosis*) of the disease.
malignant: condition that becomes progressively worse.
metastatic: disease that spreads from one place (*static*) to the next (*meta*).
prognosis: having knowledge (*gnosis*) of the course of a disease beforehand (*pro*); prediction of a disease's process.
sign: observable, measurable occurrence that indicates a disease; examples: fever, rash, or swelling.
symptom: subjective indication of something that occurs with a particular disease; example: feelings of pain or nausea.
syndrome: set of signs and symptoms that usually occur together; example: respiratory distress syndrome is a group of signs and symptoms that result from respiratory disturbance.
systemic: involving systems; disease affects systems of the body as a whole.

The term used to indicate the treatment of a disease or a pathological condition is therapy; therapeutics is a branch of medicine concerned with the applications of remedies and the treatment of disease. Two general categories of treatment in the field of medicine are surgery and internal medicine. Surgery is the art and practice of treating disease, injuries and deformities through surgical techniques. Internal medicine is the medical specialty that diagnoses disease using thorough history, complete physical, and laboratory and other diagnostic studies.

Disease

There are basically four sources from which a disease may receive its name. A disease may be named for:

1. an organism that caused it. For example, streptococcal or gonococcal infections are named for staphyloccus and gonococcus organisms. The *-al* word terminals turn them into adjectives. In this example, the organisms are members of the coccus bacterial group.
2. a portion of the anatomy. Take the terms appendicitis and urethritis, for example. The suffix *-itis* means inflammation and in these examples there is an inflammation of anatomical parts—the appendix and the urethra.
3. the person who first described it as a disease. Hansen's Disease, Bell's Palsy, and Buerger's Disease are three examples.
4. a special condition or characteristic of the disease. For example, mumps was named for the fact that the disease causes swollen glands resulting in mumbling speech. Its appearance may also give the source of its name; for example, the terms erethema multiforme and acne vulgaris give some hint as to their appearance.

Naming diseases can become confusing. Research may reveal the true cause of a disease differs from what was originally believed at the time the disease was named. New understanding may render a descriptive name incorrect. For example, erythroblastosis fetalis means a condition in which immature red blood cells cause the death of a fetus. It is now known that this condition is not due to red blood cells but rather to the Rh factor that results in a clumping of cells. An Rh+ donor should never contribute blood to an Rh+ sensitive recipient (a person with Rh− blood). The existence of the Rh factor was unknown when the disease was named.

Another area of confusion is that rare name that describes the thing itself rather than the condition. For example, tuberculosis was once called consumption or phthisis (pronounced thesis), which means wasting away, a description of what happens to the person with tuberculosis.

Some selected terms relating to diseases are:

agenesis: condition in which a body structure was not (*a*) produced (*genesis*).
bacterial: disease caused by bacteria.
congenital: condition or defect that a child has at birth (*genital*).
degenerative: disease characterized by a breakdown in structure.
endemic: disease occurring in (*en*) a population of people (*demic*).
epidemic: disease occurs above (*epi*) the expected level of that disease in people (*demic*).
exacerbation: disease becomes increasingly severe; disease comes out (*ex*) in a harsh (*acer*) way.
iatrogenic: disease that is a side effect of treatment prescribed by a physician (*iatro*).
idiopathic: disease (*pathic*) that is peculiar (*idio*) to one person; of unknown cause.
infectious: disease that spreads from one person to (*in*) another.
neoplastic: disease in which new (*neo*) cells are formed (*plastic*); referred to as cancer. Cancer is a malignant invasive growth that was thought to spread like the legs of a crab (cancer).
pandemic: disease that spreads over all (*pan*) the people (*demic*).
sepsis: infections; organisms or poisons capable of producing a breakdown of body tissues.
trauma: wound.

In multiple-system diseases, a target organ may be involved, but as the disease advances and symptoms develop, other organs become progressively affected. This is particularly true of many infections, such as those that begin with a skin rash or that initially involve the respiratory or gastrointestinal system.

X-rays often reveal disease in organs in addition to the organ primarily affected. In cases that come to autopsy, disease processes may be evidenced in many body structures far removed from the primary focus. It is not unusual for autopsies performed on stillborn infants and those dying shortly after birth to find a number of anomalies incompatible with life. There may be gross malformations of organs or heart defects that are not detected at birth.

Diagnoses of multiple-system diseases have been made possible by new and improved laboratory and x-ray procedures and the use of radioisotopes and electromyography. These techniques, and other advances in diagnostic medicine, have made it possible to trace the involvement of multiple organs in systemic diseases.

Cancer Grading and Cancer Staging

There are two methods used to categorize malignant tumors: grading and staging. These methods are based on different aspects of tumor growth and appearance.

Pathologists grade tumors by describing the microscopic appearance of their cells; specifically, their degree of anaplasia (alteration). From this, tumors are assigned one of four grades. Grade I tumors closely resemble the normal parent tissues of origin. Grade IV tumors are so anaplastic that even recognition of their tissues of origin may be difficult. Grade II and III tumors are intermediate in appearance, either moderately or poorly differentiated rather than well differentiated (Grade I) or dedifferentiated (Grade IV).

Grading aids in cancer prognoses; patients with Grade I tumors have a high survival rate, while patients with Grades II, III, and IV tumors have poorer survival rates. Grading is also used in evaluating precancerous cells, such as those of the uterine cervix (Pap Smear), trachea, or stomach.

Staging is determined by the progression of tumor growth and development. It is based on the fact that tumors follow stages of growth and so, they are judged within each staging category in addition to being graded by appearance. An example of a staging system is the TNM (Tumor, Nodes, Metastasis) system, usually applied to malignancies such as breast and lung cancer: T refers to tumor size and degree of local extension; N refers to the number of regional lymph nodes invaded by the tumor; and M refers to the presence or absence of tumor cell metastases. The following abbreviations refer to this system:

TNM Staging System

Abbreviation	Description
Tumor	
T0	No evidence of a primary tumor
TIS	Carcinoma in situ
T1, T2, T3, T4	Progressive increase in tumor size and involvement
TX	Tumor unassessable
Nodes	
N0	Regional lumph nodes not abnormal
N1, N2, N3, N4	Increasing degrees of abnormal lymph nodes
NX	Regional lymph nodes unassessable
Metastasis	
M0	No evidence of distant metastasis
M1, M2, M3	Degrees of distant metastasis
MX	Minimum requirements to assess the presence of distant metastasis cannot be met

Word Roots Relating to Cancer

16.1 **benign-** mild; favorable for recovery

This word is used in phrases to describe the relative severity of a disease.

EXAMPLES:

benign psychosis—psychosis that is not life threatening

benign malaria—malarial condition having good prognosis

The principal use of this term is to designate the absence of cancerous tumors, as in a benign tumor versus a carcinoma.

16.2 **carcin-** cancer; malignant growth

Cancer is the name used to designate a mass of tissue cells that grow rampantly, spreading throughout the body.

EXAMPLES:

carcinous (carcin/ous)—pertaining to cancer; cancerous

carcinoma (carcin/oma)—malignant growth that infiltrates surrounding tissues

carcinosis (carcin/osis)—spread of cancer throughout the body; advanced metastatic disease

adenocarcinoma (aden/o/carcin/oma)—malignant tumor composed of gland-like cells

16.3 **malign-** bad; harmful

EXAMPLES:

malignant (malign/ant)—condition that gets progressively worse and results in death

malignancy (malign/ancy)—tendency to spread; used for cancerous growths that progressively invade body tissues

The terms malignant and benign have opposite meanings.

16.4 **onco-** mass; tumor; swelling

EXAMPLES:

oncology (onc/ology)—study of tumors

-oncus (-onc/us)—designation for swelling or tumor

arthroncus (arthr/onc/us)—swelling of a joint

cheiloncus (cheil/onc/us)—tumor of the lip

16.5 **scirr-** hard; hard tumor

The root *scirr-* (also *scirrh-*) denotes relationship to a scirrhus, the name for a hard, cancerous tumor.

EXAMPLES:

scirrhus (scirrh/us)—name for a hard, cancerous tumor

scirrhous (scirrh/ous)—pertaining to a scirrhus

mastoscirrhus (mast/o/scirrh/us)—hard cancer of the breast

dacryadenoscirrhus (dacry/aden/o/scirrh/us)—hard cancerous tumor (scirrhus) of the lacrimal (tear) gland

Diseases Relating to Body Systems

The remainder of this chapter presents disease terminology associated with the various body systems. Terms are defined by breaking them down into their elemental forms.

Diseases of the skeletal system

Disease conditions of the skeletal system include:

achondroplasia: condition (*ia*) in which there is a lack of (*a*) growth (*plas*) at the ends of long bones covered with cartilage (*chondr*); may produce a form of dwarfism.

bunion: protrusion on the surface of the foot near the joint of the big or small toe.
callus: new, hard (*callus*) bone formation at the site of a bone fracture.
coxa plana: disease condition in which the head of the femur, part of the hip (*coxa*) joint, becomes flattened (*plana*).
exostosis: condition (*osis*) in which there is excessive (*ex*) formation of bone (*ost*), forming a protuberance.
fibrous dysplasia: abnormal (*dys*) formation (*plasia*) in which fibrous tissue (*fibrous*) replaces bone tissue.
genu varum: genu (knee) varum (turned); bowlegged.
multiple myeloma: multiple tumors (*oma*) of the bone marrow (*myel*), which replace normal bone cells.
osteitis deformans: inflammation (*itis*) of bone (*oste*), that results in deformity (*deformans*) of bony structures.
osteoarthritis: inflammation (*itis*) of bone (*osteo*) at the joint (*arthr*).
osteochondritis: inflammation (*itis*) of bone (*osteo*) and cartilage (*chondr*).
osteoclasia: condition (*ia*) in which bone (*osteo*) is destroyed (*clas*); surgical fracture of bone to remedy deformity.
osteogenesis imperfecta: disease in which production (*genesis*) of bone (*osteo*) is imperfect (*imperfecta*).
osteogenic sarcoma: tumor (*oma*) of connective tissue (*sarc*) arising (*genic*) in bone (*osteo*).
osteoma: tumor (*oma*) in bone (*osteo*).
osteomalacia: bones (*osteo*) become soft (*malacia*).
osteomyelitis: bones (*osteo*) and bone marrow (*myel*) are inflamed (*itis*).
osteoporosis: condition (*osis*) in which bone (*osteo*) becomes porous (*por*).
spondylitis: inflammation (*itis*) of the spine (*spondyl*).
syndactylism: condition in which the fingers or toes (*dactyl*) have grown together.
talipes calcaneus: condition in which the foot touches the floor only at the heel bone (*calcaneus*).
talipes valgus: joints of the foot are turned outward (*valgus*).
talipes varus: joints of the foot are turned inward (*varus*).

The following terms are related to disease conditions of joints and bursae:

ankylosis: condition (*osis*) in which a joint becomes crooked (*ankyl*); abnormal fixation of a joint due to pathological changes.
arthritis: inflammation (*itis*) of the joints (*arthr*).
bursitis: inflammation (*itis*) of the bursa (*burs*).
degenerative joint disease: disease of joints that results from a deterioration of tissue.
rheumatoid arthritis: inflammation (*itis*) in a joint (*arthr*); from the humoral theory of diseases implicating a change in the flow (*rheum*) of body fluids as the cause of disease.
tendonitis: inflammation (*itis*) of a tendon (*tendon*).

Diseases of the muscular system

The following terms are related to disease conditions of muscles:

fibromyositis: inflammation (*itis*) of muscle (*myo*) and fibrous tissue (*fibro*).
hemiplegia: paralysis (*plegia*) of one-half (*hemi*) of the body, either the right or left side.
myasthenia gravis: muscle (*my*) weakness (*asthenia*) of a very grave (*gravis*) type.

muscle atrophy: lack of (*a*) muscle growth (*trophy*).
muscle hypertrophy: excessive (*hyper*) growth (*trophy*) or enlargement of muscle.
muscular dystrophy: weakening, degeneration, or abnormal (*dys*) development (*trophy*) of muscle.
polymyositis: inflammation (*itis*) of many (*poly*) muscles (*myo*).

Diseases of the integumentary system

These selected terms relate to diseases of the integumentary system and include signs and symptoms:

abrasion: scraped (*rasion*) away (*ab*) portion of the skin.
acne: pointed (*acne,* variation of *acme*), often pus-filled, eruptions on the skin.
angioma: tumor (*oma*) of blood vessels (*angi*) that appear on skin; also called hemangioma.
callus: condition in which an area of skin has hardened (*callus*).
carbuncle: small (*cle*) inflammation of the skin containing pus and reddened to a color similar to burning coal (*carbun*, variation of *carbon*).
cheilitis: inflammation (*itis*) of the lips (*cheil*).
contusion: condition in which tissue beneath skin is injured, but skin is unbroken.
cutis anserina: condition of the skin (*cutis*) in which bumps with a texture like that of a plucked goose (*anserina*) develops; also known as goosebumps.
decubitis ulcer: sore (*ulcer*) on skin of a person who has been lying down (*decub*); bed sore.
dermatitis: inflammation (*itis*) of the skin (*derma*).
ecthyma: skin condition in which fluid rushes (*thyma*) out (*ec*, variation of *ex*) of sores in the skin; also called ulcerative impetigo.
eczema: condition in which there is a flowing of fluid (*ecze*) out (*ec*, variation of *ex*) from the skin.
erysipelas: disease in which a deep red (*erysi*, variation of *erythro*) color spreads over the skin (*pelas*).
erythema: abnormal redness (*eryth*) of the skin.
erythromelalgia: condition in which the skin of the extremities (*mel*) becomes red (*erythro*) and painful (*algia*).
eschar: hard crust or scab (*eschar*) that forms after a traumatic injury.
furuncle: skin boil.
gynecomastia: condition (*ia*) in which the male breast (*mast*) resembles the breast of a female (*gyneco*).
hidradenitis: inflammation (*itis*) of a sweat (*hidr*) gland (*aden*).
hives: condition of skin characterized by the appearance of itchy areas.
hyperhidrosis: condition (*osis*) in which there is excessive (*hyper*) sweating (*hidr*).
hypertrichosis: condition (*osis*) in which there is an excessive (*hyper*) amount of hair (*trich*).
ichthyosis: condition (*osis*) in which skin is scaly like the skin of a fish (*ichthy*).
icterus: condition in which skin becomes yellow (*icteric*), another name for jaundice.
impetigo: skin invaded by bacteria, resulting in eruptions.
intertrigo: dermatitis between (*inter*) folds of skin caused by rubbing (*trigo*); chafing.
laceration: process (*tion*) in which a wound or irregular tear (*lacera*) of the skin or flesh occurs.

macula: spot (*macula*) or blotch that is flat and less than one-half centimeter in diameter.
melanoma: tumor (*oma*) involving the melanocyte (*melan*) cells in skin.
nevus: mark on the skin; includes various types of birthmarks (*nevus*) and all types of moles.
onychomycosis: disease (*osis*) of the nails (*onych*), due to fungus (*myc*).
pediculosis: condition (*osis*) in which there is an infestation of lice (*pedicul*).
pediculosis pubis: lice in the pubic (*pubis*) hair.
pediculosis capitis: head (*capitis*) lice.
pediculosis corporis: body (*corporis*) lice.
petechia: small hemorrhage under the skin that appears as a small spot (*petechia*).
plantar keratosis: condition (*osis*) in which there is hardening (*kerat*) of skin on the sole (*plantar*) of the foot.
psoriasis: chronic skin disease (*iasis*) characterized by scaly, itchy (*psor*) patches.
pustule: small (*ule*), circumscribed elevation of the skin containing pus (*pust*).
scabies: skin disease caused by parasitic mites that burrow under the skin and cause itchiness (*scabies*).
scleroderma: condition characterized by hardening (*sclera*) of skin (*derma*).
seborrheic dermatitis: inflammation (*itis*) of the skin (*derma*) in which there is an excessive flow (*orrh*) of sebum (*seb*).
suppuration: process (*tion*) in which pus is produced (*suppur*).
telangiectasia: condition (*sia*) in which the ends (*tel*) of blood vessels (*angi*) are dilated (*ectasis*); especially the capillaries of the nose and face.
tinea: skin disease caused by fungus; also known as ringworm (*tinea*).
verruca: small, flat growths commonly known as warts (*verruca*).
vitiligo: smooth, white patches of skin and hair (*vitiligo*) caused by loss of pigmentation.

Diseases of the cardiovascular system

The following are selected terms relating to disease conditions of the cardiovascular system:

aneurysm: dilation or widening (*eury*) of (*an*, variation of *ana*) a blood vessel caused by weakness in its wall.
arteriosclerosis: disease (*osis*) characterized by hardening (*scler*) of walls of arteries (*arterio*).
atherosclerosis: fatty substances (*athero*) deposited in and between layers lining arteries.
avascular necrosis: condition in which there is death of tissues (*necrosis*) due to lack (*a*) of blood supply through blood vessels (*vascular*).
bacterial endocarditis: inflammation (*itis*) of the inner (*endo*) lining of the heart (*card*) caused by bacteria.
cardiomyopathy: disease (*pathy*) of the heart (*cardio*) muscle (*myo*).
congestive heart failure: condition in which the heart fails to pump blood adequately, resulting in congestion of blood in the lungs.
coronary occlusion: obstruction (*occlusion*) in circulation to the heart.
embolus: ball (*bolus*) of clotted blood, and possibly other substances, carried in (*em*) the bloodstream. floating clot
hematoma: tumor (*oma*) or swelling that contains blood (*hemat*).
hemorrhoid: dilated vein filled with blood (*hemo*) in the area of the anal sphincter.
hypertension: elevation (*hyper*) of blood pressure (*tension*) above normal limits.

* **hypotension:** condition of low (*hypo*) blood pressure (*tension*).
* **myocardial infarction:** death (*infarct*) of a portion of the heart (*cardial*) muscle (*myo*).
myocardial insufficiency: action of the muscle (*myo*) of the heart (*cardial*) is not (*in*) adequate (*sufficient*).
* **myocardial ischemia:** decrease (*isch*) in the blood (*hemia*) supply to the muscle (*myo*) of the heart (*cardial*).
phlebitis: inflammation (*itis*) of a vein (*phleb*).
pulmonary stenosis: condition (*osis*) in which there is constriction or narrowing (*sten*) of the main blood vessel to the lungs (*pulmonary*).
shock: inadequate tissue perfusion.
anaphylactic shock: reaction from severe allergy to foreign substance; shock occurs because the person is not (*an*) protected (*phylactic*) from that substance.
cardiogenic shock: shock that is produced (*genic*) from failure of the heart (*cardio*).
neurogenic shock: shock that is produced (*genic*) from a failure of the nervous system (*neuro*).
cardiac tamponade: condition in which fluid accumulates in the pericardial sac around the heart muscle so that the heartbeat is impaired and the flow of blood is blocked (*tampon*).
thromboangiitis obliterans: inflammation (*itis*) of a blood vessel (*angi*) that results in formation of a blood clot (*thrombo*) obstructing (*obliterans*) the flow of blood.
thrombophlebitis: inflammation (*itis*) of a vein (*phleb*) that results in formation of a blood clot (*thrombo*).

Diseases of the blood

The following terms relate to diseases of the blood and include changes in blood caused by diseases:

agranulocytosis: condition (*osis*) in which there is a lack (*a*) of granulocytes.
anemia: condition in which there is a lack (*an*) of blood (*emia*).
aplastic anemia: anemia characterized by lack (*a*) of blood cell formation (*plast*).
hemolytic anemia: anemia resulting from breakdown (*lytic*) of blood (*hemo*) cells.
hypochromic microcytic anemia: anemia characterized by decrease (*hypo*) in the normal color (*chromic*) of blood cells (*cytic*) that are smaller (*micro*) than normal; usually due to iron deficiency or chronic disease.
iron-deficiency anemia: anemia caused by lack of (*deficiency*) iron needed to produce normal red blood cells.
macrocytic anemia: anemia characterized by appearance of large (*macro*) red blood cells (*cytic*).
pernicious anemia: anemia that may lead to (*per*) death (*nici*, variation of *necro*).
sickle-cell anemia: anemia characterized by sickle-shaped red blood cells.
anisocytosis: condition (*osis*) in which red blood cells (*cyt*) are unequal or dissimilar (*aniso*).
anoxia: deficiency (*an*) of oxygen (*oxia*) in blood.
acidosis: condition (*osis*) in which blood is too acidic.
alkalosis: condition (*osis*) in which blood is too alkaline (*alkal*).
dyscrasia: blood condition (*ia*) that refers to defective or abnormal (*dys*) mixtures (*cras*) of formed blood elements.
embolus: clump that acts as a stopper (*bolus*) inside (*em*) a blood vessel; floats in the blood until it lodges in a blood vessel too small for it to pass through.

erythrocytosis: condition (*osis*) in which there is an excess of red blood cells (*erythrocyt*).
erythropenia: deficiency (*penia*) of red blood cells (*erythro*).
granulocytopenia: condition in which there is a decrease (*penia*) in the number of granulocytes.
hemolysis: breaking down (*lysis*) of red blood (*hemo*) cells.
hemophilia: hereditary blood disease in which the time it takes blood to coagulate is prolonged, as though there was a love (*philia*) of blood (*hemo*).
hemostasis: stoppage or stagnation (*stasis*) of blood (*hemo*), usually normal blood clotting.
hyperglycemia: excessive (*hyper*) amount of glucose (*glyc*) in blood (*emia*).
hypoglycemia: decrease (*hypo*) in the amount of glucose (*glyc*) in blood (*emia*).
hypoxia: condition (*ia*) in which there is a decrease (*hyp*) in the amount of oxygen (*ox*) in blood.
leukemia: condition (*ia*) characterized by presence of abnormally high numbers of white blood cells (*leuk*) in the blood (*em*, a form of *hem*).
leukopenia: abnormal decrease (*penia*) in the number of white blood cells (*leuko*).
pancytopenia: reduction (*penia*) in all (*pan*) cellular (*cyto*) elements of the blood.
poikilocytosis: condition (*osis*) in which red blood cells (*cytes*) have varied or irregular (*poikilo*) shapes.
polycythemia: excess (*poly*) of blood (*hemia*) cells (*cyt*).

Diseases of the lymphatic system

Terms relating to diseases of the lymphatic system, including signs and symptoms of diseases, are:

dependent edema: swelling (*edema*) occurring as a result of the hanging down (*dependent*) of the legs; lymph does not drain, resulting in an accumulation of fluid (*edema*).
elephantiasis: disease (*iasis*) condition in which lymph collects in a limb or genitalia, causing it to swell to a point where it resembles an elephant's skin, usually due to infection from a filarial worm.
lymphadenitis: inflammation (*itis*) of lymph (*lymph*) glands (*aden*).
lymphadenopathy: general term meaning disease (*pathy*) of the lymph (*lymph*) glands (*adeno*).
lymphatic metastasis: condition in which disease moves from one place (*stasis*) to another (*meta*) by way of the lymph system.
lymphoma: tumor (*oma*) of the lymph (*lymph*) nodes; one type is Hodgkin's disease.
lymphosarcoma: malignant (*sarc*) tumor (*oma*) of the lymph (*lympho*) nodes.

Diseases of the respiratory system

The following terms relate to diseases of the respiratory system and include signs and symptoms of disease:

apnea: absence (*a*) of breathing (*pnea*).
atelectasis: incomplete (*atel*) dilation (*ectasis*) of lung tissue.
bronchiectasis: excessive dilation (*ectasis*) of bronchi (*bronchi*) characterized by the accumulation of mucus.
bronchitis: inflammation (*itis*) of bronchi (*bronch*).
dyspnea: difficult (*dys*) breathing (*pnea*).

emphysema: condition (*ma*) in which alveoli of the lungs have been blown (*physe*) in (*em*); lungs are permanently overinflated.
hemoptysis: spitting (*ptysis*) of blood (*hemo*) from the respiratory tract.
hemothorax: condition in which there is blood (*hemo*) in the thoracic cavity (*thorax*).
hyperventilation: excessive (*hyper*) breathing (*ventilation*).
laryngitis: inflammation (*itis*) of the larynx.
laryngospasm: sudden contraction (*spasm*) of the larynx (*laryngo*).
orthopnea: condition in which breathing (*pnea*) is easier when person is positioned upright, or straight (*ortho*).
pleurisy: inflammation (*isy*, variation of *itis*) of the pleura (*pleur*).
pneumonia: disease condition (*ia*) of the lungs (*pneumon*).
pneumoconiosis: lung (*pneumo*) condition (*osis*) caused by inhalation of various types of dust particles (*coni*).
pneumothorax: air (*pneumo*) in thoracic cavity (*thorax*) outside the lungs.
pulmonary edema: excessive fluid (*edema*) in the lungs (*pulmonary*).
pyothorax: pus (*pyo*) in thoracic cavity (*thorax*) between pleura.
sinusitis: inflammation (*itis*) of the paranasal sinuses.
tachypnea: rapid (*tachy*) breathing (*pnea*).

Diseases of the digestive system

The following terms relate to diseases of the digestive system and its accessory organs and includes signs and symptoms of disease:

anorexia: condition (*ia*) in which there is a loss of (*an*) desire for food.
borborygmus: rumbling or gurgling sounds made by movement of gas in the intestine.
cholecystitis: inflammation (*itis*) of the gallbladder (*cholecyst*).
choledocholithiasis: condition in which there are stones (*lithiasis*) in the bile (*chole*) ducts (*docho*).
cholelithiasis: condition in which there are bile (*chole*) stones (*lithiasis*) in the gallbladder; may also be in the duct.
cirrhosis: condition (*osis*) of the liver that causes a dark yellowish (*cirrh*) color.
diarrhea: condition in which the intestinal contents flow (*rrhea*) rapidly through (*dia*) the digestive system.
diverticulosis: condition (*osis*) in which a small (*cul*) tubular projection turns (*verti*) or grows out from (*di*, variation of *de*) the inside surface of the intestinal tract.
dysentery: disease or difficulty (*dys*) in the intestines (*enteron*).
dyspepsia: condition (*ia*) in which there is difficulty (*dys*) in digestion (*peps*).
dysphagia: difficulty (*dys*) in swallowing (*phagia*).
emesis: action in which the contents of the stomach are sent forth (*eme*, variation of *emit*), or vomited.
eructation: belching of air from the stomach; burping.
gastritis: inflammation (*itis*) of the stomach (*gastr*).
hematemesis: vomiting (*emesis*) of blood (*hemat*).
hepatitis: inflammation (*itis*) of the liver (*hepat*).
hernia: protrusion of an organ from its usual location.
- ***femoral hernia:*** organ passes through the femoral ring under the inguinal ligament.
- ***hiatal hernia:*** protrusion of the stomach into the thoracic cavity through an opening (*hiatal*) in the diaphragm.

inguinal hernia: hernia in the groin (*inguin*) above the inguinal ligament.
umbilical hernia: protrusion at the navel; also called ***omphalocele.***
incisional hernia: protrusion at the site of an earlier incision.
strangulated hernia: protruding part is squeezed to the point where circulation is cut off (*strangulated*).

intussusception: slipping (*susception*) of one section of the intestine into (*intus*) another section.
jaundice: condition in which skin takes on a yellow (*jaundice*) color caused by an excess of bile in the bloodstream; also called icterus (*yellow*).
malocclusion: condition in which teeth of the upper and lower jaws do not (*mal*) close (*occlusion*) together.
perforated viscus: condition in which a hole develops in (*perforate*) a hollow organ (*viscus*).
periodontal disease: disease in the area around (*peri*) the teeth (*dontal*).
proctitis: inflammation (*itis*) of the rectum (*proct*).
prolapse of the rectum: weakened walls of the rectum fall (*lapse*) outward (*pro*) or downward.
pruritus ani: excessive itchiness (*pruritis*) around the anus (*ani*).
pyorrhea: flowing (*rrhea*) of pus (*pyo*) from infected gums.
rectocele: outpouching (*cele*) of the rectum (*recto*).
steatorrhea: flow (*rrhea*) of undigested fat (*steato*) through the digestive system.
stomatitis: inflammation (*itis*) of the mouth (*stomat*).
tenesmus: straining (*tenesmus*) or feeling an urgent need to defecate, without success.
volvulus: small (*ulus*) twisting or turning (*volv*) of the intestine, creating an obstruction.

Diseases of the genitourinary system

The following terms relate to diseases of the urinary tract:

anuria: absence (*an*) of urine (*uria*).
cystitis: inflammation (*itis*) of the urinary bladder (*cyst*).
enuresis: involuntary (*en*, variation of *in*) passing of urine (*uresis*).
glomerulonephritis: inflammation (*itis*) of the glomeruli (*glomerulo*) of the kidneys (*nephr*).
glycosuria: sugar (*glycos*) in the urine (*uria*).
hematuria: blood (*hemat*) in the urine (*uria*).
hydroureter: overdistention of the ureter (*ureter*) from the backup of water (*hydro*), or urine.
incontinent: lack of (*in*) ability to contain (*continent*) or hold urine.
kidney agenesis: absence (*a*) of one or both kidneys at birth (*genesis*).
nephrolithiasis: stones (*lithiasis*) in the kidney (*nephro*); renal calculi.
nephroptosis: kidney (*nephr*) has dropped (*ptosis*) from its normal place; floating kidney.
neurogenic bladder: decreased functioning of the bladder caused by (*genic*) injury of the nerves (*neuro*) to the bladder muscle.
nocturia: frequent urination (*uria*) during the night (*noct*).
nocturnal enuresis: involuntary urination that occurs at night, bedwetting.
oliguria: scant or small amounts (*olig*) of urine (*uria*) are produced.
polyuria: urinating (*uria*) many times (*poly*).
polydipsia: excessive (*poly*) thirst (*dips*) that usually accompanies polyuria.

pyelonephritis: inflammation (*itis*) of the kidney (*nephr*) pelvis (*pyelo*).
uremia: urea normally found in urine (*ur*) is not filtered through the kidney and remains in the blood (*emia*).
ureteral colic: pain (*colic*) from a stone or blood clot in the ureter.
ureteritis: inflammation (*itis*) of the ureter.

The following terms relate to conditions and diseases of the male reproductive system:

anorchism: condition (*ism*) in which testes (*orch*) are absent (*an*).
balanitis: inflammation (*itis*) of the glans penis (*balan*).
cryptorchism: condition (*ism*) in which testes (*orchid*) remain in the pelvic cavity and thus are hidden (*crypt*); undescended testicles.
epididymoorchitis: inflammation (*itis*) of the epididymis and testes (*orch*).
eunuchoidism: condition (*ism*) in which the male develops characteristics like (*oid*) those of a eunuch; castrated male.
hydrocele: outpouching (*cele*) of testes caused by an accumulation of fluid (*hydro*).
hypogonadism: condition (*ism*) in which there is undersecretion (*hypo*) of the sex-related (*gonad*) hormones.
impotence: condition characterized by lack of (*im*, variation of *in*) sexual power (*potence*); male who is unable to experience an erection.
inguinal hernia: protrusion (*hernia*) of abdominal contents through the inguinal canal into the region of the scrotum above the inguinal ligament.
oligospermia: condition (*ia*) in which only a small amount (*oligo*) of sperm is produced.
orchitis: inflammation (*itis*) of the testes (*orch*).
paraphimosis: condition (*osis*) in which the foreskin is tightly constricted (*phim*) around (*para*) the penis behind the glans.
phallitis: inflammation (*itis*) of the penis (*phall*).
phimosis: condition (*osis*) in which the foreskin is tightly constricted (*phim*) and cannot be retracted over the glans.
spermatocele: condition characterized by bulging (*cele*) of the epididymis containing sperm (*spermato*).
varicocele: bulging (*cele*) due to swelling of the veins (*varico*) of the testes.

Conditions or diseases of the female reproductive system are divided into two categories: gynecological and obstetrical. Gynecological conditions are those that relate to the female reproductive system; the term gynecologic means: the study (*ologic*) of the female (*gynec*) reproductive system. Obstetrical conditions are those that relate to birth and pregnancy; the term obstetric means: woman (*tric*) who stands (*ste*) before (*obs*) another giving birth.

The following terms relate to conditions and diseases of the female reproductive system:

anovulation: ovulation does not (*an*) occur.
cervicitis: inflammation (*itis*) of the cervix (*cervic*).
cystocele: wall of the urinary bladder (*cyst*) protrudes (*cele*) or bulges into the vagina.
dyspareunia: situation (*ia*) in which a woman experiences pain (*dys*) during coitus with a partner (*pareun*).
endocervicitis: inflammation (*itis*) of the lining inside (*endo*) the cervix (*cervic*).
endometriosis: condition (*osis*) in which endometrial (*endometri*) tissue grows in the abdominal cavity in unusual locations, causing irritation.

fibromyoma: tumor (*oma*) consisting of uterine muscle (*myo*) and fiber (*fibro*).
kraurosis of the vulva: condition (*osis*) in which the external reproductive organs (*vulva*) become dry (*kraur*).
leukorrhea: flow (*rrhea*) of white (*leuko*) mucus from the vagina.
menstrual disorder:
amenorrhea: lack of (*a*) menstrual (*meno*) flow (*rrhea*).
dysmenorrhea: difficult (*dys*) or painful menstrual flow (*menorrhea*).
hypomenorrhea: menstrual flow (*menorrhea*) is decreased (*hypo*).
menorrhagia: menstrual (*meno*) flow (*rrhagia*) is excessive.
metrorrhagia: flow (*rrhagia*) of blood from the uterus (*metro*) at irregular intervals.
oligomenorrhea: menstrual flow (*menorrhea*) decreases in frequency; woman has fewer (*oligo*) menses.
postmenopausal bleeding: recurrence of bleeding after (*post*) menstrual cycles (*meno*) have ceased (*pausal*).
premenstrual: group of symptoms that occur before (*pre*) menses (*menstrual*) in which the person may feel a degree of discomfort and irritability (*PMS*).
prolapsed uterus: uterus slips (*lapse*) outward (*pro*) through the vagina.
rectocele: wall of the rectum (*recto*) protrudes (*cele*) or bulges into the vagina.
uterine retroflexion: uterus bends (*flexion*) backward (*retro*).
vaginismus: condition (*ismus*) characterized by painful spasms of the vagina (*vagin*).
vaginitis: inflammation (*itis*) of the vagina.
vulvitis: inflammation (*itis*) of the vulva (*vulv*).
vulvovaginitis: inflammation (*itis*) of the vulva (*vulvo*) and vagina (*vagin*).

Diseases of the endocrine glands

Diseases of the endocrine glands and subsequent symptoms are often interrelated. For example, a condition of the pituitary may also affect the thyroid, adrenal, and gonads. Since the hormones in the body are so delicately balanced, undersecretion or oversecretion of any hormones may cause abnormal conditions.

Terms relating to disease conditions of the endocrine system, including terms relating to signs and symptoms of endocrine diseases, are:

acromegaly: condition in which the ends (*acro*) of the extremities become enlarged (*megal*).
diabetes insipidus: disease in which large amounts of clear urine, without distinctive qualities (*insipid*), are passed (*betes*) through (*dia*) the kidneys.
diabetes mellitus: disease in which sugar (*mellitus*) passes (*betes*) through (*dia*) the urine.
exophthalmic goiter: type of goiter characterized by the protrusion of the eyes (*ophthalmic*) outward (*ex*).
goiter: enlargement of the throat (*goiter*) caused by enlargement of the thyroid gland.
hyperadrenocorticism: condition (*ism*) in which there is oversecretion (*hyper*) of hormones from the adrenal (*adreno*) cortex (*cortic*).
hyperthyroidism: condition (*ism*) in which there is oversecretion (*hyper*) of thyroid (*thyroid*) hormones.
hypothyroidism: condition (*ism*) in which there is undersecretion (*hypo*) of thyroid (*thyroid*) hormones.
myxedema: condition resulting from hypothyroidism in which there is swelling (*edema*) caused by mucus (*myx*) deposits in the skin.

pheochromocytoma: tumor, usually of the adrenal medulla, in which cells (*cyt*) become dusky (*pheo*) in color (*chroma*).

Diseases of the nervous system

Diseases of the nervous system affect almost every other system of the body. The muscular system, however, is the system most directly affected since it involves movement and muscular control. Terms relating to diseases involving the nervous system include:

amyotrophic lateral sclerosis: progressive atrophy (*a*) of muscles (*myo*) resulting from a condition (*osis*) characterized by hardening (*scler*) of nerve tissues on the sides (*lateral*) of the spinal cord.
cerebral aneurysm: sac (*aneurysm*) formed by dilation of a blood vessel in the cerebrum (*cerebral*).
cerebral palsy: form of paralysis (*palsy*) caused by cerebral (*cerebral*) defect.
cerebral vascular accident: sudden interference (*accident*) in brain function (*cerebral*) resulting from interruption of blood flow (*vascular*) in the brain; a stroke.
encephalitis: inflammation (*itis*) of the brain (*encephal*).
encephalopathy: general term meaning disease (*pathy*) in the brain (*encephalo*).
meningitis: inflammation (*itis*) of the meninges.
meningocele: protrusion (*cele*) of the meninges (*meningo*) through an opening in the skull or spinal column.
microcephalus: head (*cephalus*) is small (*micro*).
multiple sclerosis: condition (*osis*) caused by hardening (*scler*) of many (*multiple*) tissue patches in the central nervous system.
myotonic dystrophy: increased muscle (*myo*) tension (*tonic*) that causes wasting away (*dystrophy*).
narcolepsy: frequent and uncontrollable need for sleep; person is seized (*lepsy*) by sleep (*narco*).
neurofibroma: tumor (*oma*) of the connective tissue (*fibr*) of a nerve (*neuro*).
paralysis agitans: disease that produces rigid shaking tremors (*agitans*) that may lead to paralysis; Parkinson's disease.
sciatica: severe pain in the leg along the course of the sciatic (*sciatic*) nerve.
spina bifida: split (*bifida*) in the wall of the spine (*spina*) through which a part of the spinal cord protrudes.
subarachnoid hemorrhage: flow of blood (*hemorrhage*) into the subarachnoid space.
subdural hematoma: localized collection of blood (*hematoma*) in the subdural space.
transection of the cord: traumatic injury that cuts (*section*) across (*trans*) the spinal cord.
transient ischemic attacks: sudden (*attack*) decrease in blood supply (*ischemic*) to the brain that lasts only a short time (*transient*).

Diseases of the eye

The following terms relate to diseases or abnormal conditions of the eye:

amblyopia: dull (*ambly*) vision (*opia*); called lazy eye because it results in disuse (lazy) of the eye.
ametropia: general term denoting a refractive disorder.
anisometropia: focusing ability differs causing unequal (*aniso*) vision (*opia*).

anopia: condition (*ia*) in which there is no (*an*) vision (*op*); usually in only one eye.
aphakia: no (*a*) lens (*phakia*) in the eye.
arcus senilis: appearance of a ring (*arcus*) around the cornea found in elderly persons.
astigmatism: condition (*ism*) in which light rays do not (*a*) converge to a point (*stigmat*).
blepharitis: inflammation (*itis*) of the eyelid (*blephar*).
blepharoptosis: drooping (*ptosis*) eyelids (*blepharo*); usually shortened to ***ptosis***.
cataract: lens becomes opaque as if flooded (*cataract*) and the amount of light that passes through it is diminished.
conjunctivitis: inflammation (*itis*) of the membrane surrounding eye and lining the eyelid (*conjunctiv*).
corneal ulcers: sores (*ulcers*) on the cornea (*corneal*).
dacryoadenitis: inflammation (*itis*) of the tear (*dacryo*) gland (*aden*).
detached retina: retina is pulled (*tach*) away (*de*) from the choroid and is floating in the vitreous humor.
diplopia: condition (*ia*) in which there is double (*di*) vision (*op*).
ectropion: eyelid is turned (*tropion*) out (*ec*) and does not protect the eye.
enophthalmia: inward (*en*) or sunken-in condition (*ia*) of the eye (*ophthalm*).
epicanthus: vertical fold of skin covers over (*epi*) the inner angle (*canthus*) of the eye.
epiphora: excessive (*epi*) tearing of the eye.
episcleritis: inflammation (*itis*) of the tissue over (*epi*) the sclera (*scler*).
esotropia: cross-eyed; turning (*tropia*) in (*eso*) of the eyes.
exophthalmia: outward (*ex*) or protruding condition (*ia*) of the eye (*ophthalm*).
exotropia: turning (*tropia*) out (*exo*) of the eyes.
glaucoma: increase of pressure within the eye that causes swelling (*oma*) and nerve damage that appears gray (*glau*).
hemianopia: condition (*ia*) of loss (*an*) of vision (*op*) in one-half (*hemi*) of the visual field.
hyperopia: distance to focused images from the lens is greater (*hyper*) than the length of the eye (*opia*) so that the images are focused in back of the retina; far-sighted.
hypopyon: presence of pus (*pyo*) under (*hypo*) the cornea in the anterior chamber.
iridocyclitis: inflammation (*itis*) of the iris (*irido*) and the ciliary body (*cycl*).
iridodialysis: splitting (*lysis*) through (*dia*) of the iris (*irido*); circular rings of the iris (*irido*) broken or split (*lysis*) through (*dia*).
keratitis: inflammation (*itis*) of the cornea (*kerat*).
keratoconjunctivitis: inflammation (*itis*) of the cornea (*cerato*) and conjunctiva (*conjunctiv*).
mydriasis: dilated pupil.
myopia: condition in which the objects being viewed are focused in front of the retina; squinting (*my*) of the eye (*op*) to see distant objects; near-sighted.
myosis: small (*myo*) or constricted pupil.
nebula: faint, cloud-like (*nebula*) opacity of the cornea.
nyctalopia: condition (*ia*) in which there is blindness or poor (*al*) vision (*op*) at night (*nyct*); night blindness.
nystagmus: involuntary oscillation or swinging movement of the eyeball, usually from side to side.
optic neuritis: inflammation (*itis*) of the optic nerve (*neu*).
ophthalmoplegia: paralysis (*plegia*) of one or more muscles of the eye (*ophthalm*).

photophobia: intolerance or dread (*phobia*) of light.
presbyopia: refractive disorder of the eye (*opia*) associated with older (*presby*) persons.
proptosis: falling (*optosis*) forward (*pro*) of the eyeball; bulging eye.
pterygium: small (*ium*), wing-like (*pteryg*) fold of conjunctiva extending laterally from the inner corner of the eye.
retinitis: inflammation (*itis*) of the retina.
retinopathy: general term for diseases (*pathy*) of the retina (*retino*).
scotoma: loss of vision in part of the visual field; blind spot or dark spot (*scotoma*) is seen.
strabismus: vision disorder due to turning of the eyes so that neither is aimed in the same direction.
trachoma: disease in which rough (*trach*) swellings (*oma*) appear on the surface of the eye.
trichiasis: condition (*iasis*) in which the hairs (*trich*) of the eyelid grow inward.

Diseases of the ear

The following terms relate to diseases of the ear and include signs and symptoms of disease:

endolymphatic hydrops: condition characterized by an abnormal accumulation of fluid (*hydrops*) inside the membranous labyrinth (*endolymph*) of the inner ear; Meniere's disease.
eustachian salpingitis: inflammation (*itis*) of the tube (*salping*) from the middle ear to the nasopharynx (*eustachian*).
external otitis: inflammation (*itis*) of the external ear (*ot*).
impacted cerumen: condition in which wax (*cerumen*) is tightly packed (*impacted*) in the ear canal.
mastoiditis: inflammation (*itis*) of the mastoid process of the temporal bone.
myringitis: inflammation (*itis*) of the tympanic membrane.
otalgia: pain (*algia*) in the ear (*ot*).
otitis media: inflammation (*itis*) of the middle (*media*) ear (*ot*) chamber.
otorrhagia: bursting (*rrhagia*) of blood vessels in the ear (*oto*); bleeding from the ear.
otorrhea: discharge (*rrhea*) of fluid from the ear (*oto*).
otosclerosis: condition (*osis*) in which hard (*scler*) new bone develops around the oval window of the ear (*oto*).
preauricular node: presence of a lump (*node*) in front of (*pre*) the ear (*auricular*).
tinnitus: sensation of noises in the ear, including hissing, ringing, buzzing, thumping, whistling, and roaring.
vertigo: dizziness.

Terminology Trivia

Radiology

The x-ray was discovered by Roentgen (1845–1923) in 1895. It was first used in diagnosis of fractures, diseases, and the presence of foreign bodies. Later it was used in the study of internal organs, then as a treatment for cancer, and today has progressed to the technical sophistication of computerized axial tomography (*CAT*) scan. The *CAT* scan is used to simulate accurate cross-sectional views of the body.

Pronunciation and Meaning of New Terms

adenitis (ad″ ĕ ni′ tis) Inflammation of a gland.

adenocarcinoma (ad″ ĕ no kar″ sĭ no′ mah) Cancerous tumor of a gland.

angioma (an″ je o′ mah) Tumor of a vessel.

ankylosing spondylitis (ang′ kĭ lo sing spon″ dĭ li′ tis) Inflammation of the spine marked by stiffening of the spinal joints and ligaments, so that movement becomes increasingly painful and difficult. It is a form of rheumatoid arthritis that affects the spine, and affects males almost exclusively.

ankylosis (ang″ kĭ lo′ sis) A stiff condition.

arrhythmia (ah rith′ me ah) Irregularity of the pulse.

arteriopathy (ar″ te re op′ ah the) Any disease of the arteries.

arteriosclerosis (ar te″ re o sklĕ ro′ sis) Thickening and loss of elasticity of the walls of the arteries.

atherosclerosis (ath″ er o″ skle ro′ sis) A form of arteriosclerosis with fatty degeneration of the walls of the arteries.

auscultation (aws″ kul ta′ shun) Listening for sounds within the body, usually to ascertain the condition of the thoracic or abdominal viscera and to detect pregnancy.

blepharedema (blef″ ar e de′ mah) Swelling of the eyelids.

blepharitis (blef″ ah ri′ tis) Inflammation of the eyelid.

cachexia (kah kek′ se ah) A profound state of general ill health and malnutrition.
pituitary c., profound ill health due to hyposecretion of the pituitary gland.

carcinogen (kar sin′ o jen) Any substance that produces cancer.

carcinogenic (kar″ sĭ no jen′ ik) Pertaining to that which causes cancer.

carcinoma (kar″ sĭ no′ mah) A malignant tumor; cancerous tumor.
basal cell c., an epidermoid carcinoma common on the face in the elderly and having a low degree of malignancy.

colitis (ko li′ tis) Inflammation of the large intestine.

cervicitis (ser″ vĭ si′ tis) Inflammation of the cervix.

cervicocolpitis (ser″ vĭ ko kol pi′ tis) Inflammation of the cervix uteri and the vagina.

cheilitis (ki li′ tis) Inflammation of the lip.

curettage (ku″ rĕ tahzh′) Scraping of a cavity.

decubitus ulcer (de ku′ bĭ tus) A bedsore or ulceration due to prolonged pressure from lying too still in bed for too long a time.

diabetes mellitus (di″ ah be′ tēz mel′ it us) A disorder of carbohydrate metabolism that is characterized by hyperglycemia and glycosuria. The disorder is a result of inadequate production or utilization of insulin.

diaphoresis (di″ ah fo re′ sis) Sweating or perspiration, especially profuse perspiration.

dysuria (dis u′ re ah) Difficult or painful urination.

encephalitis (en″ sef ah li′ tis) Inflammation of the brain.

encephalomyelitis (en sef″ ah lo mi″ ĕ li′ tis) Inflammation involving both the brain and the spinal cord.

endocarditis (en″ do kar di′ tis) Inflammation of the inner lining of the heart.

endometriosis (en″ do me″ tre o′ sis) Ectopic endometrium located in various places, usually in the pelvic cavity.

expectorate (ek spek′ to rate) To cough up and spit out material from the lungs, bronchi, and trachea.

fibroma (fi bro′ mah) A tumor composed mainly of fibrous tissue.

gastroduodenitis (gas″ tro du od″ e ni′ tis) Inflammation of the stomach and duodenum.

hemangioma (hē man″ je o′ mah) A benign tumor composed of newly formed blood vessels.

hematocrit (he mat′ o krit) A laboratory test in which the red blood cells are separated from the plasma by centrifugation and the volume percentage of red cells in whole blood is determined.

hematoma (hem″ ah to′ mah) Any localized collection of blood, usually clotted, in an organ, tissue, or space.

hemorrhoid (hem′ o roid) A varicose dilation of a vein of the anal canal inside or just outside the rectum that causes pain, itching, and bleeding.

hemothorax (he″ mo tho′ raks) A collection of blood in the chest cavity.

impotence (im′ po tense) Inability to copulate.

infarction (in fark′ shun) The formation of a localized area of necrosis due to insufficient blood supply, produced by an occlusion.

laryngitis (lar″ in ji′ tis) Inflammation of the voice box.

laryngotracheitis (lah ring″ go tra″ ke i′ tis) Inflammation of the larynx and the trachea.

lymphadenitis (lim fad″ e ni′ tis) Inflammation of a lymph node.

lymphadenoma (lim fad e no′ mah) A tumor of a lymph node.

lymphangitis (lim″ fan ji′ tis) Inflammation of a lymphatic vessel.

malignant (mah lig′ nant) Tending to grow worse and threatening to produce death.

megalogastria (meg″ ah lo gas′ tre ah) Enlargement or abnormally large size of the stomach; gastric hypertrophy.

midsagittal (mid saj′ i tal) The plane vertically dividing the body through the midline into right and left halves.

mycodermatitis (mi″ ko der″ mah ti′ tis) Inflammation of the skin due to a fungus.

mycosis (mi ko′ sis) Any condition due to fungi.

myelencephalitis (mi″ e len sef″ ah li′ tis) Inflammation of the brain and spinal cord; myeloencephalitis.

myeloma (mi e lo′ mah) A tumor made up of cells normally found in the bone marrow.

multiple m., a neoplastic disease characterized by infiltration of the bone and bone marrow by multiple tumor masses.

myocarditis (mi″ o kar di′ tis) Inflammation of the heart muscle.

narcolepsy (nar′ ko lep″ se) Sudden attacks of sleep occurring at intervals.

nasopharyngitis (nä zo far″ in ji′ tis) Inflammation of the nasopharnyx.

nephritis (nĕ fri′ tis) Inflammation of the kidney.

neuroma (nu ro′ mah) A tumor made up of nerve cells and nerve fibers.

nephrolith (nef′ ro lith) A kidney stone.

oophorosalpingitis (o of″ o ro sal″ pin ji′ tis) Inflammation of an ovary and uterine tube.

ophthalmitis (of″ thal mi′ tis) Inflammation of the eye.

ophthalmodynia (of thal″ mo din′ e ah) Pain in the eye.

orchiopathy (or″ ke op′ ah the) Any disease of the testes.

orchiditis (or″ kĭ di′ tis) Inflammation of a testicle.

osteoarthritis (os″ te o ar thri′ tis) Degenerative joint disease characterized by degeneration of the articular cartilage, hypertrophy of bone at the margins, and changes in the synovial membrane.

osteochondritis (os″ te o kon dri′ tis) Inflammation of the bone and cartilage.

osteomalacia (os″ te o mah la′ she ah) A skeletal disorder characterized by a disturbance in bone metabolism; softening of the bone.

osteogenesis (os″ te o jen′ e sis) The formation of bone.

otitis (o ti′ tis) Inflammation of the ear.
o. media, inflammation of the middle ear.

pancreatitis (pan″ kre ah ti′ tis) Inflammation of the pancreas.

pathogenic (path o jen′ ik) Disease-causing.

periadenitis (per″ e ad″ e ni′ tis) Inflammation of tissues around a gland.

pericolitis (per″ i ko li′ tis) Inflammation around the large intestine.

pharyngitis (far″ in ji′ tis) Inflammation of the throat.

phrenitis (frĕ ni′ tis) Inflammation of the diaphragm.

pneumonia (nu mo′ ne ah) Inflammation of the lung.

pneumothorax (nu″ mo tho′ raks) Air or gas in the pleural space that may occur spontaneously (*spontaneous p.*) or as a result of trauma or disease process, or may be introduced deliberately (*artificial p.*).

prognosis (prog no′ sis) Prediction of the probable outcome of a disease.

prophylaxis (pro″ fi lak′ sis) Protection against disease.

pyelitis (pi″ ĕ li′ tis) Inflammation of the renal pelvis.

pyuria (pi u′ re ah) The presence of pus in the urine.

salpingitis (sal″ pin ji′ tis) Inflammation of a uterine tube.

sarcoma (sar ko′ mah) A tumor composed of substance like the embryonic connective tissue, and often highly malignant.

sclerosis (skle ro′ sis) Hardening, applied chiefly to hardening of the nervous system or to hardening of the blood vessels.

scoliosis (sko″ le o′ sis) Lateral curvature of the vertebral column.

septicemia (sep″ tĭ se′ me ah) A morbid condition due to the presence of bacteria and their toxins in the blood.

spondylarthritis (spon″ dil ar thri′ tis) Inflammation of joints between the vertebrae.

spondylitis (spon″ dĭ li′ tis) Inflammation of a vertebra.
ankylosing s., rheumatoid arthritis with stiffening of the spinal joints and ligaments.

thrombophlebitis (throm′ bo fle bi′ tis) Inflammation of a vein due to a blood clot.

toxemia (tok se′ me ah) A general intoxication due to absorption of bacterial toxins; a group of pathological conditions, essentially metabolic disturbances, occurring in pregnant women.

ureteropyelitis (u re″ ter o pi ĕ li′ tis) Inflammation of a ureter and renal pelvis.

urethritis (u″ rĕ thri′ tis) Inflammation of the urethra.

urethrocystitis (u re″ thro sis ti′ tis) Inflammation of the urethra and the bladder.

vaginitis (vaj″ ĭ ni′ tis) Inflammation of the vagina.

ventriculitis (ven trik″ u li′ tis) Inflammation of a ventricle, especially a cerebral ventricle.

xeroderma (ze″ ro der′ mah) A disease characterized by rough, dry skin.

xerophthalmia (ze″ rof thal′ me ah) An eye disease characterized by an abnormally dry condition of the eyeball.

Self-test

1. The term physical refers to the exam**. The physical exam includes the following:**

a. inspection
b. palpation
c. auscultation
d. percussion
e. ~~vital signs~~ measurements

2. Vital signs include the following signs:

a. T
b. P
c. RR
d. BP

3. For each set, match Column A with Column B.

Column A

___ acute
___ anomaly
___ benign
___ chronic
___ diagnosis
___ malignant
___ metastatic
___ prognosis
___ sign
___ syndrome
___ systemic
___ atrophy

Column B

a. to know beforehand
b. favorable for recovery; a mild disease
c. sufficient knowledge of a disease to distinguish it from another
d. signs and symptoms that usually occur together
e. irregular; deviation from normal
f. sudden condition
g. becoming progressively worse
h. involves the whole body
i. condition that lasts a long time
j. observable, measureable occurrence
k. disease that spreads from one place to another
l. wasting away of an organ or part; without growth

4.

Column A

___ endemic
___ epidemic
___ pandemic
___ iatrogenic
___ idiopathic

Column B

a. disease of unknown cause
b. constantly present disease occurring in a particular group of people
c. disease that is the side effect of treatment prescribed by physician
d. spread over a large group of people in a particular area
e. widespread epidemic disease

5.

Column A

___ benign
___ M0
___ oncology
___ Grade I tumor
___ T3
___ Grade IV tumor
___ neoplastic
___ carcinosis
___ malignant

Column B

a. tumor advanced in size and involvement
b. mild
c. advanced metastatic disease
d. highly altered, difficult to recognize parent tissues
e. a disease in which new cells are formed
f. metastasis not evident
g. tumors resembling parent tissues
h. progressively worsening condition
i. study of tumors

6.

Column A

____ tendonitis
____ osteoclasia
____ fibromyositis
____ angioma
____ contusion
____ exostosis
____ spondylitis
____ furuncle
____ osteoma
____ eschar
____ abrasion
____ icterus
____ nevus
____ petechia
____ tinea

Column B

a. a bony protuberance
b. inflammation of the spine
c. inflammation of a tendon
d. tumor of blood vessels that appears on skin
e. hard crust or scab
f. skin boil
g. bone tumor
h. jaundice
i. skin scraped away
j. mark on the skin; moles and some birthmarks
k. tissue damage beneath skin with skin unbroken
l. surgical fracture to remedy a deformity
m. inflammation of muscle and fibrous tissue
n. ringworm
o. small hemorrhage under skin that forms a small spot

7.

Column A

____ myocardial ischemia
____ shock
____ anoxia
____ cardiomyopathy
____ leukemia
____ lymphoma
____ apnea
____ dyspnea
____ hemorrhoid
____ orthopnea
____ proctitis
____ eructation
____ hernia
____ dyscrasia
____ thrombophlebitis

Column B

a. disease of the heart muscle
b. anal varicose vein
c. decrease in the blood supply to the heart muscle
d. inadequate tissue perfusion
e. inflammation of a vein forming a blood clot
f. deficiency of oxygen in blood
g. defective or abnormal mixtures of blood elements
h. abnormally high numbers of white blood cells
i. absence of breathing
j. inflammation of the rectum
k. burping
l. breathing is easier when standing
m. protrusion of an organ from its original position
n. difficulty in breathing
o. tumor of lymph nodes

8.

Column A

____ cystitis
____ anorchism
____ varicocele
____ dyspareunia
____ vaginismus
____ myxedema
____ encephalitis
____ sciatica
____ otitis media
____ enuresis
____ oligouria
____ nebula
____ diplopia
____ menorrhagia
____ hydrocele

Column B

a. involuntary passing of urine
b. inflammation of the urinary bladder
c. passing small amounts of urine
d. accumulation of fluid causing extension of testes
e. excessive menstrual flow
f. painful vaginal spasms
g. varicose veins of the testes
h. inflammation of the brain
i. double vision
j. absence of testes
k. cloud-like opacity of the cornea
l. inflammation of the middle ear
m. severe pain in the leg
n. swelling caused by mucus deposits in the skin
o. painful intercourse in women

Seventeen
Pharmacology

It is an almost universal belief that certain chemical substances have the power to heal, cure, and promote well-being. When a drug (a chemical substance) is believed to be effective, but that belief has not yet been proven or disproven, the belief can be called a theory. Science was born when people began to test theory by experiment and observation; a process called empirical research.

Belief confirmed by empirical evidence is called knowledge; belief contradicted by empirical evidence is called superstition. We judge knowledge to be more valid than superstition, but belief in the curative powers of certain medicines covers a wide range and may or may not be justified. To determine the validity or danger of drugs is the charge and challenge of pharmacology.

Pharmacology is the field of medicine that studies drugs—their natures, origins, and effects on the body. It is a broad medical specialty that contains many subdivisions, including:

Chemotherapy—the study of drugs used in treatment of disease.
Medicinal chemistry—the study of new drug synthesis and the relationship between chemical structure and biological effects.
Molecular pharmacology—the study of the interaction of drugs with cells or subcellular entities. This field works toward revealing the mechanisms of drug actions.
Pharmacodynamics—the study of the ways in which drugs are absorbed, metabolized, and excreted by the body.
Pharmacokinetics—the measurement of drug concentrations in tissues and blood over a period of time.
Toxicology—the study of harmful chemicals and their effects on the body. It includes the search for antidotes to harmful effects; antidotes are given to neutralize or reverse unwanted effects.

Drugs are chemical substances used in the treatment or prevention of diseases. While it is recognized that drugs are used in ways outside this definition, this book restricts its discussion of drugs to those associated with legal medical use.

Most drugs that were used in early societies were derived from plants. They were either prepared as teas, swallowed, inserted, applied, inhaled, or administered in any other way possible. Many drugs were initially tried because of some inherent characteristic, such as color, shape, or source (sometimes superstitious); only later was it discovered that they indeed worked. Whether the cause and effect relationship of the drugs was real or psychological, belief in them was established. Many substances were found to be effective only through trial and error. Other substances, though ineffective, continued to be used because of the beliefs associated with them.

Many early drugs have survived the scrutiny of modern science. Quinine, for example, was found to have the actual medicinal properties assigned to it by primitive medicine. Belladonna was originally used to enlarge the pupils of the eyes because at one time people believed larger pupils were cosmetically attractive. A modified form of this drug is used today to enlarge pupils so eyes can be examined with an ophthalmoscope. The foxglove plant was originally boiled as a tea and consumed to treat chest pain. It is from this plant that the drug digitalis, used to treat heart disorders, is extracted today.

Animals provide another source of drugs in the form of hormones and glandular secretions. Prednisone and methotrexate, anticancer drugs, are examples of synthesized substances, another source of medicinal drugs.

Drugs are grouped into three main categories:

1. *Nonprescription* drugs, which may be sold "over the counter" since they are judged safe for use without medical supervision.
2. *Prescription* drugs, which are considered unsafe for use except under supervision and are, therefore, dispensed only by order of practitioners licensed by law to administer them; *i.e.,* physicians, veterinarians, and dentists.
3. *Illegal* drugs, which have no medical use and are banned by the FDA (Food & Drug Administration) for the public's protection.

Drugs may also be classified *generically* to signify a chemical relationship among a group of drugs; such as sulfonamides, local anesthetics, sedatives, and so forth. Generic classification focuses attention on the pharmacologic similarities among the members of a class as a whole. Usually, attention is directed within the group to one or two drugs chosen as representatives of the entire class. Procaine, for example, is commonly used to represent drugs classified as local anesthetics.

Problems in drug terminology arise when naming individual therapeutic agents. Not only is there an overwhelming number of agents available for use, but each of these agents has at least three names. Every drug has a chemical name, a nonproprietary (generic) name, and a trade name.

The chemical name of a drug is a precise description of its chemical constitution and indicates its arrangement of atoms or atomic groups. For example, one of the most popular drugs used for the treatment of anxiety is *7–chloro–2–methylamino–5–phenyl–3H–1,4–oxide*. Although descriptive, it is a little too unwieldy for most people to use. Chemical names are rarely used except for the simplest compounds, such as sodium bicarbonate.

The nonproprietary or generic name is the name assigned to a drug when it is found to be of demonstrated or potential therapeutic usefulness. This name usually becomes the legal name of the drug when it is finally admitted to an official compendia, such as The United States Pharmacopeia or The National Formulary.

The generic names selected for many drugs often defeat the purpose for which they were originally established. These names are usually too long, difficult to pronounce or spell, and hard to remember. For example, chlordiazepoxide is the generic name given to the drug mentioned earlier (by its unwieldy chemical name) for the treatment of anxiety. The trade name selected by the manufacturer is Librium. The trade name is usually shorter, more euphonious, and may be associated with the condition it is intended to treat. As a result, the trade name is the one usually remembered and used.

Confusion concerning trade names arises from the fact that a single drug will have as many trade names as there are drug manufacturers producing it. Unlike the single generic or official name, which is public property, the trade name is registered and its use restricted to the owner of the copyright. Even when a drug is new and is protected by a patent, it may be licensed for use by a number of companies; it will then appear under a variety of trade names. Patents expire after seventeen years and then a single agent may be marketed under a whole new set of trade names. A useful drug that has no successors may have as many as twenty trade names.

Drug Groups

The nation's basic drug law divides drugs into two legal categories: over-the counter (*OTC*) drugs and prescription drugs.

Over-The-Counter Drugs

Over-the-counter drugs are those that can be used safely without medical supervision, if the directions on the labels are followed. These drugs are not curative, but rather may provide relief or alleviate symptoms. Some examples of *OTC* drugs are analgesics; antacids; antidiarrheals; antihistamines (some mild ones); cough preparations; decongestants; emetics; and hypnotics.

These drugs can be purchased without a prescription unless they are combined with restricted drugs to produce synergistic (enhanced) effects. For example, if a cough medicine contains codeine (a narcotic) it is considered a different product and is classified as a prescription drug.

Prescription Drugs

There are many types of prescription drugs. The following is a summary of some of the more common prescription drug groups, some examples of drugs contained within these groups, and their medical uses:

Neuropharmacologic drugs

Neuropharmacologic drugs are those that act on the body's nervous system. There are two types of these drugs—*autonomic* drugs and *central nervous system* drugs. The autonomic drugs are given this name because they influence the body in ways similar to the autonomic nervous system. Drug groups that fall within the autonomic nervous system category are:

sympathomimetics (sym/path/o/mimet/ics)—These drugs work like adrenalin to increase both heart rate and blood pressure. An example of a sympathomimetic drug is *epinephrine*, used to treat allergies, shock, cardiovascular failure, and respiratory failure.

sympatholytics (sym/path/o/lytics)—These drugs are antagonistic to the sympathomimetics because they lower both heart rate and blood pressure. Some examples of sympatholytic drugs are *methyldopa, reserpine*, and *trimethaphan*, all used either to lower blood pressure or to depress the central nervous system.

parasympathomimetics (para/sym/path/o/mimet/ics)—These drugs mimic the action of the neurotransmitter, acetylcholine, produced by the parasympathetic nerves. Some examples of parasympathomimetic drugs are *bethanechol* and *pilocarpine,* used either to decrease heart rate, to contract smooth muscles or pupils of the eyes, or to increase excretions.

parasympatholytics (para/sym/path/o/lytics)—These drugs block the passage of impulses that move through the parasympathetic nerves. They dilate pupils, relax smooth muscles, and increase heart rate. Some examples of parasympatholytic drugs are *atropine, belladonna,* and *scopolamine,* used either to dilate pupils for ophthalmoscopic evaluations, to treat gastrointestinal diseases, or to treat enuresis.

The central nervous system drugs are so named because they influence the body in ways similar to the central nervous system. Drug groups that fall within the central nervous system category are:

stimulants—As the name implies, these drugs stimulate the metabolic processes. They increase alertness and decrease hyperactive behaviors. Some examples of stimulants are *amphetamines, diethylpropion hydrochloride,* and *phendimetrazine tartrate,* used either as an aid in control of appetite, as a preventative from narcolepsy, or as a diuretic.

depressants—Depressants depress the central nervous system and range in effects from mild sedation to general anesthesia. Included within this group are analgesics, sedatives and hypnotics, anticonvulsants or antispasmotics, traquilizers, and anesthetics. There are two groups of analgesics: narcotic and nonnarcotic analgesics. Examples of narcotic analgesics are *codeine, meperidine, morphine,* and *methadone*, all used to raise the threshold of pain and help suppress anxiety. Some nonnarcotic analgesics include *methotrimeprazine, pentazocine, propoxyphene,* and *darvon*. These drugs have the same uses as narcotic analgesics. The sedative-hypnotic group of drugs are commonly known as barbituates. Some examples of these drugs are *phenobarbital, pentobarbital, thiamylal,* and *secobarbital.* These drugs have a relaxing, calming effect on the body. Anticonvulsant drugs are used to treat epilepsy or brain lesions without affecting brain function; an example is *phenytoin* (or *dilantin*). Drugs of the tranquilizer group may be minor or major drugs. Minor tranquilizers include *chlordiazepoxide, meprobamate,* and *hydroxyzine*, and are used to treat neuroses, psychosomatic disorders, anxiety, and tension; major tranquilizers include *chlorpromazine, thioridazine, haloperidol,* and *rauwolfia*. The major tranquilizers are used to treat severely disturbed patients who have hallucinations and delusions. Anesthetics produce a loss of sensation, both general and local; drugs in this group include *procaine, lidocaine,* and *ether*. The neuropharmacologic drugs and their divisions are shown in Figure 17–1.

Antihistamines

The body responds to antigens (foreign proteins) by producing histamines. These cause allergic reactions such as hives, asthma, and anaphylactic shock. Antihistamines, such as *diphenhydramine* (*benadryl*) and *chlorpheniramine*, are used for relief of these allergy symptoms.

Adrenocorticosteriods

This group of drugs affects the kidneys and immune system of the body. They have the ability to reduce inflammation. Drugs in this group include *hydrocortisone, methylprednisolone,* and *prednisolone*, used to treat gout, bursitis, and connective tissue trauma.

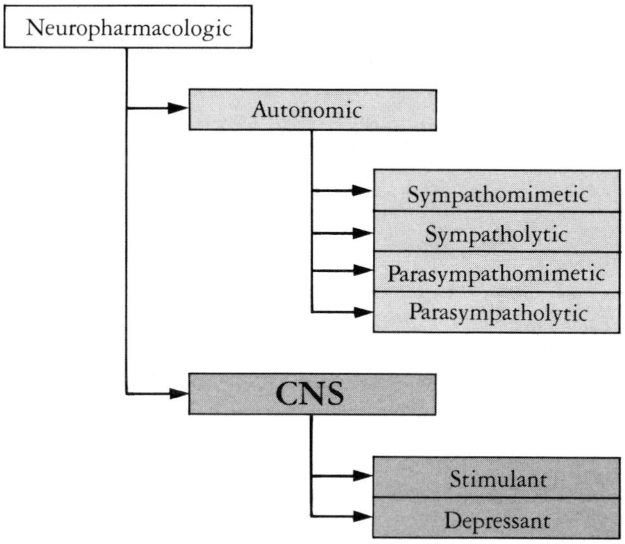

Figure 17–1 The neuropharmacologic drugs and their divisions.

Cardiovascular drugs

This group of drugs acts on the heart and affects blood pressure and blood clotting. It includes antianemics, antilepemias, antiarrhythmics, digitalis, anticoagulants, and diuretics. Major groupings of the cardiovascular drugs are shown in Figure 17–2.

antianemics (anti/anem/ics)—These drugs aid in the synthesis of hemoglobin and in the formation of red blood cells. Some examples of antianemic drugs include *ferrocholinate, ferrous sulphate,* and *polyferose.*

antilipemics (anti/lip/emics)—These drugs are used to decrease cholesterol and triglyceride levels in the blood. Some examples of antilipemic drugs include *cholestyramine, clofibrate,* and *estrogens.*

antiarrhythmics (anti/a/rrhythm/ics)—These drugs are used to prevent or eliminate abnormal heart contractions or rhythms. Some examples of antiarrhythmic drugs include *diphenylhydantoin sodium, quinidine sulfate,* and *procainamide hydrochloride.*

digitalis (digit/al/is)—These drugs are used to treat congestive heart failure and other heart disorders indicated by irregular rhythms. Some examples of drugs in this group include *digitalis, digotoxin,* and *digoxin.*

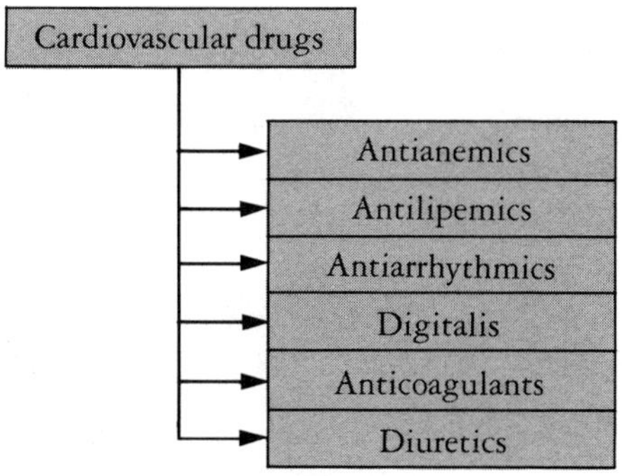

Figure 17–2 The major groupings of the cardiovascular drugs.

anticoagulants (anti/coagul/ants)—These drugs are used to prevent the formation of blood clots. Some examples of anticoagulants include *acenocoumarol, heparin sodium,* and *warfarin sodium.*

diuretics (di/uret/ics)—These drugs are used to prevent or relieve high blood pressure. Some examples of diuretics include *hydrochlorothiazide, mannitol,* and *spironolactone.*

Antibiotics

Antibiotics either stop the growth (biostatic) of or destroy (biocidal) micro-organisms. The antibiotics include penicillin, sulfonamides, streptomycin, and tetracycline; these are shown in Figure 17–3.

penicillin (pen/i/cillin)—These drugs are used to treat infections through bacteriocidal action. Some examples of penicillin include *ampicillin, penicillin G,* and *penicillin V.*

sulfonamides (sulf/on/amides)—These drugs are used to combat urinary tract infections through bacteriostatic action. Some examples of sulfonamides include *sulfa-methoxazole* and *sulfisoxazole.*

streptomycins (strep/to/mycins)—These drugs are used to treat conditions caused by gram-positive and acid-fact bacteria. Some examples of streptomycins include *gentamicin* and *kanamycin.*

tetracyclines (tetra/cyclines)—These drugs are used to inhibit growth of a wide variety of microorganisms through bacteriostatic action. Examples of tetra-cyclines are *tetracycline, chlortetracycline,* and *oxytetracycline.*

Gastrointestinal drugs

These drugs are used as palliative treatment for potentially dangerous symptoms. They include antidiarrheals, antinauseants, cathartics, and emetics, as shown in Figure 17–4.

antidiarrheals (anti/diarrhea/ls)—These drugs are used to relieve diarrhea and to decrease the rapid movement of the bowels. Some examples of antidiarrheals include *kaopectate* and *lomotil.*

antinauseants (anti/nausea/nts)—These drugs are used to relieve nausea and vomiting and to overcome motion sickness. Some examples of antinauseants include *antivert, compazine,* and *dramamine.*

cathartics (cath/ar/tics)—These drugs are used to relieve constipation and to promote defecation. Some examples of cathartics include laxatives and purgatives such as *castor oil* and *cascara sagrada.*

emetics (emet/ics)—These drugs are used to chemically induce vomiting. Examples of emetics are *ipecac, sodium chloride,* and *apomorphine.*

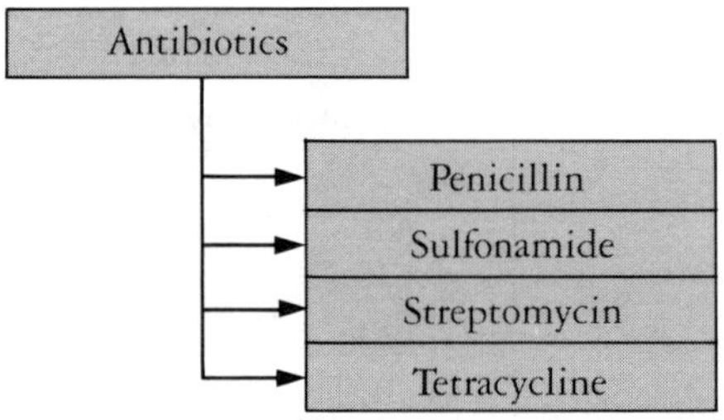

Figure 17–3 The antibiotic drugs.

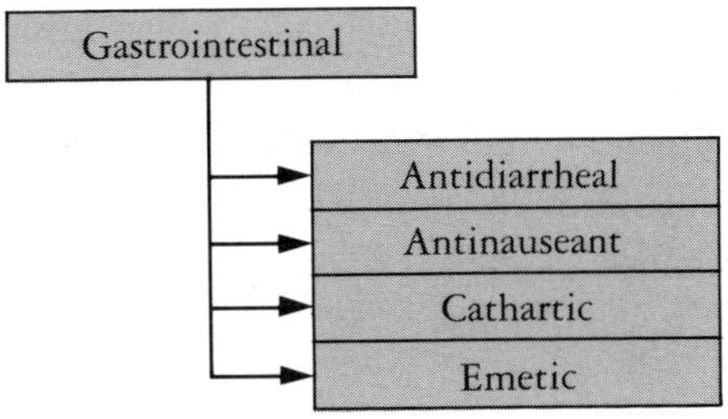

Figure 17–4 The gastrointestinal drugs.

Antineoplastic drugs

These anticancer drugs are used to treat advanced cases that cannot be controlled through either surgery or radiation. Some examples of antineoplastic drugs include *cyclophosphamide, dactinomycin,* and *methotrexate*, all used to suppress the growth and spread of malignant cells.

Drug Treatments and Functions

Drugs serve a wide variety of purposes. Earlier in this chapter, it was explained that primitive societies used drugs for curative purposes. While this still holds true today, the role of drugs in medicine is far greater than simply curative. The following is a list of the uses to which drugs are applied in modern medical care:

1. ***Curative Use:*** Drugs that exert curative actions are chemotherapeutic agents directed toward the treatment of diseases. Due mainly to the use of these drugs, communicable diseases are no longer the threat they once were in the past. Bacterial septicemias, tuberculosis, and meningitis, once considered wide-spread threats, are now easily and routinely cured.
2. ***Corrective Use:*** With corrective treatment, drugs act directly on the body to help correct physiological or biochemical abnormalities. They are not capable of curing diseases, but can terminate or reverse biological processes. Corrective drugs include general and local anesthetics, hypnotics, anticonvulsants, antipsychotics, antidepressants, antihistamines, antihypertensives, diuretics, anti-inflammatories, and neuromuscular blocking agents. The prefix *anti-* means against (the pathological process).
3. ***Palliative Use:*** With palliative treatment, drugs are used to treat symptoms. They contribute to the comfort of patients without curing biochemical or physiological abnormalities. Palliative treatment may be seen as inadequate when compared with curative action, but this type often makes a major contribution to a patient's recovery. Some palliative drugs are used for relief of minor pain and discomfort, while others block pain caused by major problems such as burns and cancers.
4. ***Substitutive Use:*** Substitutive drugs are used for treatment of diseases associated with deficiencies, many of which are endocrine- or hormone-related. For example, hypothyroid patients can be treated with thyroid extract or synthetic thyroid hormones. Similarly, patients with adrenal insufficiency can receive synthetic corticosteroids.
5. ***Prophylactic (Preventive) Use:*** Prophylactic action is taken to prevent the occurrence of disease. The best-known drugs in this category are those biological

preparations specifically used to counter communicable disease; vaccines and immunizations, for example. The use of penicillin as a treatment to prevent recurrence of strep throat and subsequent rheumatic heart disease is a good example of the prophylactic role of an antibiotic.

6. ***Restorative Use:*** Restoratives are drugs used to help the body return to a normal state. These drugs are used during convalescence to aid in the reconstructive process and to reduce the chances of relapse. Vitamins and electrolytes are examples of restorative treatments.
7. ***Supportive Use:*** Supportive treatment is used to sustain patients until other measures can be instituted to either cure or alleviate their conditions. Tranquilizers, vitamins, and antibiotics are examples of supportive treatments. The body's normal recuperative powers will overcome most illnesses, but these agents enable it to do so more efficiently and effectively.
8. ***Diagnostic Use:*** Diagnostic use of drugs is not itself a treatment, but it is included here because it provides a function that otherwise would not be acknowledged. Drugs used as aids in determining causation of symptoms are known as diagnostics. They not only help physicians determine reasons for patients' illnesses, but also help locate affected areas. For example, swallowing an inert substance, such as barium sulfate, will reveal abnormalities in the digestive tract because this substance can be observed by roentgenograms (x-ray).

Drug Actions

Drug actions occur after drugs have entered the bloodstream. The words used to describe this phenomena include:

synergistic action (potentiation)—The term synergistic action means that combining certain drugs can cause an effect greater than the sum total of the individual effects of each drug. For example, aspirin and caffeine combined are more effective than aspirin by itself. This relationship also holds true in producing a toxic effect; the common example of toxicity is the combination of alcohol and barbituates.

tolerance—The term tolerance means that drug doses of increasing amounts must be given to produce the same effect. The progressive escalation of addictive drugs serves as a good example. Ironically, aspirin does not have a tolerance effect even though many people escalate their dose levels based on the magnitude and frequency of discomfort.

cumulation—The term cumulation means that the concentration of drugs increases in body tissues with each successive dose. Successive doses of a drug may be given to enhance a certain systemic level necessary to produce a desired effect; an example of this type of therapy is found in digitalis administration.

additive—The term additive means that the effects of two similar drugs are equal to the sum of the effects of each. Two drugs may be administered at low levels to reduce unpleasant side effects obtained with a higher dosage of only one drug. If the drugs were synergistic in action, the effects of combining them would be greater than the sum total and would produce the wanted result.

Toxicity

Toxicity refers to the potentially harmful qualities inherent in drugs. Thus, by definition, all drugs have toxic qualities. Side effect is the term used for those toxic reactions that occur with drug use; these may range from unnoticeable effects to very pronounced effects, such as shock and even death. Most usually, however, side effects occur with even normal therapeutic dosage and are tolerable. If the side effects are not tolerable, an alternate drug is sought and, if one is not available, the discomfort produced by side effects must be weighed against the problem the drug is intended to treat. For example, if aspirin causes gastrointestinal distress for a patient, buffered aspirin or discontinuation of aspirin treatment would be considered. If a chemotherapeutic drug is used in cancer treatment and there is no alternate treatment available, the patient may have to tolerate nausea, vomiting, and alopecia; relatively mild discomforts weighed against the alternative of progressive disease.

Contraindications are characteristics of drug takers that may pose some degree of danger if consuming particular drugs; taking these drugs would be ill advised for these people. For example, women with histories of cardiovascular problems should not take oral contraceptives. In this case, use of oral contraceptives is contraindicated for patients having cardiovascular conditions.

Iatrogenic disorders are those caused by the treatment itself. Idiopathic disorders are those that are of unknown causation and are peculiar to one person.

Methods of Drug Administration

The ways in which drugs are administered determine their rate and degree of absorption into the bloodstream, as well as the speed and duration of their action. These factors are critical in determining a drug's effectiveness, so drugs are manufactured in forms that facilitate the most effective and desirable action. But, due to the variability both in people and in medications, drugs may be manufactured in more than one form. Tablets or capsules, injections, and suppositories imply different routes of entry into the body and separate methods of administration.

Some drugs may be administered orally. Drugs given by mouth are absorbed into the bloodstream through the intestinal wall. This method, though convenient, has a disadvantage in that the drug may be altered or destroyed by digestive fluids. There is also the risk that it may not be accepted by the stomach (causing vomiting) and that it may not be absorbed through the intestinal mucosa.

Drugs may also be administered sublingually. With this method, the drug is placed under the tongue and is allowed to dissolve in the saliva. Absorption is rapid for agents such as nitroglycerin tablets used to treat angina pain.

Some medications are administered rectally. Suppositories and aqueous solutions are examples of substances inserted into the rectum. Drugs may be given rectally when oral administration is difficult or undesirable, as when nausea or vomiting is present.

Other medications are administered parenterally. Injections may be given under the skin, in a muscle, in a vein, or in a body cavity. Obviously, this is the most rapid method of introducing a drug into the bloodstream, but it is also the most dangerous. While the other methods allow the body to reject a drug before it reaches toxic levels, this method does not.

There are also some drugs that may be administered through inhalation. Gases and aerosols (drugs suspended in air and compressed) are absorbed into the bloodstream thorugh the thin walls of air sacs found in the lungs.

Selected Drug Terms

The following terms are used to describe the drug groups and categories:

adenocorticosteroid: hormone (*steroid*) derived from the adrenal (*aden-*) cortex (*corti*).
analgesic: medication to relieve, or be without (*an*), pain (*algia*).
anesthesia: condition (*ia*) in which a person is without (*an*) feeling (*esthes*).
anorectic: appetite suppressant; without (*an*) mouth (*or*).
antianemic: against (*anti*) being without (*an*) blood (*hemia*).
antiarrhythmic: against (*anti*) a condition (*ic*) that causes a person to be without (*a*) rhythmical (*rhythm*) heartbeat.
antibiotic: against (*anti*) living forms (*bio*) of microorganisms.
anticoagulant: against (*anti*) clotting (*coagulation*).
anticonvulsant: against (*anti*) convulsions (*convulsions*).
antidiarrheal: against (*anti*) flowing (*rrhea*) through (*dia*).
antihistamine: against (*anti*) the action of histamines (*histamine*).
antilipemic: against (*anti*) fat (*lip*) in the bloodstream.
antinauseant: against (*anti*) nausea (*nausea*).
antineoplastic: against (*anti*) new (*neo*) growth (*plastic*), such as tumors.
cathartic: purification (*catharsis*) by purging.
diuretic: passing urine (*ure*) through (*dia*).
emetic: to cause vomiting (*emesis*).
narcotic: capable of causing sleep (*narco*).
parasympatholytic: chemicals produced by breaking up (*lysis*) those produced by parasympathetic nerves.
parasympathomimetic: mimicking (*mime*) the action of the parasympathetic (*parasympatho*) nerves.
sympatholytic: chemicals produced by breaking up (*lysis*) those produced by the sympathetic (*sympatho*) nerves.
sympathomimetic: mimicking (*mime*) the action of the sympathetic (*sympatho*) nerves.

The following terms relate to drugs that affect the nervous system:

analeptic: drug that acts as a stimulant, such as caffeine and amphetamines, takes away (*an*) sleep (*lep*).
analgesic: drug that takes away (*an*) pain (*alges*).
anticonvulsant: drug that works against (*anti*) convulsions (*convuls*).
antiepileptic: drug that works against (*anti*) epileptic seizures (*epilept*).
antipyretic: works against (*anti*) fever (*pyretic*).
-mimetic: imitates the action of a nervous system.
narcotic: drug capable of producing sleep or stupor (*narco*).

The following terms relate to anesthetic drugs and their uses:

anesthetic: drug capable of taking away (*an*) sensation (*esthet*).
general anesthetic: drug capable of producing a total (*general*) loss of sensation and consciousness.
local anesthetic: drug that causes a loss of sensation in a specific or local area.
saddle block: local anesthetic that deadens the area that comes in contact with a saddle.
topical: anesthetic agent applied to the surface (*top*) of the skin so that it is absorbed in that area.

Terms used in Prescription Writing

Abbreviation	Original Word or Phrase	English Equivalent
a.c.	ante cibum	before meals
ad	ad	to, up to
ad lib	ad libitum	freely
bib	bibe	drink
b.i.d.	bis in die	twice weekly
b.i.n.	bis in noctus	twice a night
c̄	cum	with
cap	capsula	capsule
h.	hora	an hour
h.s.	hora somni	bedtime
I.M.	intra muscularis	into the muscle
I.V.	intra venous	into the vein
min		minute
m	minim	minimum
non rep.	non repetatur	don't repeat
noxt	nocte; noxte	at night
nunc	nunc	now
O.D.	oculus dexter	right eye
O.S.; O.L.	oculus sinister; oculus laevus	left eye
os	os; ora	mouth
p.c.	post cibum	after meals
per		through or by
pil	pilula	pill
p.o.	per os	by mouth
p.r.	per rectum	by rectum
qAM	quaque ante meridien	every morning
qd	quaque dies	every day
qh	quaque hora	every hour
q 2h		every two hours
qod	quaque o. die	every other day
qPM	quaque post meridien	every evening
q.i.d.	quader in die	four times a day
s̄	sine	without
sig.	signa	write
s.l.	sub lingual	under the tongue
stat.	statim	immediately
sub Q; s.c.	subcutaneous	under the skin
suppos.	suppositoria	suppository
T	temperatura	temperature
tab	tabella	tablet
t.i.d.	ter in die	three times daily
tsp		teaspoon
tbsp		tablespoon
u		units
ung	unguentum	ointment
#		number
ī		one
īī		two
īīī		three

Physician's Desk Reference (*PDR*)

The Physician's Desk Reference can be found in all physicians' offices, clinics, and hospitals. It is an extremely valuable reference guide that is updated every year. The following should help you use this reference.

The *PDR* is published by Medical Economics Company with the cooperation of the manufacturers whose products are described in the "Product Information" (white) section of the book. The purpose of the "Diagnostic Products Information" (green) section is to make available essential prescription information on major pharmaceutical products. It is intended primarily for physicians' use.

The *PDR* contains the latest available information on approximately 2,500 drug products. Inside the front cover are instrucitons for using the book and a suggested method to alert the reader to revisions in a particular product's monograph.

Product descriptions appearing in the *PDR* have been prepared by the manufacturers and are edited and approved by the manufacturers' medical departments, medical directors, and/or medical consultants. Manufacturers suggest headings under which their products should be listed in the "Product Classification Index" (blue section) and in the "Generic and Chemical Name Index" (yellow section).

The products that appear in the "Product Identification" Section carry page numbers that refer to the "Alphabetical Index" (pink section), "Product Classification Index," and "Generic and Chemical Name Index." Additionally, this section contains page numbers that refer to the "Product Information" section and the "Diagnostic Products Information" section.

If only one number appears with a product, it refers the reader to the "Product Information" (white) section. If two numbers are given, the first of which is in the 400 series, that first number refers the reader to the "Product Identification" section. Page numbers from 500 to 1999 refer the reader to the "Product Information" section and products in the 2000 series can be found in the "Diagnostic Products Information" (green) section.

The products described in the *PDR* have official package circulars and must be in full compliance with Food and Drug Administration regulations. Consequently, it is a highly regulated and accurate reference. It also contains a list of Poison Control Centers found in the United States.

Since it is published annually, it is continuously revised in format. The authors have exhibited wisdom, however, in their decision to maintain the consistent use of colors in the coded sections. You may find that future publications differ slightly from the description given here.

Terminology Trivia

Anesthesia

Oliver Wendell Holmes was the first person to suggest the use of anesthetics during surgical operations. Anesthetics were America's greatest contribution to medicine during the early nineteenth century. Davy discovered the properties of nitrous oxide gas, referred to as "laughing gas," and in 1844, a dentist, Wells (1815–1848), was the first person to extract teeth using this gas. Long (1815–1878), a country practitioner in Georgia, used ether for the first time in a surgical procedure. The success of ether anesthesia spread throughout the world within a month after its initial use. Anesthetics were used for the first time in warfare during the Civil War. For about 100 years, anesthetists (nuns, medical students, and even hospital orderlies) had only the size of the pupil of the eye and respiration rate to guide them in administering anesthetics.

Surgical infections were rampant during the early nineteenth century. Celsus, a distinguished medical writer (14–37 A.D.) recommended the use of urine and vinegar to cleanse wounds. This type of antiseptic was also recommended by Hippocrates, who additionally recommended the use of dry dressings. Today in backwood areas of the United States, urine is often poured into the eye as treatment of a sty. Surgeons, during the thirteenth century, used wine to cleanse wounds.

Lister (1827–1912) was struck by the number of fatalities following amputations (often as high as forty-five percent) and the presence of gangrene and demanded cleanliness in his surgical wards. Encouraged by the work of Pasteur (1822–1895), Lister reasoned that if bacteria were destroyed, wounds would heal. He employed various antiseptic solutions, including carbolic acid, toward this end and received encouraging results. While Lister advocated antisepsis for cleansing of wounds, Pasteur first suggested sterilization of scalpels by passing them through flames.

Patent Medicines

Few proprietary medicines, especially during their heyday in the latter half of the nineteenth century, were actually patented. The reason is simple enough: in order to obtain a patent, the "inventor" would be required to list the ingredients of his "medicine," and few if any of the nostrums sold then could survive such a revelation.

Pronunciation and Meaning of New Terms

adrenocorticosteroids (add′ reno kortiko″ steer oids) A drug group whose members affect the kidneys and immune system.

antianemics (anti″ a′ neem′ iks) Curing or preventing anemia.

antiarrhythmetics (anti″ arith′ met iks) Preventing or eliminating abnormal heart contractions.

antihistamine (anti″ his′ tah mean) Any medication that counteracts the effect of histamine.

antilipemics (anti″ lip′ e miks) Any medication used to reduce fat in the blood.

antineoplastics (anti″ neo′ plas tiks) Drugs that are used in cancer chemotherapy.

cathartics (kath″ art′ iks) A purgative used to induce bowel movements.

iatrogenic (i″ at′ row jen ik) A condition induced by treatment for another condition.

idiopathic (ideo′ path ik) Condition with an unknown cause.

palliative (pall i a″ tiv) An agent that alleviates or eases.

parasympatholytic (pār a sim patho lit ik) Having a destructive effect or blocking parasympathetic nerves.

parasympathomimetic (pār a sim patho mimet ik) Producing effects similar to those produced by the parasympathetic nervous system.

prophylactic (pro′ fil ak tik) Warding off or preventing disease.

quinine (kwi′ nine) A white crystalline alkaloid used as an analgesic.

rauwolfia (rō wolf i a) Extract of a dried root that is a potent hypertensive agent.

sulfonamides (sull′ fon″ am ides) A group of bacteriostatic compounds consisting of amides of sulfanilic acid.

sympatholytic (simp″ ath o′ lit ik) A group of neuropharmacologic drugs that are antagonistic to the sympathomimetic drugs.

synergistic (sin′ er jist′ ik) The harmonious action of two drugs to produce an effect that neither could produce alone.

tetracycline (tet ra si klein) A group of broad spectrum antibiotics.

Self-test

1. For each set, match Column A with Column B.

Column A	*Column B*
___ analeptic	a. controls convulsions
___ analgesic	b. controls Parkinson's disease
___ anticonvulsant	c. controls fever
___ antiepileptic	d. restores wakefulness
___ antiparkinsonian	e. takes away pain
___ antipyretic	f. controls epilepsy
___ narcotic	g. has action similar to cutting of a parasympathetic nerve
___ narcotic antagonist	h. has action similar to cutting of a sympathetic nerve
___ parasympatholytic	i. capable of producing stupor
___ parasympathomimetic	j. imitates action of a sympathetic nerve
___ sympatholytic	k. reverses action of a narcotic
___ sympathomimetic	l. has action similar to action of parasympathetic nerves

2.

Column A

___ general
___ topical
___ infiltration
___ nerve block
___ spinal
___ epidural

Column B

a. injected near a nerve to block all sensations
b. capable of producing loss of consciousness
c. injected so it can filter through area to be operated
d. put on the surface
e. injected into subarachnoid space
f. also known as caudal anesthesia

3.

Column A

___ antidepressant
___ hallucinogen
___ hypnotic
___ psychostimulant
___ psychotropic
___ sedative
___ tranquilizer

Column B

a. causes sleep
b. change mental activity
c. produces feeling of well-being
d. causes illusions
e. ability to calm and induce sleep
f. increases activity of the mind
g. used to control depression

4.

Column A

___ sublingual administration
___ side effects
___ pharmacokinetics
___ nonproprietary name
___ contraindication
___ stimulant
___ trade name
___ sympatholytics
___ tetracycline
___ potentiation
___ heparin
___ pharmacodynamics

Column B

a. ever-present, common, unintended toxic effect of a drug
b. drug that speeds up vital processes
c. study of how drugs exert effects on the body
d. patient factors that make a drug ill-advisable to use
e. mathematical description of drug disposition in the body
f. autonomic drug group
g. drug placed under the tongue
h. broad-spectrum antibiotic
i. registered name owned by a pharmaceutical company
j. drug used to prolong blood-clotting time
k. two drugs taken together affect metabolism of one
l. name assigned when drug is found functional

Appendix One
Answers to Self-Test Questions

This appendix contains the answers to all the self-tests that appear at the end of each chapter. You should have your answers written out before looking at the answers so that you can benefit from this experience. Repeat the self-tests until you obtain at least an 80% mastery (8 out of 10 correct). Use the glossary in the back of the book or a dictionary rather than guessing. Count an answer wrong if you have to look it up.

Chapter 2

1.

Column A		*Column B*
d	ante-	a. beyond, over, between, change
g	gen-	b. night
a	meta-	c. together, union
b	noct(i)-	d. before
b	nyct-	e. first
f	post-	f. after
d	pre-	g. beginning, origin
e	prim-	
e	proto-	
c	sym-	
c	syn-	

2.

Column A		*Column B*
d	acro-	a. on, upon, over
h	anti-	b. within
e	contra-	c. above, excessive, beyond
g	ecto-	d. extremity, tip
b	endo-	e. opposite, against
a	epi-	f. before, in front of
f	fore-	g. outside, misplaced
c	hyper-	h. against

3.

Column A

m infra-
m inter-
g intra-
i medi-, meso-
d para-
a peri-
k schisto-
e sub-
b,j super-
j supra-
l trans-

Column B

a. around
b. excessive, extreme
c. between parts
d. beside, beyond
e. below
f. excessive
g. within a part
h. beneath
i. middle
j. above, over
k. split, divided
l. across, through
m. situated, formed or occurring between

4.

Column A

c a-, an-
a,k ambly-
h andro-
j angi(o)-
e ankyl(o)-
b auto-
d brady-
g co-, com-, con-
f cryo-
i dys-

Column B

a. dull
b. self
c. without
d. slow
e. crooked, bent
f. cold
g. with
h. male
i. difficult, abnormal
j. vessel, duct
k. dullness

5.

Column A

b eu-
c gyno-
a hetero-
h homo-
g hydra-, hydro-
i iso-
d mal-
f neo-
k ortho-

Column B

a. other, different
b. good, normal
c. female
d. bad
e. peculiar to the individual
f. new, strange, separate, distinct
g. water
h. same
i. equal
j. broad, wide
k. straight, normal

6.

Column A		*Column B*
a	path(o)-	a. disease
d	phag(o)-	b. fast
g	pseudo-	c. malformed, monster
h	scler-	d. eat, consume
k	steno-	e. rough
b	tachy-	f. heat, warmth
c	terato-	g. false
f	thermo-	h. hard
l	toxic-	i. behind, backward
e	trachy-	j. straight, erect
		k. contracted, narrowing
		l. poison

7.

Column A		*Column B*
c	ab-	a. away, not, down
e	ad-	b. forward, anterior
a	de-	c. away from
f	dextro-	d. against, into, toward
k	e-	e. to, toward
g	ex-	f. right
h	im-, in-	g. away from, out
d	ir-	h. in, inside, within
i	levo-, sinistro-	i. left
l	pro-, proso-	j. behind, backward
j	retro-	k. out
		l. before, in front of

8.

Prefix	*Meaning*
a. demi-	**one half**
b. mono-	**one**
c. pan-	**all**
d. bi-	**two**
e. tetr(a)-	**four**
f. semi-	**one half**
g. null(i)-	**none**
h. quadr(i)-	**four**
i. poly-	**many**
j. uni-	**one**
k. tri-	**three**
l. hemi-	**one half**
m. brachy-	**short**
n. lepto-	**small**
o. micr-	**small**
p. macro-	**large**
q. olig(o)-	**little, small**
r. alb-	**white**
s. xantho-	**yellow**
t. leuko-	**white**
u. rube-	**red**
v. cyano-	**blue**
w. erythro-	**red**
x. melan-	**black**
y. chloro-	**green**
z. cirrh-	**yellow**

Chapter 3

1.

Column A		*Column B*
e	-centesis	a. setting free, dissolution
k	-ectomy	b. creation of a mouth or opening
a	-lysis	c. fixation
b	-ostomy	d. an instrument for cutting
g	-otomy	e. puncture of a cavity
c	-pexy	f. looking at, examining
j	-plasty	g. cut into
h	-rrhaphy	h. closure by suturing, repair
f	-scope, -scopy	i. rubbing, crushing
d	-tome	j. to mold or shape
i	-tripsy	k. excision, cutting out

2.

Suffix	*Meaning*
a. -agra	**severe pain**
b. -algia	**pain**
c. -atresia	**abnormal closure**
d. -cele	**swelling**
e. -cyst	**bladder-like sac**
f. -dynia	**pain**
g. -ema	**swelling**
h. -ia	**diseased**
i. -iasis	**condition**
j. -itis	**inflammation**
k. -malacia	**softening**
l. -oma	**tumor**
m. -osis	**diseased**
n. -pathy	**disease**
o. -penia	**deficiency**
p. -philia	**love of**
q. -phobia	**fear of**
r. -ptosis	**drooping**
s. -rrhage	**bursting forth**
t. -rrhea	**flow**
u. -stasis	**stop**
v. -tonia	**stretch**

Chapter 4

1.

Terminal	*Meaning*
pyro*genic*	a. **producing**
circ*ular*	b. **pertaining to**
flacc*id*	c. **condition**
lymph*oid*	d. **resembles**
osteo*genesis*	e. **producing**
cura*tive*	f. **the quality or nature**
compli*ance*	g. **act of**

2.

Singular	*Plural*
-a	a. **-ae**
-ies	b. **-ietes**
-nx	c. **-nges**
-u	d. **-ua**
-x	e. **-ces, -cis**
-en	f. **-ina**
-is	g. **-es**
-on	h. **-a**
-um	i. **-a**
-ex	j. **-ices**
-ma	k. **-mata**
-s	l. **-tes**
-us	m. **-i, -era, -ora**

Chapter 5

1.

Column A		*Column B*
f	histo-	a. space between the cells
c	cyto-, cyte	b. fat in the blood
d	plasmo	c. cell
e	intracellular	d. cell substance
b	lipemia	e. inside the cell
a	interstitial	f. tissue

2.

1. The word root for a sheet of fibrous tissue is **fascia** .
2. Foramen is the word root meaning **opening** .
3. The type of tissue that covers the body surfaces is called **epithelial** tissue.
4. The tissue that holds the body together is called **connective** .
5. The tissue of the body involved in movement is called **muscle** tissue.

3.

Column A		*Column B*
d	collum	a. supporting structure
f	duct	b. cavity; passageway; curved space
c	foramen	c. opening or hole
g	hilum	d. neck-like part
h	node	e. definite region; series of related parts
b	sinus	f. tube-like structure that transports fluid or air
a	stem	g. place where blood vessels, nerves, or ducts enter
e	tract	h. small mass of tissue

4.

Column A		*Column B*
d	ampulla	a. body of an organ
a	fundus	b. middle or inner part
e	cortex	c. organ opening
i	fascia	d. a dilated portion of a duct
c	aperture	e. outside part, thick outer layer
h	meatus	f. layer of connective tissue
b	medulla	g. small, belly-like space in an organ
g	ventricle	h. opening or channel
		i. sheet of fibrous tissue

5.

Column A		*Column B*
c	apex	a. body
h	base	b. roundish projection of an organ
a	corpus	c. tip or point
e	fascicle	d. mouth-like opening
f	labium	e. small bundle of tissue
b	lobe	f. lip-like part
d	orifice	g. nipple-like projection from a surface
g	papilla	h. part of an organ nearest its attachment
i	viscera	i. organs of the body; usually abdominal organs

6.

Column A		*Column B*
c	anatomical	a. standing position
a	erect	b. lying horizontally on either the right or left side
d	supine	c. standing straight with arms to the side and palms facing forward
e	prone	d. lying horizontally face up
b	laterally recumbent	e. lying face down
f	internal	f. inner part or surface
i	external	g. far beneath the surface
g	deep	h. walls of a part
j	superficial	i. outer part or surface
h	parietal	j. close to the surface

7.

1. **cervical**
2. **thoracic**
3. **lumbar**
4. **sacral**
5. **coccyx**

8.

Column A		*Column B*
c	coronal	a. divides body into right and left sections
a	sagittal	b. divides body into top and bottom sections
b	horizontal	c. divides body into front and back sections
c	frontal	
a	median	
b	transverse	

9.

Term	*Direction*
superior	a. **above, upward**
inferior	b. **below, downward**
medial	c. **middle**
lateral	d. **sides**
peripheral	e. **around**
cephalad	f. **head**
caudad	g. **tail**
proximal	h. **closest**
distal cavity	i. **farthest**
ventral cavity	j. **front**
dorsal	k. **back**
volar	l. **palm**
plantar	m. **sole**
varus	n. **bent in**
valgus	o. **bent out**
dextral	p. **right**
sinistral	q. **left**
anterior	r. **front**
posterior	s. **back**

10.

Column A		*Column B*
d	lips	a. skeletal
d	nipple	b. cardiovascular and lymph
a	tendon	c. special senses
e	bronchi	d. integumentary
c	eye	e. respiratory
b	vein	
d	eyelash	

Chapter 6

1.

Column A		*Column B*
c	bucca-	a. word root meaning tongue
g	cheil-	b. grape-like structure at the back of the mouth
a	glossa-, lingua-	c. inside of the cheek
f	labia	d. roof of the mouth
e	os-, ora-	e. opening into the mouth
d	palate	f. the lips
h	stoma-	g. word root meaning lip
i	tonsil	h. mouth
b	uvula	i. oval mass of tissue on each side of the throat

2.

Column A		*Column B*
b	alveol-	a. word root meaning gum
e	cementum	b. bony sockets for the teeth
f	plaque	c. tooth
h	denti-	d. narrow portion of the tooth
c	odont-	e. tissue holding tooth in place
a	gingiv-	f. deposit of hard material
g	gum	g. firm, fleshy tissue covering the alveolar parts of the jaw
d	neck	h. word root meaning tooth
i	periodontal	i. fibrous connective tissues around the tooth

3.

Column A		*Column B*
c	duodenum	a. opening between ileum and cecum
b	ileum	b. distal portion of small intestine
a	ileocecal foramen	c. first section of small intestine
j	appendix	d. the last section of colon
i	cecum	e. ring-like opening at the end of alimentary tract
g	descending colon	f. word root meaning anus or rectum
d	sigmoid colon	g. section of bowel that moves downward
h	rectum	h. distal portion of the large intestine
e	anus	i. part of colon with blind pouch
f	procto-	j. organ hanging down from the cecum

4.

Column A		*Column B*
a	chole-	a. word root meaning bile
c	gall	b. word root meaning liver
b	hepat-	c. bile
d	cholecyst	d. gallbladder
f	hepatic duct	e. membrane covering abdominal organs
i	cystic duct	f. tube from the liver
g	common bile duct	g. tube formed from joining of ducts
h	pancreatic duct	h. tube from the pancreas
e	omentum	i. tube from the gallbladder

5.

Column A		*Column B*
d	anorexia	a. inflammation of gallbladder
g	appendicitis	b. difficulty in digestion, indigestion
k	colic	c. small tubular projections in the intestines
h	labiology	d. loss of appetite
a	cholecystitis	e. flow through of undigested food
i	cholelithiasis	f. sore in the duodenum
j	cirrhosis	g. inflammation of the appendix
e	diarrhea	h. study of lip movement
c	diverticulosis	i. bile stones
f	duodenal ulcer	j. disease in which liver becomes dark yellow
b	dyspepsia	k. acute abdominal pain

6.

Column A		*Column B*
e	emesis	a. protrusion of an organ from its normal place
c	proctoplasty	b. blockage in the intestinal tract
f	gastritis	c. surgical repair of the anus
g	hemorrhoids	d. erosion of stomach or duodenum
h	hepatitis	e. vomiting
i	hyperacidity	f. inflammation of the stomach
b	intestinal obstruction	g. dilated veins near the anus
j	jaundice	h. inflammation of the liver
k	malocclusion	i. high acid content
d	peptic ulcer	j. disease in which skin becomes yellow
		k. teeth not coming together when jaws are closed

7.

Column A

d abdominocentesis
h analplasty
b appendectomy
f cholecystectomy
g colectomy
a colostomy
c esophagectomy
i exodontia or extraction
e proctitis

Column B

a. formation of a permanent opening into the colon
b. removal of the appendix
c. removal of the esophagus
d. puncture of abdominal wall
e. inflammation of the rectum
f. removal of the gallbladder
g. removal of the colon
h. repair of the anal region
i. removal of teeth

8.

Column A

g gastrectomy
e gastroscopy
c gastrostomy
b glossectomy
a herniorrhaphy
f ileostomy
d intestinal anastomosis

Column B

a. repair of a hernia
b. removal of the tongue
c. making a somewhat permanent opening into the stomach
d. two ends of intestinal tract sewn together
e. visualizing the inside of the stomach
f. opening into the ileum
g. removal of the stomach

9.

Column A

c pancreatectomy
d pancreaticojejunostomy
e endoscopic papillotomy
b polypectomy
a proctoscopy
f sigmoidoscopy
i antacid
k antidiarrhetic
g antiemetic
j cathartic
h digestant

Column B

a. visualization of anal and rectal regions
b. removal of a polyp
c. removal of the pancreas
d. opening into jejunum for the pancreatic duct
e. viewing device passed inside body to enlarge the ampulla
f. visualization of sigmoid colon
g. drug used to control vomiting
h. drug used to aid digestion
i. drug used to control acid condition
j. substance used to cleanse bowel
k. drug used to control diarrhea

Chapter 7

1.

Column A		*Column B*
a	nephr-	a. word root meaning kidney
c	Bowman's capsule	b. pertaining to the kidney
b	renal	c. collecting unit surrounding glomerulus
f	ureter	d. tubule plus capillaries—the functioning unit of the kidney
e	glomerulus	e. ball of capillaries in nephron
d	nephron	f. tube that transports urine from kidney to bladder
j	bladder	g. urinary bladder
i	urinary meatus	h. reproductive and urinary organs
g	vesical	i. opening of tube from bladder to the outside
h	genitourinary	j. receptacle for urine
k	urethra	k. tube leaving the bladder

2.

Column A		*Column B*
a	urethrocele	a. prolapse of the urethra
b	dysuria	b. difficulty in urination
c	enuresis	c. involuntary urination
g	glomerulonephritis	d. blood in the urine
d	hematuria	e. kidney stones
e	nephrolithiasis	f. dropped kidney
f	nephroptosis	g. inflammation of the renal glomeruli
h	nocturia	h. frequent urination at night
m	oliguria	i. opening between bladder and nearby organs
k	pyelonephritis	j. waste products remaining in the blood
p	polyuria	k. inflammation of the kidney pelvis
n	nephrectomy	l. inflammation of the ureter
e	renal calculi	m. scant or small amounts of urine
j	uremia	n. removal of a kidney
l	ureteritis	o. frequent urination
i	vesical fistulas	p. excessive urinary output

3.

Column A		*Column B*
a	anorchism	a. absent testes
f	cryptorchism	b. inflammation of epididymis and testes
g	epididymitis	c. collection of fluid around the testes
b	epididymoorchitis	d. removal of one or both testes
c	hydrocele	e. undersecretion of sex-related hormones
e	hypogonadism	f. undescended testicles
l	oligospermia	g. inflammation of epididymis
j	orchitis	h. removal of all or part of the prostate gland
h	prostatectomy	i. abnormal discharge of the prostate
o	prostatitis	j. inflammation of the testes
n	spermatocele	k. inflammation of the penis
m	vasectomy	l. small amount of sperm produced
i	prostatorrhea	m. removal of a section of the vas deferens
		n. cystic distention of the epididymis
		o. inflammation of prostate gland

4.

Column A		*Column B*
c	cervicitis	a. painful intercourse in women
f	vaginitis	b. white patches on external reproductive organs
a	dyspareunia	c. inflammation of the cervix
g	endocervicitis	d. endometrial tissue found in various locations of the pelvic cavity
d	endometriosis	e. inflammation of external female genitalia
e	vulvitis	f. inflammation of the vagina
b	leukoplakia of the vulva	g. inflammation of the lining of the cervix
j	amenorrhea	h. bleeding after menses have ceased
i	dysmenorrhea	i. painful menstruation
k	menorrhagia	j. lack of menstrual flow
l	metrorrhagia	k. excessive menstrual flow
h	postmenopausal bleeding	l. flow of blood from uterus at irregular intervals

5.

a. birth control
b. colpectomy
c. colpocleisis
d. colporrhaphy
e. dilation and curettage
f. endometrial biopsy
g. pelvic examination

1. The action taken to prevent the birth of a child is called __**a**__ .
2. __**e**__ is a procedure to widen the opening of the cervix and scrape the lining of the uterus.
3. __**d**__ is the repair of the vaginal walls.
4. __**f**__ is an examination of tissue from the lining of the uterus.
5. The removal of the vagina is called __**b**__ .
6. The procedure to close the vagina with sutures is called __**c**__ .
7. The procedure in which the internal female reproductive organs are examined is called a __**g**__ .

6.

Column A		*Column B*
b	hysterectomy	a. removal of the vulva
f	oophorectomy	b. removal of the uterus
c	salpingectomy	c. removal of uterine tubes
e	salpingo–oophorectomy	d. repair of uterine tubes
d	salpingorrhaphy	e. removal of uterine tubes and ovaries
a	vulvectomy	f. removal of ovaries

7.

a. abruptio placenta
b. ectopic
c. spontaneous abortion
d. hyperemesis gravidarum
e. intrauterine death
f. placenta previa
g. premature

1. A pregnancy that develops in other than its normal place is called (a) an ___**b**___ pregnancy.
2. Labor that starts before the full term of pregnancy is complete is ___**g**___ labor.
3. ___**d**___ means excessive vomiting during pregnancy.
4. ___**a**___ is a situation in which the placenta prematurely separates from the uterus.
5. ___**f**___ means the placenta is nearer to the uterine outlet than is the baby.
6. The loss of the fetus from natural, unplanned causes is called a ___**c**___ .
7. When a child dies before it is born, an ___**e**___ has occurred.

8.

a. amnionitis
b. dystocia
c. eclampsia
d. stillborn
e. toxemia

1. A difficult labor is called ___**b**___ .
2. The condition in which harmful substances are existent in the blood of the mother is called ___**e**___ .
3. A sudden development of convulsions in pregnancy is called ___**c**___ .
4. Inflammation of the amnion is called ___**a**___ .
5. A child who is born dead is called ___**d**___ .

9.

Column A		*Column B*
d	gravida two, para one	a. woman who has given birth more than once
a	multipara	b. woman giving birth to her first child
c	nullipara	c. woman who has never had children
b	primipara	d. woman who has been pregnant twice and has one living child

Chapter 8

1.

Column A		*Column B*
b	cerebrum	a. small, round mass located in posterior section of cranium
e	mesencephalon	b. largest portion of the brain
a	cerebellum	c. column of nervous tissue running down center of vertebrae
d	pons	d. bridge-like structure
c	spinal cord	e. the midbrain

2.

Column A		*Column B*
d	cordotomy	a. recording of electrical activity of the brain
b	cephalagia	b. headache
g	subdural	c. cutting into a lobe of the brain
f	neuron	d. cutting into the spinal cord
a	electroencephalogram	e. inflammation of the brain
c	lobotomy	f. nerve cell
e	encephalitis	g. external to the dura mater
i	neurolysis	h. removal of a piece of a sympathetic nerve
k	neurotripsy	i. cutting of nerve tissue
j	dura mater	j. outermost covering of the central nervous system
h	sympathectomy	k. crushing a nerve tissue

Chapter 9

1.

Column A		*Column B*
e	superior vena cava	a. main artery of the body
b	pulmonary artery	b. blood vessel carrying blood to the lungs
f	right pulmonary vein	c. sugar in the blood
a	aorta	d. valve on the right side of the heart between the atrium and ventricle
d	semilunar valve	e. drains blood from upper part of the body to the heart
c	glycemia	f. returns blood from right lung
i	angi-	g. hair-thin blood vessel
g	capillary	h. word root meaning vein
h	phleb-	i. vessel
j	venule	j. small vein

2.

Column A		*Column B*
a	angina pectoris	a. pain in the chest
c	angiogram	b. slow heart rate
f	vasodilation	c. x-ray of blood vessels including arteries and veins
d	arteriography	d. x-ray of arteries
e	arteritis	e. inflammation of an artery
b	bradycardia	f. widening the diameter of blood vessels
g	cardiomyopathy	g. disease of the heart muscle
k	cardiomegaly	h. record of electrical activity of the heart
i	bacterial endocarditis	i. inflammation inside the heart
h	electrocardiogram	j. swelling of parts of the body
j	edema	k. enlarged heart
l	neutrophils	l. a type of leukocyte

3.

Column A		*Column B*
g	thrombus	a. inadequate heart muscle action
h	hemangioma	b. inflammation of a vein
e	hematoma	c. dilated vein containing blood in anal area
c	hemorrhoid	d. low blood pressure
f	hypertension	e. swelling containing blood
d	hypotension	f. high blood pressure
b	phlebitis	g. clot of blood obstructing blood vessels
a	myocardial insufficiency	h. tumor consisting of blood vessels
i	phlebotomy	i. incision of a vein

4.

Column A		*Column B*
b	erythrocytes	a. blood fluid
c	leukocytes	b. red blood cells
a	plasma	c. white blood cells
d	hemoglobin	d. red coloring in red blood cells
g	albumin	e. protein substance that becomes spherical in solution
e	globulin	f. protein that produces fiber
f	fibrinogen	g. protein substance that coagulates like an egg white when heated
h	prothrombin	h. protein that is involved in blood clot production

5.

Column A		*Column B*
f	agranulocytosis	a. unequal size of red blood cells
e	anemia	b. blood more acid than normal
a	anisocytosis	c. blood more alkaline than normal
d	anoxia	d. deficiency of oxygen in blood
b	acidosis	e. reduced erythrocytes, hemoglobin, or packed red cells
c	alkalosis	f. lack of granulocytes

6.

Column A		*Column B*
e	hemostasis	a. disease of lymph glands
c	lymphadenitis	b. neoplasm of lymphatic tissues
a	lymphadenopathy	c. inflammation of lymph glands
g	lymphatic metastasis	d. elevated blood sugar
b	lymphoma	e. stopping of blood
f	splenomegaly	f. enlargement of the spleen
d	hyperglycemia	g. the spread of disease through the lymphatic system

Chapter 10

1.

Column A		*Column B*
c	apnea	a. excessive breathing
f	dyspnea	b. condition in which breathing is easier in upright position
a	hyperventilation	c. absence of breathing
e	laryngotracheobronchitis	d. inflammation of the pleura
b	orthopnea	e. inflammation of larynx, trachea, and bronchi
i	pneumoconiosis	f. difficulty breathing
g	pneumothorax	g. air in thoracic cavity outside lungs between two pleura
j	pulmonary edema	h. fast rate of breathing
k	tracheotomy	i. lung condition caused by inhalation of dust particles
h	tachypnea	j. excessive fluid in lungs
		k. cutting into the trachea

Chapter 11

1.

Column A		*Column B*
b	myelo-	a. bone cell
c	osteoblasts	b. marrow
e	osteal	c. cells that form bone
a	osteocytes	d. process of bone-cell production
d	ossification	e. bony

2.

Column A		*Column B*
f	osteoarthritis	a. inflammation of bone and cartilage
a	osteochondritis	b. group of diseases in which there are growth disturbances
i	osteochondroma	c. decrease in bone mass
k	osteochondrosis	d. condition in which bone is destroyed
d	osteoclasia	e. bone tumor
b	osteodystrophies	f. inflammation of bone joint
e	osteoma	g. inflammation of bone and marrow
h	osteomalacia	h. softened bones
g	osteomyelitis	i. tumor of tone and cartilage covering the bone
c	osteopenia	j. porous bones
j	osteoporosis	k. group of diseases affecting growth centers of bone and articular cartilage

3.

Column A		*Column B*
i	cranium	a. back of skull
f	frontal	b. pertaining to the face
a	occipital	c. sieve-like bone
k	temporal	d. upper jaw
g	sphenoid	e. sides and roof of skull
c	ethmoid	f. bone in front of skull
b	facial	g. wedge-shaped bone
j	nasal	h. cheekbones
h	zygomatic	i. enclosing the brain
e	parietal	j. pertaining to the nose
m	palatine	k. bones at the temples
d	maxilla	l. lower jaw
l	mandible	m. roof of the mouth

4.

Column A		*Column B*
j	spondylous	a. five vertebrae of the loin
f	cervical vertebrae	b. vertebra that allows head to turn
b	axis	c. toward the lower portion of the spinal column
d	thoracic vertebrae	d. twelve vertebrae of back and chest
a	lumbar vertebrae	e. breastbone
i	sacral vertebrae	f. seven bones of the neck
k	coccygeal vertebrae	g. cervical vertebrae that may be felt
e	sternum	h. spinal column
h	rachis	i. five fused vertebrae
c	caudal	j. pertaining to vertebrae or spinal column
		k. four fused vertebrae of the tailbone

5.

Column A		*Column B*
f	clavicle	a. single bone of upper arm
g	scapula	b. bones in fingers and thumb
a	humerus	c. small bone in forearm on the thumb side
d	ulna	d. larger bone in forearm
c	radius	e. bones of the wrist
e	carpal bones	f. collarbone
h	metacarpal bones	g. shoulder blade
b	phalanges	h. bones in the hand

6.

Column A		*Column B*
b	pelvis	a. place where pubic bones grow together
c	ilium	b. shaped like a basin
a	symphysis pubis	c. superior portion of hip
f	femur	d. kneecap
d	patella	e. anklebone
i	tibia	f. thighbone
g	fibula	g. outer, thinner bone of lower leg
e	tarsal bones	h. bones of the foot
h	metatarsal bones	i. inner, larger bones of the lower leg

7.

Column A		*Column B*
a	carpectomy	a. removal of wrist bones
b	hallux valgus	b. great toe displaced toward other toes
c	diskectomy	c. removal of intervertebral cartilage
f	osteoclasis	d. joint taken apart, and limb removed
e	osteoplasty	e. reconstruction or repair of bone
g	osteotomy	f. surgical breaking of bone
i	dactylion	g. cutting into bone
h	spinal fusion	h. two or more vertebrae joined together
k	chondroma	i. union of fingers
j	arthrotomy	j. incision of a joint
l	tenotomy	k. tumor of cartilage
		l. incision of a tendon

Chapter 12

1.

Column A		*Column B*
c	origin	a. end of a muscle attached to bone that moves
e	belly	b. fibrous cord by which a muscle is attached
a	insertion	c. end of muscle attached to bone that does not move
d	fascia	d. layer of thin fibrous tissue between muscles and enclosing muscles
b	tendon	e. long extension of a muscle
h	agonist	f. muscle that works against a contracting muscle
f	antagonist	g. word root meaning motion
g	kine-	h. contracting muscle, the prime mover
i	sthen-	i. word root meaning strength
j	synergist	j. muscle that works with other muscles

2.

Column A		*Column B*
b	maximus	a. smallest
a	minimus	b. largest
c	major	c. larger
f	minor	d. long
d	longus	e. short
e	brevis	f. smaller
i	cuneiform	g. feather-like, pennate
o	deltoid	h. four-sided
m	fusiform	i. wedge-shaped
g	penniform	j. four-sided with opposite sides parallel
k	platy-	k. flat
h	quadrilateral	l. saw-like edge
j	rhomboid	m. spindle-shaped
l	serratus	n. four-sided with two parallel and two nonparallel sides
n	trapezoid	o. triangular
		p. kite-shaped

3.

Column A		*Column B*
a	bipennate	a. joining a tendon from both sides
d	curved	b. slanted or angled arrangement
b	oblique	c. extends in same direction and does not cross
c	parallel	d. bent arrangement
e	rectus	e. straight
j	adductor	f. muscle that straightens
k	flexor	g. muscle that tightens a part
f	extensor	h. muscle that moves a part away from midline
i	depressor	i. muscle that lowers a part
g	tensor	j. muscle that moves a part toward midline
		k. muscle that bends a part

4.

Column A		*Column B*
g	smooth muscles	a. muscle weakness
a	myasthenia gravis	b. abnormal development of muscles
d	muscle hypertrophy	c. inflammation of many muscles
b	muscular dystrophy	d. excessive growth; muscle enlargement
i	myospasmia	e. motion sickness
j	skeletal muscles	f. breakdown of striated muscle
e	kinesia	g. involuntary muscles
c	polymyositis	h. lack of growth; muscle shrinkage
		i. muscle rigidity
		j. voluntary muscles

Chapter 13

1.

Column A

d sebaceous glands
b sebum
a lunula
c cuticle
e paronychial

Column B

a. moon shaped
b. oily, glandular secretion
c. small area of dead skin around base of nail
d. glands that open into hair follicles or directly onto surface of skin
e. area around the nail

2.

a. areola
b. galact or lacto
c. mammary gland
d. mast- or mamm-
e. theli-
f. lactation

1. The word root for tip or point of the breast is **e** .
2. The small area of color around the nipple is called the **a** .
3. The breast of the female is sometimes called the **c** .
4. The process of producing milk is called **f** .
5. The word root for milk is **b** .
6. The word root for breast is **d** .

3.

a. hyperhidrosis
b. hypertrichosis
c. hypomastia
d. laceration
e. macula
f. melanoma
g. epithelioma
h. mottled skin
i. depilation

1. The process for removing hair is **i** .
2. Another name for a spot or blotch is **e** .
3. A wound in which there is an irregular tear is called a **d** .
4. An excessive amount of sweating is called **a** .
5. A term meaning very small, underdeveloped breasts is **c** .
6. A tumor of the skin is **g** .
7. A condition in which there is excessive amount of hair is called **b** .
8. A condition in which there is variation in the color of skin produced by underlying blood vessels is called **h** .
9. A tumor of the melanocyte cells is called a **f** .

4.

Column A		*Column B*
g	scleroderma	a. scraping skin to remove acne scars
a	dermabrasion	b. preparation used to soften skin
c	depilatory	c. chemical preparation for removal of hair
f	sebaceous cyst	d. inflammation of a nipple
b	emollient	e. liquid preparation used to break down a hard layer of skin
e	keratolytic lotion	f. a sac-like structure filled with sebum
d	thelitis	g. hardening of the skin
h	mammography	h. x-ray examination of breasts
i	mammoplasty	i. plastic surgery on breasts
j	mastectomy	j. removal of a breast

Chapter 14

1.

Column A		*Column B*
a	blepharoptosis	a. drooping upper eyelid
c	canthus	b. discharge of pus from lacrimal gland
i	caruncle	c. corner of the eyelid
b	dacryopyorrhea	d. eyelashes
e	lacrimal gland	e. tissue that secretes tears
f	lacrimal duct	f. small canals that transport tears from eyes to nose
h	lacrimal sac	g. tube that carries tears down the nose
g	nasolacrimal duct	h. pouch-like area at beginning of duct in the nose
		i. small, fleshy eminence

2.

Column A		*Column B*
c	amblyopia	a. no vision, usually in one eye
e	ametropia	b. paralysis of the iris sphincter
h	anisometropia	c. dull vision; lazy eye
a	anopia	d. softening of the iris
b	iridoplegia	e. general term meaning a refractive disorder
g	blepharitis	f. drooping eyelid
f	blepharoptosis	g. inflammation of the eyelid
d	iridomalacia	h. different focusing ability in each eye

3.

Column A		*Column B*
f	conjunctivitis	a. inflammation of tear gland
a	dacryoadenitis	b. inside lining of eye pulled away
d	dacryocystitis	c. fold of skin over corner of the eye
b	detached retina	d. inflammation of tear sac
g	diplopia	e. eye appearing to be sunken into the orbit
e	enophthalmia	f. inflammation of the outer lining of the eye
c	epicanthus	g. double vision
k	esotropia	h. farsightedness
j	exophthalmia	i. turning out of the eyes
i	exotropia	j. protruding eyes
l	phakitis	k. turning in of the eyes; cross-eyed
h	hyperopia	l. inflammation of the eye lens
n	keratitis	m. inflammation of cornea and conjunctiva
m	keratoconjunctivitis	n. inflammation of the cornea

4.

Column A		*Column B*
a	leukoma	a. dense, white opacity of cornea
d	nyctalopia	b. paralysis of eye muscles
c	optic neuritis	c. inflammation of optic nerve
b	ophthalmoplegia	d. night blindness
e	proptosis	e. bulging eye
i	retinitis	f. noninjured eye suffering with the injured eye
s	retinopathy	g. hairs of eyelid growing inward
j	scleritis	h. bleeding under conjunctiva
h	subconjunctival hemorrhage	i. inflammation of the retina
f	sympathetic ophthalmia	j. inflammation of the sclera
g	trichiasis	k. general term meaning disease of the retina

5.

Column A		*Column B*
d	bilateral otitis media	a. inflammation of auditory tube
a	eustachian salpingitis	b. tympanic membrane
f	external otitis	c. injury to the ear due to a change in air pressure
b	myringa	d. middle ear inflammation in both ears
e	mastoiditis	e. inflammation of the bony process of the temporal bone
i	malleus	f. inflammation of the external ear
j	myringitis	g. last bone of the middle ear
l	otosclerosis	h. bleeding from the ear
k	otalgia	i. first bone of the middle ear
h	otorrhagia	j. inflammation of tympanic membrane
m	otorrhea	k. pain in the ear
g	stapes	l. spongy bone replacing the hard bone of the labyrinth
		m. discharge from the ear

Chapter 15

1.

Column A

- __b__ acromegaly
- __c__ adrenogenital syndrome
- __d__ exophthalmic goiter
- __a__ goiter
- __e__ hyperadrenocorticism
- __j__ hyperthyroidism
- __g__ hypothyroidism
- __f__ parathyroid tetany
- __h__ thyroiditis
- __k__ thyrotoxicosis

Column B

a. enlargement of the thyroid gland
b. enlarged extremities
c. hyperformation of adrenal cortex; includes symptom of early development of the reproductive organs
d. condition characterized by eyes protruding from their sockets
e. oversecretion of hormones from adrenal cortex
f. severe muscle contractions due to hormone deficiency
g. undersecretion of thyroid hormones
h. inflammation of thyroid gland
i. abnormal mucus deposits under the skin
j. oversecretion of thyroid hormones
k. toxicity caused by oversecretion of the thyroid gland

Chapter 16

1. The term physical refers to the **exam**. The physical exam includes the following:

a. **inspection**
b. **palpation**
c. **percussion**
d. **auscultation**
e. **measurements**

2. Vital signs include the following signs:

a. **temperature**
b. **pulse**
c. **respiratory rate**
d. **blood pressure**

3.

Column A

- __f__ acute
- __e__ anomaly
- __b__ benign
- __i__ chronic
- __c__ diagnosis
- __g__ malignant
- __k__ metastatic
- __a__ prognosis
- __j__ sign
- __d__ syndrome
- __h__ systemic
- __l__ atrophy

Column B

a. to know beforehand
b. favorable for recovery; a mild disease
c. sufficient knowledge of a disease to distinguish it from another
d. signs and symptoms that usually occur together
e. irregular; deviation from normal
f. sudden condition
g. becoming progressively worse
h. involves the whole body
i. condition that lasts a long time
j. observable and measurable occurrence
k. disease that spreads from one place to another
l. wasting away of an organ or part; without growth

4.

Column A

- __b__ endemic
- __d__ epidemic
- __e__ pandemic
- __c__ iatrogenic
- __a__ idiopathic

Column B

a. disease of unknown cause
b. constantly present disease occurring in a particular group of people
c. disease that is the side effect of treatment prescribed by physician
d. spread over a large group of people in a particular area
e. widespread epidemic desease

5.

Column A

- __b__ benign
- __f__ M0
- __i__ oncology
- __g__ Grade I tumor
- __a__ T3
- __d__ Grade IV tumor
- __e__ neoplastic
- __c__ carcinosis
- __h__ malignant

Column B

a. tumor advanced in size and involvement
b. mild
c. advanced metastatic disease
d. highly altered, difficult to recognize parent tissues
e. a disease in which new cells are formed
f. metastasis not evident
g. tumors resembling parent tissues
h. progressively worsening condition
i. study of tumors

6.

Column A		*Column B*
c	tendonitis	a. a bony protuberance
l	osteoclasia	b. inflammation of the spine
m	fibromyositis	c. inflammation of a tendon
d	angioma	d. tumor of blood vessels that appears on skin
k	contusion	e. hard crust or scab
a	exostosis	f. skin boil
b	spondylitis	g. bone tumor
f	furuncle	h. jaundice
g	osteoma	i. skin scraped away
e	eschar	j. mark on the skin; moles and birthmarks
i	abrasion	k. tissue damage beneath skin with skin unbroken
h	icterus	l. surgical fracture to remedy a deformity
j	nevus	m. inflammation of muscle and fibrous tissue
o	petechia	n. ringworm
n	tinea	o. small hemorrhage under skin that forms a small spot

7.

Column A		*Column B*
c	myocardial ischemia	a. disease of the heart muscle
d	shock	b. anal varicose vein
f	anoxia	c. decrease in the blood supply to the heart muscle
a	cardiomyopathy	d. inadequate tissue perfusion
h	leukemia	e. inflammation of a vein forming a blood clot
o	lymphoma	f. deficiency of oxygen in blood
i	apnea	g. defective or abnormal mixtures of blood elements
n	dyspnea	h. abnormally high numbers of white blood cells
b	hemorrhoid	i. absence of breathing
l	orthopnea	j. inflammation of the rectum
j	proctitis	k. burping
k	eructation	l. breathing is easier when standing
m	hernia	m. protrusion of an organ from its original position
g	dyscrasia	n. difficulty in breathing
e	thrombophlebitis	o. tumor of lymph nodes

8.

Column A		*Column B*
b	cystitis	a. involuntary passing of urine
j	anorchism	b. inflammation of the uninary bladder
g	varicocele	c. passing small amounts of urine
o	dyspareunia	d. accumulation of fluid causing extension of testes
f	vaginismus	e. excessive menstrual flow
n	myxedema	f. painful vaginal spasms
h	encephalitis	g. varicose veins of the testes
m	sciatica	h. inflammation of the brain
l	otitis media	i. double vision
a	enuresis	j. absence of testes
c	oligouria	k. cloud-like opacity of the cornea
k	nebula	l. inflammation of the middle ear
i	diplopia	m. severe pain in the leg
e	menorrhagia	n. swelling caused by mucus deposits in the skin
d	hydrocele	o. painful intercourse in women

Chapter 17

1.

Column A		*Column B*
d	analeptic	a. controls convulsions
e	analgesic	b. controls Parkinson's disease
a	anticonvulsant	c. controls fever
f	antiepileptic	d. restores wakefulness
b	antiparkinsonian	e. takes away pain
c	antipyretic	f. controls epilepsy
i	narcotic	g. has action similar to cutting of a parasympathetic nerve
k	narcotic antagonist	h. has action similar to cutting of a sympathetic nerve
g	parasympatholytic	i. capable of producing stupor
l	parasympathomimetic	j. imitates action of a sympathetic nerve
h	sympatholytic	k. reverses action of a narcotic
j	sympathomimetic	l. has action similar to action of parasympathetic nerves

2.

Column A		*Column B*
b	general	a. injected near a nerve to block all sensations
d	topical	b. capable of producing loss of consciousness
c	infiltration	c. injected so it can filter through area to be operated
a	nerve block	d. put on the surface
e	spinal	e. injected into subarachnoid space
f	epidural	f. also known as caudal anesthesia

3.

Column A		*Column B*
g	antidepressant	a. causes sleep
d	hallucinogen	b. change mental activity
a	hypnotic	c. produces feeling of well-being
f	psychostimulant	d. causes illusions
b	psychotropic	e. ability to calm and induce sleep
e	sedative	f. increases activity of the mind
c	tranquilizer	g. used to control depression

4.

Column A		*Column B*
g	sublingual administration	a. ever-present, common, unintended toxic effects of a drug
a	side effects	b. drug that speeds up vital processes
e	pharmacokinetics	c. study of how drugs exert effects on the body
l	nonproprietary name	d. patient factors that make a drug ill-advisable to use
d	contraindication	e. mathematical description of drug disposition in the body
b	stimulant	f. autonomic drug group
i	trade name	g. drug placed under the tongue
f	sympatholytics	h. broad-spectrum antibiotic
h	tetracycline	i. registered name owned by a pharmaceutical company
k	potentiation	j. drug used to prolong blood-clotting time
j	heparin	k. two drugs taken together affect metabolism of one
c	pharmacodynamics	l. name assigned when drug is found functional

Appendix Two Glossary

A glossary is a listing of specialized words with explanations, comments, and in this case, pronunciations. It is not a dictionary and should not discourage or substitute for use of a dictionary. Medical dictionaries give comprehensive lists of words and word elements; they also give entymologic information about words (parts and their origins), pronunciations, some synonyms, and parts of speech (nouns, verbs, adverbs, adjectives, and prepositions).

This glossary contains words introduced in the text, as well as other medical words, to allow as comprehensive a list as possible. Certain compound words that are easily pronounced and have a logical constructable meaning are not listed, but their component elements are. For example, cecoileostomy is not listed, but cecum and ileum are and the suffix *-ostomy* is a commonly used element that means to make a new opening. This omission is intentional to encourage the practice of word building and interpretation, a skill that contributes both to learning and to intellectual growth.

If a word has more than one meaning, each is given and separated from the others by a semicolon. For example, the term cephalad appears as:

cephalad (sef″ ah lad) Referring to the head; toward the head.

As you can see, the term has two meanings separated by a semicolon. When appropriate, a semicolon will also separate a synonym. For example, in the listing:

bifurcate (bi fur′ kāt) Divide into two branches; fork

the synonym, fork, follows the semicolon.

The glossary also contains some secondary word definitions. The primary word is the first word that appears in combination words. For example, in the term adrenal cortex, adrenal is the primary word and cortex is the secondary word. The meaning and pronunciation of adrenal is given and then listed under this is the secondary word (or words) preceded by the first letter of the primary word. The example would appear as:

adrenal (ah dre′ nal) A flattened body above each kidney that secretes steroid hormones. . . .
a. cortex, the outer portion of the adrenal, which makes up the bulk of the gland.

The *a.* stands for adrenal; the secondary word, *cortex,* is then given with its meaning.

Each time you look up a word in this glossary, use the guide to pronunciation that appears in parentheses after the word. Each word is broken down into syllables and spelled phonetically. A macron above a letter (as in the word, sāt) gives it a long sound. The symbol (″) tells you which syllable to emphasize and the symbol (′) also emphasizes a syllable, but to a lesser degree. So, a word like cephalgia is followed by (sef″ al′ je ah). Emphasize the first syllable, *sef,* and briefly pause at the next, *al,* to give it notice to the listener. Pronounce the other syllables as they are spelled. The word, cartilage (kar′ ti lij) is a more common term, so its pronunciation is a little easier to follow. Emphasize the syllable *kar,* then pronounce *ti* and *lij* as they are phonetically spelled.

As with other languages, there are both local and regional variations in pronunciation, called accents. So, words pronounced by others may have slightly different sounds due to different emphases, dependent on the speaker's origin. When this occurs, we suggest you use the local preference over the one presented here.

The authority and validation for this glossary is *Taber's Cyclopedic Medical Dictionary* (12th ed.) Philadelphia: F.A. Davis Company, 1975.

abdominocentesis (ab dom″ i no sen te′ sis) Surgical puncture of the abdomen.

abduction (ab duk′ shun) Drawing away from the median plane or drawing away the digits from the axial line of a limb.

abductor (ab duk′ tor) Any muscle that makes movement away from the midline of the body.

abscess (ab′ ses) A localized collection of pus in a cavity that is formed by disintegration of tissues.

acidosis (as″ i do′ sis) An abnormal condition resulting from accumulation of acid or loss of base from the body.

acrocyanosis (ak″ ro si ah no′ sis) Blue condition of the hands and feet.

acrodermatitis (ak″ ro der″ mah ti′ tis) Inflammation of the skin of the hands or feet.

acromegaly (ak″ ro meg′ ah le) A disorder in which there is abnormal enlargement of the extremities of the skeleton caused by hypersecretion of growth hormone following maturity.

acute (ah kūt′) A condition that is sudden; having symptoms lasting only a short time.

adduction (ad duk′ shun) The act of drawing toward the median plane or drawing the digits toward the axial line of a limb.

adductor (ad duk′ tor) Any muscle responsible for drawing toward the midline of the body.

adenectomy (ad″ e nek′ to me) Surgical removal of a gland.

adenitis (ad″ e ni′ tis) Inflammation of a gland.

adenocarcinoma (ad″ e no kar″ si no′ mah) Cancerous tumor of a gland.

adenoid (ad′ e noid) Resembling a gland; an enlarged mass of lymphoid tissue at the back of the pharynx.

adenoiditis (ad″ e noid i′ tis) Inflammation of the adenoid tissue of the nasopharynx.

adenoma (ad″ e no′ mah) Tumor with a gland-like structure.

adenopathy (ad″ e nop′ ah the) Enlargement of glands, especially of the lymph nodes.

adenosis (ad″ e no′ sis) Any condition of a gland.

adhesion (ad he′ zhun) The sticking together of parts.

adipose (ad′ i pōs) Pertaining to fat; fatty.

adipsia (ah dip′ se ah) Absence of thirst.

adrenal (ah dre′ nal) A flattened body above each kidney that secretes steroid hormones, epinephrine, and norepinephrine.

a. cortex, the outer portion of the adrenal, which makes up the bulk of the gland.

adrenalectomy (ah dre″ nal ek′ to me) Surgical removal of an adrenal gland.

adrenaline (ah dren′ ah lin) A hormone produced by the adrenal glands.

adrenocorticotropic (ad re″ no kor″ te ko trop′ ik) Capable of stimulating the adrenal cortex.

adrenocorticotropin (ad re″ no kor″ te ko trop′ in) Adrenocorticotropic hormone; *ACTH,* the hormone that stimulates the adrenal cortex.

adrenopathy (ad″ ren op′ ah the) Any disease of the adrenal glands.

aerosol (air o sol″) A suspension of fine particles in air or gas.

afebrile (a feb′ ril) Without fever.

afferent (af′ er ent) Conducting toward a specific site or reference.

agglutination (ah gloo″ ti na′ shun) Aggregation of suspended cells into clumps or masses; the process of union in wound healing.

albinism (al bi nizm) Congenital absence of pigment in the skin, hair, and eyes.

albumin (al bu′ min) A protein found in animal tissue; the major serum protein.

albuminuria (al″ bu mi nu′ re ah) The presence of albumin in the urine.

algesia (al je se ah) Sensitivity to pain; hyperesthesia.

alkalosis (al″ kah lo′ sis) Increased alkaline nature of body fluids due to accumulation of base.

allergen (al″ er jen) Any substance that can produce an allergy.

alveolar (al ve′ o lar) Pertaining to the alveoli.

alveolus (al ve′ o lus) A small sac-like dilation.

pulmonary a, one of a cluster of small outpocketings at the end of the bronchioles through which the exchange of carbon dioxide and oxygen takes place.

amblyopia (am″ ble′ o pe ah) Dull vision; without focus.

amenorrhea (ah men″ o re′ ah) Absence of menstruation.

amniocentesis (am″ ne o sen te′ sis) Puncture of the amnion for the purpose of removing fluid.

analgesic (an″ al je′ zik) A remedy for pain; a medication that relieves pain.

anaphylaxis (an″ ah fi lak′ sis) An unusual or exaggerated reaction to a substance that is foreign to the body.

androgen (an″ dro jen) Male sex hormone.

anemia (ah ne′ me ah) A condition in which the blood is deficient in red blood cells and (or) hemoglobin.

anesthesia (an″ es the′ ze ah) Having no feeling or sensation.

aneurysm (an′ u rizm) A sac formed by localized dilation of an artery, a vein, or the heart; a weakened dilated blood vessel wall.

angiectasis (an″ je ek′ tah sis) The dilation of a blood vessel.

angiectomy (an″ je ek′ to me) Removal or resection of a vessel.

angiitis (see angitis).

angina pectoris (an ji′ nah pek′ to res) Severe pain and constriction within the heart caused by insufficient supply of blood.

angiocarditis (an″ je o kard′ i tis) Inflammation of the large blood vessels of the heart.

angiography (an″ je og′ rah fe) Roentgenography of body vessels.

angioma (an″ je o′ mah) Tumor of a vessel.

angiopathy (an je op′ ah the) Any disease of the vessels.

angiospasm (an′ je o spazm″) Spasmodic contraction of the blood vessels.

angiostomy (an″ je os′ to me) Surgical formation of a new opening in a blood vessel.

angiotomy (an″ je ot′ o me) Incision or severing of a blood or lymph vessel.

angitis (ang′ i tis) Inflammation of a blood vessel.

anisocytosis (an ih″ so si to′ sis) A condition in which cells are not of equal size.

ankylodactylia (ang′ ki lo dak til e ah) Fusion of the bones of the fingers and toes.

ankylosed (ang′ ki lōsd) Stiffened; fused joint.

ankylosis (ang″ ki lo′ sis) A stiff condition; joint fixation due to pathological changes.

anophthalmia (an″ of thal′ me ah) A developmental abnormality characterized by absence of eyes.

anorchidism (an or′ kid izm) Absence of testes.

anorchism (an or′ kizm) Congenital absence of the testes, either unilaterally or bilaterally.

anorectic (an″ or ek′ tik) An appetite suppressant.

anorexia (an′ o rek′ se ah) Lack or loss of appetite for food.

a. nervosa, loss of appetite caused by emotional upset.

anorexic (an″ o rek′ sik) Pertaining to loss of appetite for food.

anotia (an o′ she ah) Congenital absence of the external ears.

anoxia (an nok′ se ah) Oxygen deficiency.

antepartum (an″ te par′ tum) Before parturition (giving birth).

anterior (an ter′ e or) Situated in front or in the forward part of an organism.

antibacterial (an″ ti bak te′ re al) Stopping the growth of bacteria.

antibiotic (an″ ti bi ot′ ik) A medication that destroys microorganisms.

antibody (an′ ti bod″ e) An immunoglobulin molecule produced by the body that interacts only with a specific antigen (protein substance).

anticoagulant (an″ ti ko ag′ u lant) Acting to prevent blood clotting; any substance that delays or prevents blood clotting.

anticonvulsive (an″ ti kon vul′ siv) An agent that suppresses convulsions.

antidepressant (an″ ti de pres′ ant) Medication used to prevent depression.

antidiuretic hormone (an′ ti dye ure etic) A hormone produced by the hypothalamus that decreases the amount of water lost in urination.

antigen (an′ ti jen) Any substance that is capable of inducing antibody formation and of reacting specifically with antibodies.

antihistamine (an″ ti his′ tah mēn) A drug that counteracts the effects of histamines produced by the body.

anti-inflammatory (an″ ti in flam′ ah to″ re)

Counteracting inflammation; an agent that relieves inflammation.

antimycotic (an″ ti mi kot′ ik) Antifungal; destructive to fungi.

antipsychotic (an″ ti si kot′ ik) Medication used in the treatment of psychoses.

antipyretic (an″ ti pi ret′ ik) Effective against fever.

antisepsis (an″ ti sep′ sis) The prevention of infection by destroying or inhibiting the growth of microorganisms.

antiseptic (an″ ti sep′ tik) A substance that will destroy or inhibit the growth of microorganisms.

antitoxin (an″ ti tok′ sin) Antibody produced in response to a toxin that neutralizes its effects.

antrum (an″ trum) The chamber inside the entrance to the duodenum.

anuria (ah nu′ re ah) Absence of urination; usually the production of less than 100 *ml.* of urine per day.

aortopathy (a″ or top′ ah the) Any disease of the aorta.

aphagia (ah fa′ je ah) Loss of the power to swallow.

aphasia (ah fa′ se ah) Defect or loss of expression by speech.

aphasic (ah fa′ zik) A person affected with aphasia.

aphonia (a fo′ ne ah) Loss of voice.

aplasia (ah pla′ zhe ah) Incomplete or defective development.

aplastic (ah plas′ tik) Having no tendency to develop new tissue; without growth.

apnea (ap ne′ ah) Absence of breathing.

appendectomy (ap″ en dek′ to me) Surgical removal of the vermiform appendix.

arachnoid (ah rak′ noid) The middle of three coverings (meninges) of the brain.

arrhythmia (ah rith′ me ah) Irregularity of the pulse.

arterial (ar te′ re al) Pertaining to an artery or arteries.

arteriectasis (ar″ te re ek′ tah sis) Dilation of an artery; usually involves lengthening.

arteriole (ar te′ re ol) One of the fine divisions of the arterial branches.

arteriopathy (ar″ te re op′ ah the) Any disease of the arteries.

arteriorrhexis (ar te″ re o rek′ sis) Rupture of an artery.

arteriosclerosis (ar te″ re o skle ro′ sis) Thickening and loss of elasticity in the walls of arteries.

arthralgia (ar thral′ je ah) Pain in a joint.

arthrectomy (ar threk′ to me) Surgical removal of a joint.

arthritis (ar thri′ tis) Inflammation of the joint(s).

arthrocentesis (ar″ thro sen te′ sis) Surgical puncture of a joint.

arthrochondritis (ar″ thro kon dri′ tis) Inflammation of cartilage and a joint.

arthroclasia (ar″ thro kla′ ze ah) Breaking down of a stiff joint to enable free movement.

arthrodesis (ar″ thro′ de sis) Surgical fusion of a joint.

arthrodynia (ar″ thro din′ e ah) Painful joint.

arthrographia (ar″ throg′ rah fea) X-ray of a joint after injection of an opaque substance.

arthrosclerosis (ar″ thro skle ro′ sis) Hardening of a joint.

arthroscope (ar′ thro skōp) An instrument for examining the interior of a joint.

arthroscopy (ar thros′ kō pe) Examination of the interior of a joint using an arthroscope.

arthrotomy (ar throt′ o me) Incision of a joint.

articular (ar tik′ u lar) Pertaining to a joint.

articulation (ar tik″ u la′ shun) The place of union between two or more bones; joint.

asepsis (a sep′ sis) Absence of infection.

asymptomatic (a″ simp″ to mat′ ik) Without symptoms.

asystole (ah sis′ to le) Cardiac arrest; absence of a heartbeat.

atelectasis (a te lek′ ta sis) Incomplete dilation of a lung.

atherosclerosis (ath″ er o″ skle ro′ sis) A form of arteriosclerosis with fatty degeneration in the walls of arteries.

atoxic (ah tok′ sik) Not poisonous; not due to a toxin (poison).

atrial (a′ tre al) Pertaining to the atrium.

atrioventricular (a″ tre o ven trik′ u lar) Pertaining to an atrium and ventricle of the heart.

atrium (a′ tre um) A chamber affording entrance to another structure or organ; the upper, smaller cavity on either side of the heart.

atrophy (at′ ro fe) A wasting away; without growth; decrease in size of an organ, tissue, or part.

auditory (aw′ di to″ re) Pertaining to the sense of hearing.

a. tube, the narrow channel connecting the middle ear and the nasopharynx; eustachian tube.

auscultation (aws″ kul ta′ shun) Listening to sounds of the body.

autopsy (aw′ top se) The postmortem examination of a body to determine the cause of death.

axilla (ak sil′ ah) The armpit.

axillary (ak′ si lar″ e) Of or pertaining to the armpit.

axon (ak′ son) A process of a nerve cell that conducts impulses away from the cell body.

bactericidal (bak tēr i″ si′ dal) Capable of killing bacteria.

bacteriostatic (bak tē″ re o stat′ ik) Stopping the growth of bacteria.

base (bās) A substance that combines with acids to form salts.

bifurcate (bi fur′ kāt) Divide into two branches; fork.

bilateral (bi lat′ er al) Pertaining to both sides.

bile (bīl) A fluid secreted by the liver into the small intestine to aid digestion.

biopsy (bi′ op se) Removal and examination, usually microscopic, of tissue from a living body.

bipara (bip′ ah rah) A female who has given birth to two children.

bladder (blad′ der) A membranous sac serving as a receptacle for secretions.

blepharadenoma (blef″ ar′ aden oma) A glandular tumor of the eyelid.

blepharal (blef′ ah ral) Pertaining to the eyelid.

blepharedema (blef″ ar e de′ mah) Swelling of the eyelids.

blepharitis (blef″ ah ri′ tis) Inflammation of the eyelid.

blepharoplasty (blef′ ah ro plas te) Plastic surgery of the eyelid.

blepharoptosis (blef″ ah ro to′ sis) Drooping of the eyelid; ptosis.

blepharospasm (blef′ ah ro spazm″) Twitching of the eyelid.

borborygmus (bor″ bor′ ig mus) Rumbling and gurgling sounds made by gas in the intestines.

brachypnea (brā key′ ne ah) Shortness of breath.

bradycardia (brād″ e kar′ de ah) Slow heartbeat; slow pulse.

bradykinesia (brād″ e ki ne′ se ah) Slow movement; sluggishness of physical or mental responses.

bradyphasia (brād′ e fa′ ze ah) Slow speech.

bradypnea (brād″ e ne′ ah) Slow breathing.

bronchiectasis (brong ke ek′ tah sis) Dilation of the bronchi.

bronchiole (brong′ ke ōl) One of the fine divisions of the bronchial tree.

bronchiolectasis (brong″ ke o lek′ tah sis) Dilation of the bronchioles.

bronchitis (brong ki′ tis) Inflammation of the bronchi.

bronchopneumonia (brong″ ko nu mo′ ne ah) Inflammation of the lungs and bronchi.

bronchus (brong′ kus) Either of the two main branches of the trachea.

bucca (bukka) Inside the cheek.

bulla (bue′ la) A large vesicle.

bursa (ber′ sah) Sacs or pouches of fluid situated in tissues where friction would otherwise occur, especially near joints.

cachexia (kah kek′ se ah) A profound state of general ill health and malnutrition.

calcaneal (kal ka′ ne al) Pertaining to the calcaneum or heel bone.

calcification (kal″ si fi ka′ shun) Process where tissue becomes hardened by a calcium deposit.

calculus (kal′ ku lus) An abnormal deposit in hollow organs or in their passages.

capillary (kap′ ill ar″ e) One of the minute vessels connecting the arterioles and venules.

carcinogen (kar sin′ o jen) Any substance that can produce cancer.

carcinogenesis (kar″ si no jen′ e sis) The origin of cancer.

carcinogenic (kar″ si no jen′ ik) Pertaining to that which causes cancer.

carcinoma (kar″ si no′ mah) A malignant tumor; cancerous cell.

basal cell c., an epidermoid carcinoma common to the face in the elderly and having a low degree of malignancy.

cardiac (kar′ de ak) Pertaining to the heart.

c. arrest, ceasing of heart activity.

c. arrhythmia, irregular heart action.

c. insufficiency, inadequate functioning of the heart.

cardiectomy (kar″ di ek′ to me) Surgical removal of the upper end of the stomach.

cardiocentesis (kar″ de o sen te′ sis) Surgical puncture of the heart.

cardiogram (kar′ de o gram″) A tracing produced by the electrical impulses of the heart.

cardiomyopathy (kar″ de o mi op′ ah the) Any disease of the heart.

cardiorrhexis (kar″ de o rek′ sis) Rupture of the heart.

cardiotomy (kar″ de ot′ o me) Incision of the heart.

carditis (kar di′ tis) Inflammation of the heart.

carpal (kar′ pal) Pertaining to the carpus or wrist.

carpectomy (kar pek′ to me) Surgical removal of the wrist bones.

carpus (kar′ pus) The wrist; the joint between the arm and hand.

cartilage (kar′ ti lij) Fibrous connective tissue.

cathartic (kath ar′ tik) A drug or action that causes purging; laxative.

catheter (kath′ e ter) A flexible tube passed through a body channel such as a blood vessel or the urethra.

cecum (se′ kum) The first part of the large intestine, extending from the ileum to the colon.

cementum (se men′ tum) The bone-like connective tissue that covers the root of a tooth.

central nervous system The brain and the spinal cord.

cephalad (sef″ ah lad) Referring to the head; toward the head.

cephalgia (sef″ al′ je ah) Headache.

cephalodynia (sef″ ah lo din′ e ah) Pain in the head; headache.

cerebellar (ser″ e bel′ ar) Pertaining to the cerebellum, the part of the brain concerned with coordination of movements.

cerebral (ser′ e bral, se re′ bral) Pertaining to the cerebrum.

c. aneurysm, a thin sac filled with blood on the wall of an artery in the brain.

c. cortex, the convoluted layer of gray matter covering each hemisphere of the brain.

c. palsy, a brain disorder characterized by paralysis and lack of muscular coordination.

cerebrovascular (ser″ e bro vas′ ku lar) Pertaining to the blood vessels of the cerebrum.

c. accident, a condition involving the blood vessels of the brain; a stroke.

cerebrum (ser′ e brum, se re′ brum) The main portion of the brain, occupying the upper part of the skull.

cervical (ser′ vi kal) Pertaining to the neck or to the cervix.

cervicocolpitis (ser″ vi ko kol pi′ tis) Inflammation of the cervix and vagina.

cervix (ser′ viks) Neck; a constricted portion of an organ.

c. uteri, the narrow lower end of the uterus.

cesarean section (se sa′ re an) Incision through the abdominal and uterine walls for the purpose of delivering a child; also called c-section.

cheilitis (ki li′ tis) Inflammation of the lip.

cheiloplasty (ki′ lo plas″ te) Surgical repair of a defect of the lip.

cheilosis (ki″ lo′ sis) Splitting and scaling of the lips and angles of the mouth.

cheilostomatoplasty (ki″ lo sto mat′ o plas″ te) Plastic surgery of the lips and mouth.

chirospasm (ki′ ro spazm) Cramping of the hand; writer's cramp.

cholecyst (ko′ le sist) The gallbladder.

cholecystectomy (ko″ le sis tek′ to me) Surgical removal of the gallbladder.

cholecystography (ko″ le sis tog′ rah fe) X-ray examination of the gallbladder.

cholelith (ko′ le lith) A gallstone.

cholelithiasis (ko″ le li thi′ ah sis) The presence of gallstones.

cholestasis (ko″ le sta′ sis) Suppression of bile flow.

chondral (kon′ dral) Pertaining to cartilage.

chondrectomy (kon drek′ to me) Surgical removal of cartilage.

chondroid (kon′ droid) Resembling cartilage.

chondrolysis (kon drol′ i sis) Destruction of cartilage.

chorion (ko′ re on) The outermost membrane that forms the fetal part of the placenta.

chronic (kron′ ik) Showing little change or slow progression over a long period of time.

chyme (kime) A liquid-like mass of food in the stomach.

cilia (sil″ e ah) A hair or hair-like projection; eyelash.

circumcision (ser″ kum sizh′ un) Surgical removal of all or part of the foreskin.

cirrhosis (sir ro′ sis) A chronic liver disease characterized by degeneration and hardening of liver cells.

clitoris (klit′ o ris) A small erectile body in the female that is sensually homologous to the male penis.

coagulation (ko ag″ u la′ shun) Formation of a clot.

coccyx (kok′ siks) The tail bone; the small bone that forms the distal end of the vertebral column.

colic (kol′ ik) Painful spasm of the large intestine.

colitis (ko li′ tis) Inflammation of the large intestine.

mucus c., colitis; also called spastic colitis, irritable colon, or functional bowel distress.

ulcerative c., a chronic ulceration in the colon.

colon (ko′ lon) The part of the large intestine extending from the cecum to the rectum.

colopexy (ko′ lo pek″ se) Surgical fixation of the large intestine to the abdominal wall.

coloproctitis (ko″ lo prok ti′ tis) Inflammation of the large intestine and rectum.

coloptosis (ko″ lop to′ sis) Downward displacement of the colon.

colostomy (ko los′ to me) Surgical formation of a new opening from the large intestine.

colostrum (ko los′ trum) The thin, milky fluid secreted by the mammary gland the first few days following birth.

colpitis (kol pi′ tis) Inflammation of the vagina; vaginitis.

colpodynia (kol″ po din′ e ah) Vaginal pain.

colpohysterectomy (kol″ po his″ ter ek′ to me) Surgical removal of the uterus by way of the vagina.

colporrhagia (kol″ po ra′ je ah) Vaginal hemorrhage.

colporrhaphy (kol por′ ah fe) Suture of the vagina.

coma (ko′ mah) A profound unconsciousness from which the patient cannot be aroused.

commissure (ko′ miss′ ure) Coming together of two structures.

concussion (kon kush′ un) An injury resulting

from impact with an object; loss of function associated with a blow or fall.

congenital (kon jen′ it al) Present or existing from the time of birth.

congestive (kon jes′ tiv) Pertaining to or associated with abnormal accumulation of blood in a body part.

c. heart failure, a condition characterized by weakness, breathlessness, and edema in lower portions of the body.

contraindication (kon′ trah in″ di ka′ shun) Any condition that renders some particular line of treatment improper or undesirable.

contusion (kon′ tu shun) A condition in which tissue beneath the skin is injured but the skin is not broken.

contralateral (kon″ trah lat′ er al) Associated with a particular part on an opposite side.

corium (ko′ re um) The dermis; the layer of skin lying under the epidermis.

coronary (kor′ o na re) Encircling in the manner of a crown or corona, especially the arteries of the heart.

corpus (kor pus) A column.

c. cavernosum, a long column of erectile tissue on each side of the penis.

c. spongiosum, a column of erectile tissue forming the urethra.

cortex (kor teks) The outer layer of an organ.

adrenal c., the outer portion of the adrenal gland that makes up the bulk of this gland.

cerebral c., the convoluted layer of gray matter covering each cerebral hemisphere.

costal (kos′ tal) Pertaining to the ribs.

costalgia (kos tal′ je ah) Pain in the ribs.

costectomy (kos tek′ to me) Removal of a rib.

craniectomy (kra″ ne ek′ to me) Excision of a skull segment.

craniocele (kra′ ne o sēl) Protrusion of the brain through a defect in the skull.

craniotomy (kra″ ne ot′ o me) Cutting into the skull.

cranium (kra′ ne um) The skull.

cretinism (kre′ tin izm) A condition, due to congenital lack of thyroid secretion, that causes arrested physical and mental development.

cryosurgery (kri″ o sur′ jer e) Destruction of tissue through application of extreme cold.

cryotherapy (kri″ o ther′ ah pe) Treatment of tissue using cold temperatures.

cryptorchidism (krip tor′ kid izm) A developmental defect in which the testicles remain in the abdominal cavity; undescended testicles.

curettage (ku′ rē tahzh′) Scraping of a cavity; curettement; commonly referred to as D&C—D is short for dilation.

cutaneous (ku ta′ ne us) Pertaining to the skin.

cyanoderma (si″ ah no der′ mah) Blueness of the skin; also cyanosis (si″ ah no′ sis).

cyanopia (si″ ah no′ pe ah) A visual defect in which all objects appear blue.

cyanotic (si ah not′ ik) Pertaining to a blue skin condition.

cyst (sist) Any sac containing a fluid that develops abnormally in the body.

cystectomy (sis tek′ to me) Excision of a cyst.

cystitis (sis ti′ tis) Inflammation of the bladder.

cystocele (sis′ to sēl) Herniation of the urinary bladder into the vagina.

cystoclysis (sis″ tok′ li sis) Irrigation of the bladder.

cystorrhexis (sis″ to rek′ sis) Rupture of the bladder.

dacryocyst (dak′ re o sist″) The lacrimal sac; tear sac.

dacryocystitis (dak″ re o sis ti′ tis) Inflammation of the lacrimal sac.

dactylitis (dak″ ti li′ tis) Inflammation of a finger or toe.

dactylospasm (dak′ ti lo spazm) Cramp or twitching of the fingers or toes.

decalcification (de″ kal si fi ka′ shun) The loss of calcium.

decubitus ulcer (de ku′ bi tus) A bedsore or ulceration due to prolonged pressure from lying too still in bed for too long a time.

defibrillator (de fib″ ri la′ tor) An apparatus used to stop fibrillation through brief electro-shocks to the heart.

dehydrate (de hi′ drāt) To remove water.

dementia (de men′ she ah) Loss of intellectual function due to organic brain disease.

dendrite (den′ drīt) One of the thread-like extensions of the cytoplasm of a neuron.

dentalgia (den tal′ je ah) Toothache.

dentin (den′ tin) The chief substance of the teeth that surrounds the tooth pulp and is covered by enamel on the crown and by cementum on the roots.

depression (de presh′ un) A hollow or lowered area; a decrease of functional activity; a sense of dejection or melancholy.

dermabrasion (der mah bra′ shun) A surgical procedure that uses an abrasive disk or other mechanical method to plane the skin.

dermatitis (der″ mah ti′ tis) Inflammation of the skin.

dermatoma (der mah to′ mah) Tumor of the skin.

dermatosis (der″ mah to′ sis) Any skin condition.

dermis (der′ mis) The layer of skin that lives beneath the outermost layer, the epidermis.

diabetes mellitus (di″ ah be′ tēz mel′ it us) A disorder of carbohydrate metabolism that is a result of inadequate production or utilization of insulin.

dialysis (di al′ i sis) The artificial diffusion of blood across a semipermeable membrane to remove toxic materials and to maintain proper balances of fluid and blood electrolytes.

diaphoresis (di″ ah fo re′ sis) Sweating or perspiring, usually profusely.

diaphragm (di′ ah fram) The muscular partition that separates the chest and abdominal cavities; also a contraceptive device worn over the cervix.

diaphysis (di af′ i sis) The elongated, cylindrical portion (shaft) of a long bone.

diarrhea (di″ ah re′ ah) Abnormal frequency and softness of fecal discharge due to its rapid passage through the bowel.

diastole (di as′ to le) The period of relaxation of the heart.

diathermy (di′ ah ther″ me) A treatment in which heat is passed through body tissues.

diencephalon (di″ en sef′ ah lon) The portion of the brain that consists of the hypothalamus and the thalamus.

digit (dij′ it) A finger or toe; a number less than 10.

dilation (di la′ shun) The condition of being dilated or stretched beyond normal dimensions.

dilation and curettage A surgical procedure in which the uterine wall is scraped (D&C).

diplegia (di ple′ je ah) Paralysis of both sides of the body.

diploid (dip′ loid) Having two sets of chromosomes, as found in the somatic cells.

diplopia (di plo′ pe ah) Perceiving two images of a single object.

disk (disk) A circular or rounded flat plane.
herniated d., rupture of an intervertebral disk.

dislocation (dis lo ka′ shun) Displacement of a bone from a joint.

distal (dis′ tal) Far or distant from the origin or point of attachment.

diuretic (di″ u ret′ ik) Increased urination or an agent (drug) that increases urination.

diverticula (di″ vert′ ik u la) Small pockets in a hollow structure such as in the intestines.

dorsal (dor′ sal) Directed toward or situated on the back surface; the opposite of ventral.

dorsalgia (dor sal′ je ah) Pain in the back.

dorsodynia (dor″ so din′ e ah) Pain in the back.

duct (dukt) A passage with well-defined walls.
hepatic d., duct that carries bile from the liver.
lactiferous d., one that drains the lobe of a mammary gland.
nasolacrimal d., duct that conveys tears from the lacrimal sac to the nasal cavity.

duodenitis (du″ od e ni′ tis) Inflammation of the duodenum.

duodenostomy (du″ od e nos′ to me) Formation of a new opening into the duodenum.

duodenotomy (du″ od e not′ o me) Incision into the duodenum.

duodenum (du″ o de′ num) The part of the small intestine that connects with the stomach.

dura mater (du′ rah ma′ ter) The outermost and toughest of the three membranes of the brain and spinal cord.

dyscrasia (dis kra′ ze ah) An abnormal state or condition.

dysfunction (dis funk′ shun) Any abnormality or difficulty in functioning.

dyskinesia (dis″ ki ne ze ah) Difficult movement.

dysmenorrhea (dis″ men or re′ ah) Painful menstruation.

dyspepsia (dis pep′ se ah) Poor digestion.

dysphagia (dis fa′ je ah) Difficulty in eating.

dysphasia (dis fa′ ze ah) Speech impairment.

dysphonia (dis fo′ ne ah) Difficulty in speaking; weak voice.

dysplasia (dis pla′ se ah) Abnormality in development; abnormal size, shape, and organization of adult cells.

dyspnea (disp′ ne ah) Difficulty in breathing.

dystrophy (dis′ tro fe) Faulty nutrition and development.

dysuria (dis u′ re ah) Difficult or painful urination.

echocardiogram (ek″ o kar′ de o gram″) Record of the heart produced by an echocardiograph from ultrasound waves that echo through the chest wall.

ectoenzyme (ek″ to en′ zīm) An enzyme that is secreted from a cell into the medium surrounding it.

ectogenous (ek toj′ ē nus) Arising from causes outside the organism; exogenous.

ectopic (ek top′ ik) Out of the usual place.
e. pregnancy, the implantation of a fertilized egg in any place other than the uterus.

eczema (ek″ zee′ mah) A skin condition in which fluid is excreted through the skin.

edema (eh de′ mah) An abnormal accumulation of fluid in intercellular spaces in the tissues.

efferent (ef′ er ent) Conveying away from a center.

effusion (e fu′ zhun) The escape of fluid into a part or tissue; an effused material.

electrocardiogram (e lek″ tro kar′ de o gram″) A tracing produced by the electrical impulses of the heart (*ECG* or *EKG*).

electroencephalogram (e lek″ tro en sef′ ah lo gram) A record produced by the electrical impulses of the brain (*EEG*).

embolectomy (em″ bo lek′ to me) Surgical removal of an embolis lodged in a blood vessel.

embolism (em′ bo lizm) The blocking of a vessel by a clot or other material brought there by the blood.

embolus (em′ bo lus) A clot or other plug brought by the blood and forced into a smaller vessel where it lodges and obstructs circulation.

emesis (em′ e sis) Vomiting.

emetic (e′ met ik) That which causes vomiting.

emphysema (em″ fi se′ mah) A pulmonary disease characterized by destruction of alveolar walls and loss of elasticity.

encephalitis (en″ sef ah li′ tis) Inflammation of the brain; sleeping sickness.

encephalocele (en sef′ ah lo sēl) Hernial protrusion of brain through a congenital or traumatic opening of the skull.

encephaloma (en″ sef ah lo′ mah) Tumor of the brain.

encephalomeningitis (en sef″ ah lo men″ in ji′ tis) Inflammation of the brain and its membranes.

encephalomyelitis (en sef″ ah lo mi″ e li′ tis) Inflammation involving both the brain and the spinal cord.

encephalomyelopathy (en sef″ ah lo mi″ e lop′ ah the) A disease involving the brain and the spinal cord.

endocardial (en″ do kar′ de al) Pertaining to the endocardium; situated or occurring within the heart.

endocarditis (en″ do kar di′ tis) Inflammation of the inner lining of the heart.

endocardium (en″ do kar′ de um) The membrane lining the inner surface of the heart.

endodontium (en″ do don′ she um) Dental pulp.

endogenous (en doj′ e nus) Produced within or caused by factors within an organism.

endometriosis (en″ do me″ tre o′ sis) Ectopic endometrium (uterine lining) usually in the pelvic cavity (causing irritation).

endometritis (en″ do me′ tri′ tis) Inflammation of the lining of the uterus.

endometrium (en do me′ tre um) The membrane lining the uterus.

enteral (en′ ter al) Pertaining to the small intestine.

enteritis (en″ ter i′ tis) Inflammation of the small intestine.

enterocele (en′ ter o sēl) Any hernia of the intestine.

enteroclysis (en″ ter ok′ li sis) Irrigation of the intestine.

enteroplegia (en″ ter o ple′ je ah) Paralysis of the intestine.

enterostasis (en″ ter o sta′ sis) The stoppage of food in its passage through the intestine.

epidermis (ep″ i der′ mis) The outermost layer of the skin.

epididymis (ep″ i did′ ē mis) The elongated structure along the posterior border of the testis.

epiglottis (ep″ i glot′ is) The lid-like structure composed of cartilage that covers the larynx during swallowing.

epinephrine (ep″ i nef′ rin) A hormone secreted by the adrenal medulla; adrenalin.

epiphysis (e pif′ i sis) Either end of a long bone.

eructation (e ruk tay shun) Belching of air from the stomach; burping.

erythema (er″ i the′ mah) Abnormal redness of the skin.

erythrocyte (e rith′ ro sīt) A red blood cell.
e. count, the number of red blood cells in a blood sample.

erythrocytopenia (e rith″ ro si″ to pe′ ne ah) A deficiency in the number of red blood cells; anemia.

erythrocytosis (e rith′ ro si to′ sis) An increase in the number of red blood cells.

erythroderma (e rith″ ro der′ mah) Abnormal redness of the skin.

erythropenia (e rith″ ro pe′ ne ah) A deficiency in the number of red blood cells.

erythropia (er″ e thro′ pe ah) A visual defect in which all objects appear to be red in color.

erythropoiesis (e rith″ ro poi e′ sis) The production of red blood cells.

eschar (es kār) A hard crust or scab that forms after a traumatic injury.

esophagomalacia (e sof′ ah go mah la′ she ah) Softening of the esophagus.

esophagus (e sof′ ah gus) A muscular canal extending from the throat to the stomach.

eupepsia (u pep′ se ah) Normal digestion.

euphoria (u fo′ re ah) A sense of well being; absence of distress.

eupnea (u ne′ ah) Normal breathing.

eustacean tube (u sta′ she an) The auditory tube extending from the middle ear chamber to the pharynx.
euthanasia (u″ thah na′ zhe ah) Painless death.
exacerbation (eks″ aser ba shun′) A disease that becomes increasingly severe.
exogenous (eks oj′ e nus) Developed or originating outside the organism.
exophthalmos (ek″ sof thal′ mos) Abnormal protrusion of the eyeball.
expectorate (ek spek′ to rate) To cough up and spit.
expiration (eks″ per a′ shun) The act of expelling air from the lungs; death.
extension (ek sten′ shun) The movement that brings the members of a limb into or toward a straight condition.
extensor (eks ten′ sor) Any muscle that extends a joint.
extracellular (eks″ trah sel′ u lar) Situated or occurring outside a cell.
extrauterine (eks″ trah u′ ter in) Outside the uterus.

fascia (fas she ah) A sheet of fibrous tissue.
fascicle (fas sickle) A small bundle of tissue.
femoral (fem′ or al) Pertaining to the femur (thigh bone).
fertilization (fer′ ti li za′ shun) Rendering gametes fertile or capable of further development.
fetus (fe′ tus) Name for the unborn offspring from seven to eight weeks after fertilization until birth.
fiberoptics (fi″ ber op′ tiks) The transmission of an image along flexible bundles of parallel glass or plastic fibers.
fibrillation (fib ri la′ shun) Involuntary muscular contraction due to spontaneous activation of single muscle cells or fibers.
ventricular f., cardiac arrhythmia marked by rapid, ineffective contractions of the ventricles.
fibrinogen (fi brin′ o jen) A protein in plasma that is essential for clotting of blood.
fibroid (fi′ broid) Resembling a fiber (a tough thread-like material); a fibroma is a small benign tumor of the uterus, usually called fibroids.
fissure (fish′ ūr) A split, cleft, or groove.
fistula (fis′ tu lah) An abnormal communication (opening between two internal organs).
flexion (flek′ shun) Being bent.
flexor (flek′ sore) Any muscle that flexes a joint.
fracture (frak′ chur) A break or rupture in a bone.
communicated f., the bone is crushed or splintered.
compound f., causing a break in the skin.
greenstick f., one side of a bone is broken, the other intact (usually in children).
impacted f., one fragment is firmly driven into the other.
oblique f., slanted, between the direction of and at a right angle to the axis of the bone.
open f., accompanied by a wound through the overlying or adjacent soft tissues, communicates with the site of the break.
transverse f., at right angles to the axis of the bone.
frontal (frun′ tal) Pertaining to the forehead; a plane that divides the body into anterior and posterior portions.
fundus (fun′ dus) The upper portion of the stomach toward the left side.

gallbladder (gawl′ blad er) The reservoir for bile on the posterioinferior surface of the liver.
ganglion (gang′ le on) A knot-like mass; a general term for a group of nerve cells located outside the central nervous system.
gastralgia (gas tral′ je ah) Pain in the stomach; stomachache.
gastrectomy (gas trek′ to me) Removal of all or part of the stomach.
gastric (gas′ trik) Pertaining to the stomach.
gastroenteritis (gas″ tro en ter i′ tis) Inflammation of the stomach and intestines.
gastrointestinal (gas″ tro in tes′ tin al) Pertaining to the stomach and the intestines.
gastromegaly (gas″ tro meg′ ah le) Enlargement of the stomach.
gastrostomy (gas tros′ to me) The creation of a new opening into the stomach.
genitalia (jen″ i tāl′ e ah) The reproductive organs.
gingiva (jin′ ji vah) The gums; the mucus membrane, with supporting and fibrous tissue, that covers the tooth-bearing portion of the jaw.
gingivitis (jin″ ji vi′ tis) Inflammation of the gum.
gingivoglossitis (jin″ ji vo gloss si′ tis) Inflammation of the gums and tongue.
gingivostomatitis (jin″ ji vo sto″ mah ti′ tis) Inflammation of the gums and mouth.
gland (gland) An aggregation of specialized cells that secrete material unrelated to their ordinary needs.
adrenal g., a flattened body above the kidneys that secretes steroid hormones, epinephrine, and norepinephrine.
endocrine g., a gland that secretes hormones directly into the blood.
lacrimal g., the gland that secretes tears.

mammary g., the milk-secreting organ.

parathyroid g., four glands that lie beside the thyroid and are responsible for secreting hormones that regulate calcium and phosphorus.

parotid g., a paired salivary gland anterior to the ear.

pituitary g., the hypophysis, a small, oval, two-lobed body at the base of the brain that regulates other glands by secreting hormones.

salivary g., glands of the oral cavity that secrete saliva.

sebaceous g., skin glands that secrete sebum to keep the skin and hair flexible.

sublingual g., salivary gland that lies under the tongue.

submaxillary g., salivary gland on each side of the jaw.

sweat g., a gland in the skin that produces perspiration.

thyroid g., a gland anterior in the neck that produces hormones for growth and metabolism.

globulin (glob′ u lin) A type of protein found in blood.

glomerulonephritis (glo mer″ u lo ne fri′ tis) A type of nephritis in which there is inflammation of the loops in the glomeruli.

glomerulus (glo mer′ u lus) A small cluster of blood vessels or nerve fibers; one of the renal glomeruli that acts as a filter.

glossal (glos′ al) Pertaining to the tongue.

glossectomy (glos sek′ to me) Surgical removal of the tongue.

glossopharyngeal (gloss″ o fah rin′ je al) Pertaining to the tongue and the throat.

glottis (glot′ tis) The vocal apparatus of the larynx.

glycemia (gli se′ me ah) The presence of sugar in the blood.

glycolysis (gli kol′ i sis) The breaking down of glycogen.

glycosuria (gli′ ko su re ah) The presence of sugar in urine.

goiter (goy′ ter) Enlargement of the thyroid gland that often gives a grotesque swelling to the neck.

exophthalmic g., goiter accompanied by a protrusion of the eyeballs, due to hyperthyroidism.

gonad (go′ nad) Ovary or testis.

grafting (graft′ ing) The implanting or transplanting of any organ or tissue.

gravid (grav′ id) Pregnant.

gravida (grav′ i dah) A pregnant woman.

gynecologic (gi″ ne ko loj′ ik) Pertaining to females.

heliotherapy (he″ le o ther′ ah pe) Treatment of disease by exposing the body to sunlight.

hemangioma (he man″ je o mah) A benign tumor composed of newly formed blood vessels that pool together.

hematemesis (hem″ ah tem′ e sis) Vomiting of blood.

hematocrit (he mat′ o krit) A lab test to determine the volume percentage of red blood cells in whole blood.

hematoma (hem″ ah to′ mah) Any localized collection of blood in an organ, tissue, or space.

hematopoiesis (hem″ ah to poi e′ sis) The formation and development of blood cells.

hematuria (hem″ ah tu′ re ah) The presence of blood in the urine.

hemiplegia (hem′ e ple′ je ah) Paralysis of one side of the body.

hemodialysis (he″ mo di al′ i sis) The process of diffusing blood through a semipermeable membrane to remove toxic substances.

hemoglobin (he″ mo glo′ bin) The oxygen-carrying red pigment of the blood.

hemolysin (he mol′ ī sin) A substance that causes destruction of red blood cells.

hemopericardium (he″ mo per″ i kar′ de um) An effusion of blood within the pericardium.

hemophilia (he″ mo fil′ e ah) An hereditary hemorrhagic disorder.

hemoptysis (he mop′ ti sis) The spitting of blood or blood-stained sputum.

hemorrhage (hem′ or ij) Bleeding.

hemorrhoid (hem′ o roid) A varicose dilation of a vein in the anus.

hemostasis (he″ mo sta′ sis) Stopping the flow of blood through coagulation or surgical means; interruption of blood flow through any vessel or to any part of the body.

hemothorax (he″ mo tho′ raks) A collection of blood in the chest.

hepatic (hep at′ ik) Pertaining to the liver.

hepatitis (hep ah ti′ tis) Inflammation of the liver, usually causing jaundice (yellowing).

hepatomegaly (hep″ ah to meg′ ah le) Enlargement and tenderness of the liver.

hernia (her′ ne ah) Protrusion of an organ, or part of it, through the wall of the cavity that houses it.

femoral h., an organ passes through the femoral ring under the inguinal ligament.

hiatal h., protrusion of any structure through the esophageal hiatus of the diaphragm.

inguinal h., hernia in the groin above the inguinal ligament.

umbilical h., protrusion at the navel; omphalocele.

incisional h., protrusion occurs at the site of an incision.

strangulated h., protruding part is squeezed to the point where circulation is cut off.

hidradenitis (hi″ drad e ni′ tis) Inflammation of a sweat gland.

hidradenoma (hi″ drad e no′ mah) Tumor of a sweat gland.

hidrosis (hi″ dro′ sis) Formation and excretion of sweat; profuse perspiration.

histolysis (his tol′ i sis) The destruction of tissue.

historrhexis (his″ to rek′ sis) The breaking down of tissues.

hives (hives) Itchy areas of the skin.

homeostasis (ho′ me o sta sis) Sameness or stability in the normal body state of an organism; equilibrium.

homologous (ho′ mol o jus) Referring to the same fundamental structure.

hormone (hor′ moan) A chemical substance produced in the body that has a specific effect on the cavity of cells or organs.

humeral (hu′ mer al) Pertaining to the humerus (bone of the upper arm).

hydrocele (hi″ dro sēl) Water hernia in a swelling, especially of the male gonads.

hydrocephaly, hydrocephalus (hi″ dro sef′ ah le) A condition due to an abnormal accumulation of cerebrospinal fluid within the skull, resulting in an enlarged head and subsequent mental retardation.

hypalgesia (hi″ pal je′ ze ah) Decreased sensitivity to pain.

hyperadrenalism (hi′ per ah dre′ nal izm) Increased activity of the adrenal glands.

hyperalgesia (hi″ per al je′ ze ah) Excessive sensitivity to pain; also hyperalgia.

hyperemia (hi″ per e′ me ah) Excessive blood flow to a part of the body.

hyperglycemia (hi″ per gli se′ me ah) An increased amount of sugar in the blood.

hyperkeratosis (hi″ per ker a to sis) Excessive growth of the horny layer of skin.

hyperlipemia (hi″ per li pe′ me ah) An increased amount of fat in the blood.

hyperpnea (hi″ per ne′ ah) An abnormal increase in depth and rate of respiration.

hypersomnia (hi″ per som ne ah) Excessive sleep.

hypertension (hi″ per ten′ shun) Increased blood pressure.

hyperthermia (hi″ per ther′ me ah) Increased body temperature.

hyperventilation (hi″ per ven″ ti la′ shun) Abnormally increased pulmonary ventilation, resulting in an imbalance of carbon dioxide metabolism.

hypoalgesia (hi″ po al je′ se ah) Decreased sensitivity to pain.

hypodermic (hi″ po der′ mik) Beneath the skin.

hypoesthesia (hi″ po es″ the′ ze ah) Abnormal decrease in sensitivity to stimuli.

hypoglossal (hi″ po glos′ al) Beneath the tongue.

hypoglycemia (hi″ po gli se′ me ah) Abnormally low blood sugar.

hypophysis (hi pof′ i sis) The pituitary gland.

hypotension (hi″ po ten′ shun) Decreased blood pressure.

hypothalamus (hi″ po thal′ ah mus) The part of the brain most concerned with moderating behavior.

hypothermia (hi″ po ther′ me ah) Low body temperature.

hypoxemia (hi″ pok se′ me ah) Deficient oxygen in the blood.

hypoxia (hi pok′ se ah) A condition of decreased oxygen.

hysterectomy (his″ ter ek′ to me) Removal of the uterus.

hysteropexy (his′ ter o pek se) Surgical fixation of the uterus.

iatrogenic (i′ a′ tro gen ik) A disease that is a side effect of a treatment.

ichthyosis (ik″ the o′ sis) Any of several generalized skin disorders marked by scaliness (like fish scales).

icterus (ik″ ter′ us) A yellow condition of the skin; jaundice.

idiopathic (id″ e o path′ ik) Occurring without known cause.

ileocecal (il″ eo se′ kal) Pertaining to the ileum and cecum.

ileum (il′ e um) The distal portion of the small intestine that extends from the jejunum to the cecum.

iliac (il′ e ak) Pertaining to the ilium (a bone of the pelvic girdle).

immunity (i mu′ ni tee) Being immune; nonsusceptible to the pathogenic effects of certain antigens.

immunoglobulin (im″ u no glob′ u lin) A system of proteins capable of acting as antibodies.

impotence (im″ put ense; im″ poat ence) Inability to experience an erection.

incise (in″ size) To cut into something.

incision (in sizh′ un) A cut or wound produced by a sharp instrument; cutting.

incontinent (in con tin ant) Unable to hold urine.

infarction (in fark′ shun) The formation of a localized area of necrosis, due to insufficient blood supply produced by an occlusion.

myocardial i., death or weakness of an area of the heart muscle, occurring as a result of oxygen deprivation.

inferior (in fēr′ e or) Situated below or directed downward; of lesser quality.

inferomedian (in″ fer o me′ de an) Situated in the middle of the underside.

infirm (in″ ferm) Weak; not well.

infracostal (in″ frah kos′ tal) Below a rib.

inguinal (ing′ gwi nal) Pertaining to the groin.

inspiration (in″ spi ra′ shun) Drawing of air into the lungs.

insulin (in′ su lin) A hormone secreted by the pancreas into the blood.

intercellular (in″ ter sel′ u lar) Between the cells.

intercerebral (in″ ter ser′ e bral) Between the two cerebral hemispheres.

intercostal (in″ ter kos′ tal) Between the ribs.

i. muscles, the muscles that move the ribs when breathing.

interstitial cells (in″ ter stish′ al) Cells located in groups between the seminiferous tubules that produce testosterone.

intervertebral (in″ ter ver′ te bral) Between two contiguous vertebrae.

i. disk, the layer of fibrocartilage between the bodies of adjoining vertebrae.

intracellular (in″ trah sel′ u lar) Within a cell.

intramyocardial (in″ trah mi″ o kar′ de al) Within the heart muscle.

intrathecal (in″ trah the′ kal) Within a sheath or within the spinal cord.

intravenous (in″ trah ve′ nus) Situated within the vein.

i. pyelogram, roentgenogram of the ureter and renal pelvis.

in vitro (in ve′ tro) In an artificial environment, such as a test tube or petri dish.

in vivo (in ve′ voh) Within the living body.

ischial (is′ ke al) Pertaining to the ischium of the pelvis.

ischium (is′ ke um) The inferior, dorsal portion of the hip.

isocyte (i″ so sīt′) A cell that is equal in size to another cell.

isocytosis (i″ so si to′ sis) A condition in which the cells are the same size, especially red blood cells.

isotonic (i″ so tōn′ ik) Equal tension; denoting a solution that has the same tonicity as another solution with which it is compared.

isotope (i′ so toap) A chemical element that has the same atomic number as another but that has a different atomic mass.

jaundice (jawn′ dis) Yellowness of the skin, sclera, and excretions usually due to bile in the blood.

jejunoileostomy (jē joo″ no il e os′ to me) Formation of a new opening between the jejunum and the ileum.

jejunum (jē joo′ num) That portion of the small intestine which extends from the duodenum to the ileum.

joint (join′ t) The site of union between two or more bones.

synovial j., a general classification of joints that have a cavity between articulating bones and are freely moveable.

karyomegaly (kar″ e o meg′ ah le) Abnormal enlargement of the cell nucleus.

keratogenesis (ker″ ah to′ jen′ e sis) The formation of horny material.

keratosis (ker″ ah to′ sis) Any horny growth; a condition of the skin characterized by the formation of horny growths.

ketonuria (ke″ to nu′ re ah) Excretion of ketones in the urine.

kinesiotherapy (ki ne″ se o ther′ ah pe) The treatment of disease by movement or exercise.

labia (la′ be ah) Fleshy edges, usually designated the labia majora and labia minora.

l. majora, a pair of elongated folds running downward from the mons pubis in the female.

l. minora, a small fold of skin located on each side between the labium majus and the opening of the vagina.

lacrimal (lak′ ri mal) Pertaining to tears.

lacrimation (lak″ ri ma′ shun) Secretion and discharge of tears; crying.

lactation (lak ta′ shun) The secretion of milk or the period of milk secretion.

lactiferous (lac tif′ er us) Producing or conveying milk.

lactogenesis (lak″ to jen′ e sis) The formation of milk.

lactogenic (lak″ to jen′ ik) Stimulating the production of milk.

l. hormone, one of the gonadotropic hormones produced by the anterior pituitary that stimulates secretion of milk.

laparocolostomy (lap″ ah ro ko los′ to me) Forming a permanent opening into the colon by an incision in the wall of the abdomen.

laparocolotomy (lap″ ah ro ko lot′ o me) Surgical incision of the colon through the abdominal wall.

laparogastrotomy (lap″ ah ro gas trot′ o me) Incision into the stomach through the abdominal wall.

laparotomy (lap ah rot′ o me) Surgical incision through the abdominal wall.

laryngalgia (lar″ in gal′ je ah) Pain in the larynx.

laryngitis (lar″ in ji′ tis) Inflammation of the voice box.

larynx (lar′ inks) The organ of voice; the air passage between the lower pharynx and the trachea.

lateral (lat′ er al) Pertaining to a side; denoting a position farther from the median plane or midline of the structure.

lavage (lah vahj) The irrigation or washing out of an organ; to wash out or irrigate.

leiomyoma (lay′ o my′ oma) A tumor composed of smooth muscle fibers.

leptodermic (lep″ to der mik) Having thin skin.

leukemia (loo ke′ me ah) A disease of the blood-forming organs characterized by a marked increase in leukocytes.

leukocyte (loo′ ko sīt) A white blood cell.

l. count, the number of white blood cells in a blood sample.

leukocytopenia (loo″ ko si to pe′ ne ah) A deficiency in the number of white blood cells.

leukocytosis (loo″ ko si to′ sis) An increase in the number of white blood cells.

leukopenia (loo″ ko pe′ ne ah) A deficiency in the number of white blood cells.

ligament (lig′ ah ment) A band of fibrous tissue that connects bones or cartilage and serves to support and strengthen joints.

lingual (ling′ gwal) Pertaining to or near the tongue.

lipid (lip′ id) A fat.

lipoid (lip′ oid) Resembling fat.

lipoma (lip″ o′ mah) A tumor composed of fatty tissue.

lipopenia (lip″ o pe′ ne ah) A deficiency of fats in the body.

lithiasis (li thi′ ah sis) A condition marked by formation of stones.

litholysis (li thol′ i sis) The dissolving of a stone.

lithotripsy (lith′ o trip″ se) Surgical crushing of a stone.

lobectomy (lo bek′ to me) Excision of a lobe, as removal of a lobe of the lung, brain, or liver.

lumbar (lum′ bar) Pertaining to the lower back.

lymphadenitis (lim fad″ e ni′ tis) Inflammation of a lymph node.

lymphadenoma (lim fad e no′ mah) A tumor of a lymph node.

lymphangioma (lim fan″ je o′ mah) A tumor composed of newly formed lymph channels.

lymphatics (lim fat′ iks) A system of vessels that collect tissue fluids from all parts of the body and return them to the blood.

lymphocyte (lim′ fo sīt) A white blood cell that is manufactured by lymphatic tissue.

lymphoma (lim fo′ mah) A lymphatic tumor.

macrocephaly (mak″ ro sef′ ah le) An excessively large head.

macrocyte (mak′ ro sīt) A very large cell, usually referring to a very large blood cell.

macrophage (mak′ ro fāj) Any of the highly phagocytic cells in the walls of blood vessels and in loose connective tissue.

macula (mak′ u la) A spot or blotch, usually on the skin.

malabsorption (mal″ ab sorp′ shun) Faulty nutritive absorption.

malacia (mah la′ she ah) A morbid softness or softening of a tissue or a part.

malaise (mal āz) A general feeling of ill health.

malignant (mah lig′ nant) Tending to grow worse and threatening to produce death.

malocclusion (mal″ o kloo zhun) Improper position of the teeth.

mammogram (mam′ o gram) A roentgenogram of the breast.

mammoplasty (mam′ o plas″ te) Surgical repair of the breast.

augmentation m., plastic surgery to increase the size of the breast.

reduction m., plastic surgery to reduce the size of the breast.

mania (ma′ ne ah) A disordered mental state of extreme excitement.

marrow (mar′ o) Soft material that fills the cavity of bones.

mastectomy (mas tek′ to me) Surgical removal of a breast.

mastitis (mas ti′ tis) Inflammation of the breast.

mastocarcinoma (mas″ to kar″ sin o mah) Malignancy of the breast.

mastoptosis (mas″ top to sis) Sagging breasts.

meatus (me ate us) An opening or channel.

medial (me″ de al) Near the midline of the body.

mediastinum (me″ de as ti′ num) A median portion; an area in the middle of the chest.

mediolateral (me″ de o lat′ er al) Pertaining to the middle and to one side.

medulla (me dul′ ah) The innermost part of an organ or structure.

adrenal m., the inner portion of the adrenal gland.

m. oblongata, the lower portion of the brain stem.

megalocardia (meg″ ah lo card e ah) Abnormal enlargement of the heart.

megalogastria (meg″ ah lo gas′ tre ah) Abnormally large stomach; gastric hypertrophy.

megalomania (meg″ ah lo ma′ ne ah) A disordered mental state characterized by delusions of grandeur.

melancholy (mel′ an ko le) A depressed and painful emotional state.

melanin (mel′ ah nin) The dark pigment found in the skin.

melanocarcinoma (mel″ ah no kar″ sin o mah) A black tumor composed of melanin-pigmented cells.

melanocyte (mel′ ah no sīt) A black cell; a cell that produces melanin.

melanoderma (mel″ ah no der′ mah) Black skin; an abnormal deposit of melanin in the skin.

melanoma (mel″ ah no′ mah) A tumor that appears black; a tumor that is composed of melanin-pigmented cells.

menarche (men ark′ ke) The beginning of the menstrual function.

meninges (me nin′ jēz) The three membranes covering the brain and spinal cord: dura mater, arachnoid, and pia mater.

meningocele (me ning′ go sēl) A hernial protrusion of meninges through a defect in the skull or vertebral column.

menopause (men′ o pawz) That period of time in a female's life when menstruation ceases.

menorrhea (men″ o re′ ah) Menstruation; very profuse menstruation.

menses (men′ sēz) Menstruation, the normal flow of blood from the female genital tract.

menstrual disorder (men″ stroo al)
- *amenorrhea,* absence of menstruation.
- *dysmenorrhea,* difficult or painful menstruation.
- *hypomenorrhea,* decreased menstrual flow.
- *menorrhagia,* excessive menstrual flow.
- *metrorrhagia,* irregular discharge of blood from the uterus.
- *oligomenorrhea,* decrease in menstrual events and flow.
- *postmenopausal bleeding,* discharge after menstrual cycle has ceased.
- *premenstrual syndrome,* discomfort and irritibility occurring prior to menstruation; *PMS.*

menstruation (men″ stroo a′ shun) The cyclic, physiologic discharge of blood and mucosal tissue through the vagina.

mesonasal (mes″ o na′ zal) Situated in the middle of the nose.

metabolic (met″ a ball ik) The sum of all chemical and physical changes in the body.

metacarpal (met″ ah kar′ pal) Pertaining to the metacarpus; one of the bones of the metacarpus.

metatarsal (met″ ah tar′ sal) Pertaining to the metatarsus; a bone of the metatarsus.

metatarsus (met″ ah tar′ sus) The part of the foot between the ankle and the toes.

metritis (me tri′ tis) Inflammation of uterine tissue.

microcardia (mi″ kro kar′ de ah) Smallness of the heart.

microcephaly (mi″ kro sef′ ah le) Abnormally small brain and skull.

microcytosis (mi″ kro si to′ sis) An increase in the number of undersized red cells.

microorganism (mi″ kro or′ gan izm) Minute living organisms that include viruses, bacteria, rickettsiae, protozoa, molds, and yeasts.

midbrain (mid′ brān) The part of the brain that connects the pons and the cerebellum with the hemispheres of the cerebrum; mesencephalon.

midsagittal (mid saj′ i tal) The plane vertically dividing the body through the midline into right and left halves.

mitral (mi′ tral) Pertaining to the mitral or bicuspid valve of the heart.

mucoid (mu′ koid) Resembling mucus.

mucosa (mu ko′ sah) Mucous membrane.

mucus (mu kus) The free slime of the mucus membranes that is composed of secretions of the glands.

multigravida (mul″ ti grav′ i dah) A woman who has been pregnant at least twice before.

multipara (mul tip′ ah rah) A female who has given birth to more than one viable child.

multiple myeloma (mul ti′ pull mi″ el′ o ma) A neoplastic disease characterized by multiple tumor masses in the bone and bone marrow.

multiple sclerosis (mul ti′ pull skle ro′ sis) A chronic disease of the central nervous system in which there is development of disseminated demyelinated glial patches, called plaques.

murmur (mur′ mur) An auscultatory sound, particularly a periodic sound of short duration of cardiac or vascular origin.

muscular dystrophy (mus′ ku lar dis′ tro fe) A genetically determined myopathy characterized by atrophy and wasting away of muscles.

myalgia (mi al′ je ah) Pain in a muscle or muscles.

myasthenia (mi″ as the′ ne ah) Muscular weakness.
- *m. gravis,* a functional abnormality characterized by muscular weakness.

mycodermatitis (mi″ ko der″ mah ti′ tis) Inflammation of the skin due to a fungus.

mycosis (mi ko′ sis) Any condition due to a fungi invasion.

myelencephalitis (mi″ e len sef″ ah li′ tis) Inflammation of the brain and spinal cord; myeloencephalitis.

myelin sheath (mi′ e lin shēth) The sheath surrounding the axon of some nerve cells.

myelitis (mi″ e li′ tis) Inflammation of the bone marrow; inflammation of the spinal cord.

myelocele (mi′ e lo sēl) Hernial protrusion of the spinal cord through a defect in the vertebral column.

myelocyte (mi′ e lo sīt) A cell found in the bone marrow.

myeloma (mi e lo′ mah) A tumor composed of cells normally found in the bone marrow.

myocardial (mi″ o kar′ de al) Pertaining to the muscular tissue of the heart.

m. ischemia (ish″ key′ me ah), decrease in blood supply to the heart.

myocarditis (mi″ o kar di′ tis) Inflammation of the heart tissue.

myocardium (mi″ o kar′ de um) The middle and thickest layer of the heart wall, made up of cardiac muscle.

myocele (mi″ o sēl) Hernia of the muscle.

myocellulitis (mi″ o sel″ u li tis) Inflammation of the cellular and muscle tissues.

myodynia (mi″ o din′ e ah) Pain in a muscle.

myofibril (mi″ o fi′ bril) One of the slender threads of a muscle fiber, composed of numerous myofilaments.

myofibroma (mi″ o fi bro′ mah) A tumor composed of muscular and fibrous elements.

myofibrosis (mi″ o fi bro′ sis) Replacement of muscle tissue by fibrous tissue.

myometrium (mi o me′ tre um) The smooth muscle of the uterus.

myopathy (mi op′ ah the) Any disease of muscle tissue.

myospasm (mi′ o spazm) Cramping of a muscle.

myringa (mi′ ring′ ah) Eardrum.

myxedema (mik″ se de′ mah) A condition resulting from hypothyroidism.

narcolepsy (nar′ ko lep″ see) Sudden attacks of sleep occurring spontaneously at variable intervals.

nares (na′ rēz) The nostrils; the external opening of the nose.

nasal (na′ zal) Pertaining to the nose.

nasolacrimal (na″ zo lak′ ri mal) Pertaining to the nose and lacrimal apparatus.

nasopharynx (na″ zo far′ inks) The upper portion of the pharynx, continuous with the nasal passages.

natal (na′ tal) Pertaining to birth.

necrophobia (nec″ ro fo′ be ah) Fear of death or dead bodies.

necropsy (nek′ rōp se) Examination of a dead body; autopsy.

necrosis (ne kro′ sis) Death of tissue.

necrotic (ne krot′ ik) Characterized by dead tissue.

neonatal (ne′ o na tal) Pertaining to a newborn child, usually designating the first four weeks after delivery.

neonate (ne′ o nāt) A newborn child.

neoplasm (ne′ o plazm) Tumor; any new and abnormal growth.

nephradenoma (nef′ rad en oma) A glandular tumor of the kidney.

nephrectasis (ne′ frek ta″ sis) Distention of the kidney.

nephrectomy (ne′ frek to me) Surgical excision of a kidney.

nephritis (ne fri′ tis) Inflammation of the kidney.

nephrocele (nef′ ro sēl) Hernia of the kidney.

nephrolith (nef′ ro lith) A kidney stone.

nephrolithiasis (nef″ ro li thi′ ah sis) A condition marked by the presence of kidney stones.

nephron (nef′ ron) The structural and functional unit of the kidney.

nephropexy (nef′ ro pek″ se) Surgical fixation of a floating kidney.

nephroptosis (nef″ rop to′ sis) Downward displacement of the kidney; floating kidney.

neuralgia (nu ral′ je ah) Pain of a nerve.

neuritis (nu ri′ tis) Inflammation of a nerve.

neuroarthropathy (nu″ ro ar throp′ ah the) Any disease of joint structures associated with diseases of the central or peripheral nervous system.

neurogenic (nu″ ro jen′ ik) Originating in the nervous system.

neuroglia (nu rog′ le ah) The supporting structure of nervous tissue.

neurolysis (nu rol′ i sis) Release of a nerve sheath by cutting it longitudinally.

neuroma (nu ro′ mah) A tumor made up of nerve cells and nerve fibers.

neuron (nu′ ron) A nerve cell.

neurosis (nu ro′ sis) A functional disorder of the nervous system having anxiety as its chief characteristic.

neutrophil (nu′ tro fil) A granular leukocyte having a three- to five-lobed nucleus and granular cytoplasm.

nevus (ne′ vus) A mark on the skin; birthmarks and some moles.

noctiphobia (nock′ ti fōb e ah) Fear of the night.

nocturia (nock′ tour e ah) Urination during the night.

nocturnal (nock′ tour nal) Occurring at night.
normocyte (nor′ mo sīt) A normal cell, usually referring to a normally sized red blood cell.
nucleoprotein (nu′ kle o pro teen) A protein found in the nuclei of cells.
nullipara (nuh lip′ ah rah) A female who has never given birth.
nyctalgia (nick″ tal′ je ah) Pain during the night.
nyctalopia (nick″ tal′ o pe ah) Night blindness.
nyctaphonia (nick″ ta fone′ e ah) Loss of voice during the night.

occlusion (o kloo′ zhun) The act of closing; the relation of the teeth of both jaws during mandibular activity.
ocular (ok′ u lar) Pertaining to the eye.
olfaction (ol fak′ shun) The sense of smell; the act of smelling.
olfactory (ol fak′ to re) Pertaining to the sense of smell.
oligodendrocyte (ol″ i go den′ dro sīt) A type of neuroglial cell that serves as a support.
oligouria (ol″ i ger e′ ah) Small amount of urine produced.
omentum (o′ men′ tum) The membraneous cover of the abdominal organs.
omphalic (om fal′ ik) Pertaining to the navel.
omphalitis (om″ fah li′ tis) Inflammation of the navel.
omphaloma (om″ fah lo′ mah) Tumor of the navel.
omphalos (om′ fah los) The navel.
oncology (ong kol′ o je) The study of tumors.
onychoma (on″ i ko mah) A tumor of the nail or nail bed.
onychomalacia (on″ i ko mah la′ she ah) Softening of the nails.
onychomycosis (on″ i ko mi ko′ sis) A disease of the nails due to a fungus.
oogenesis (o″ o jen′ e sis) The organ and formation of eggs in the female.
oophoralgia (o″ of or al′ je ah) Ovarian pain.
oophorectomy (o″ of or rek′ to me) The removal of an ovary or ovaries.
oophoritis (o″ of o ri′ tis) Inflammation of an ovary.
oophorogenous (o of″ o roj′ e nus) Derived from the ovary.
oophorohysterectomy (o of″ o ro his″ ter ek′ to me) Surgical removal of the uterus and ovaries.
oophoroma (o of″ or o′ mah) A tumor of the ovary.
oophoropexy (o of′ o ro pek″ se) Surgical fixation of the ovary.
oophorosalpingectomy (o of″ o ro sal″ pin jek′ to me) Surgical removal of an ovary and uterine tube.
oophorosalpingitis (o of″ o ro sal″ pin ji′ tis) Inflammation of an ovary and uterine tube.
ophthalmalgia (of″ thal mal′ je ah) Pain in the eye.
ophthalmic (of thal′ mik) Pertaining to the eye.
ophthalmitis (of″ thal mi′ tis) Inflammation of the eye.
ophthalmodynia (of thal″ mo din′ e ah) Pain in the eye.
ophthalmomalacia (of thal″ mo mah la′ she ah) Abnormal softness of the eye.
ophthalmopathy (of″ thal mop′ ah the) Any disease of the eye.
ophthalmoscope (of thal′ mo skōp) Any instrument used to examine the interior of the eye.
optical (op′ ti kal) Pertaining to vision.
oral (o′ ral) Pertaining to the oral cavity or mouth.
orchialgia (or″ key al′ je ah) Pain in a testis.
orchidalgia (or″ kid al′ je ah) Pain in a testis.
orchidectomy (or″ kid ek′ to me) Excision of a testicle.
orchiditis (or″ kid i′ tis) Inflammation of a testicle.
orchidopexy (or′ kid o pek″ se) Surgical fixation of a testicle.
orchidorrhaphy (or″ kid or′ ah fe) Suturing of the testicles.
orchiectomy (or″ ke ek′ to me) Excision of one or both testes.
orchiopathy (or″ ke op′ ah the) Any disease of the testes.
orchiopexy (or″ ke o pek′ se) Surgical fixation of an undescended testis in the scrotum.
oropharynx (o″ ro far′ inks) That part of the pharynx between the soft palate and the upper edge of the epiglottis.
orthopnea (or″ thop ne′ ah) A condition in which breathing is easier when the person is in an upright position.
osmatic (oz mat ik) Pertaining to the sense of smell.
osseous (os″ e us) Bony; of the nature or quality of bone.
ossification (os″ i fi ka′ shun) The formation of bone or a bony substance.
ostealgia (os″ te al′ je ah) Pain in a bone.
osteitis (os″ te i′ tis) Inflammation of a bone.
osteoarthritis (os″ te o ar thri′ tis) Degenerative joint disease characterized by degeneration of the articular cartilage, hypertrophy of bone at the margins, and changes in the synovial membrane.
osteoarthropathy (os″ te o ar throp′ ah the) Any disease of the bones and joints.

osteochondritis (os″ te o kon dri′ tis) Inflammation of the bone and cartilage.
osteoclasia (os″ te o klay she ah) Surgical fracture of a bone to repair a deformity.
osteodynia (os″ te o din′ e ah) Pain in the bone.
osteoid (os′ te oid) Resembling bone.
osteomalacia (os″ te o mah la′ she ah) A skeletal disorder characterized by a disturbance in bone metabolism; softening of the bone.
osteomyelitis (os″ to o mi″ e li′ tis) Inflammation of the bone and bone marrow.
osteotome (os′ te o tōm″) An instrument used to cut bone.
ostomy (os′ to me) A general term for surgery in which an artificial opening is formed.
otalgia (o tal′ je ah) Pain in the ear; earache.
otitis (o″ ti′ tis) Inflammation of the ear.
o. media, inflammation of the middle ear.
otodynia (o′ to din′ e ah) Pain in the ear; earache.
otorrhagia (o″ to ra′ je ah) Hemorrhage from the ear.
otorrhea (o″ to re′ ah) Discharge from the ear.
otoscope (o″ to skōp) An instrument for viewing inside the ear.
ovarian (o″ va′ re an) Pertaining to an ovary or ovaries.
ovary (o″ vah re) The female gonad; either of the paired organs in which eggs are formed.
ovulation (o″ vu la′ shun) The discharge of an egg from the ovary.
ovum (o″ vum) An egg; the female reproductive germ cell.
oxytocin (ok″ se to′ sin) A pituitary hormone that stimulates uterine contractions and milk ejection.

palate (pal′ at) The roof of the mouth separating the nasal and oral cavities.
hard p., the anterior portion of the palate.
soft p., the posterior portion of the palate.
palatine (pal′ ah tīn) Pertaining to the palate.
palpebra (pal′ pey bra) Eyelid.
palpebrate (pal′ pa brate) Wink.
palpebration (pal′ pe bray shun) Abnormal winking.
palsy (pawl′ ze) Paralysis.
pancreatectomy (pan″ kre ah tek′ to me) Excision of the pancreas.
pancreatic (pan″ kre at′ ik) Pertaining to the pancreas.
pancreatitis (pan″ kre ah ti′ tis) Inflammation of the pancreas.
pancreatography (pan″ kre ah tog′ rah fe) X-ray of the pancreas using contrast medium in the pancreatic fluid.
pancreatotomy (pan″ kre ah tot′ o me) Incision of the pancreas.
pandemic (pan″ dem ik) A disease that is widely spread throughout the world or continent.
Papanicolaou's smear (pap″ ah nik″ o la′ ooz) Collection of material from the cervix and the vagina, followed by microscopic study for observing precancerous cells; Pap test or Pap smear.
papilla (pap′ i lay) A nipple-like projection.
paracentesis (par″ ah sen te′ sis) Surgical puncture of a cavity for aspiration of fluid.
paralysis (pah ral′ i sis) Loss or impairment of motor function due to neural or muscular lesions.
paraplegia (par ah ple′ je ah) Paralysis of the legs and lower part of the body due to disease or injury to the spinal cord.
paracystitis (par ah cyst i tis) Inflammation of the tissues around the urinary bladder.
parasympathetic (par ah sim pah thet′ ik) Referring to the nerves that are part of the automatic system and work against the sympathetic nerves.
parasympathomimetic (par″ ah sim″ pah tho mi met′ ik) Producing effects resembling those of parasympathetic nerves.
parathyroid (par ah thi′ roid) Four glands situated beside the thyroid gland that secrete a hormone that regulates calcium and phosphorous.
parenteral (pah ren′ ter al) Injection into the body, not through the alimentary canal.
parotitis (par″ o ti′ tis) Inflammation of the parotid gland.
epidemic p., mumps.
parous (pa′ rous) Having given birth to a child or children.
parturition (par′ tu rish′ un) Childbirth.
patella (pah tel′ ah) The kneecap or bone situated anterior to the knee joint.
pathogen (path′ o jen) Any disease-producing agent or microorganism.
pathogenic (path o jen′ ik) Disease causing.
pathologic (path o loj′ ik) Indicating or caused by some morbid disease process.
pathosis (path′ o sis) A disease condition.
pediculosis (ped′ ik u low sis) Infested with lice.
p. capitis, head lice.
p. corporis, body lice.
p. pubis, lice in the pubic region; crabs.
pelvic (pel′ vik) Pertaining to the pelvis.
pelvimetry (pel vim′ e tre) Measurement of the dimensions and capacity of the pelvis.
pelvis (pel′ vis) The lower portion of the trunk; any basin-like structure.
renal p., in the kidney, the funnel-shaped structure at the upper end of the ureter.
penis (pe′ nis) The male organ of urination and

copulation; erectile body in the male that is sensually homologous to the female clitoris.

periadenitis (per″ e ad″ e ni′ tis) Inflammation of tissues around a gland.

pericarditis (per″ i kar di′ tis) Inflammation of the pericardium.

pericardium (per″ i kar′ de um) The sac enclosing the heart and the roots of the great vessels.

pericerebral (per″ i ser′ e bral) Around the cerebrum; around the brain.

perichondral (per″ i kon′ dral) Around the cartilage.

perichondrium (per i kon′ dre um) The layer of fibrous tissue around all cartilage except articular cartilage of synovial joints.

periodontal (per″ e o don′ tal) Around a tooth; pertaining to periodontium.

periodontitis (per″ e o don ti′ tis) Inflammation of the periodontium caused by residual food, bacteria, and tartar that collects in the space between gum and lower part of the tooth.

periosteum (per″ e os te um) A tough fibrous membrane that surrounds a bone.

peripheral nervous system (per′ if er al) The nerve process beyond the central nervous system (brain and spinal cord) that connect with receptors, muscles, and glands.

peristalsis (per″ i stal′ sis) Movement by which the alimentary canal propels its contents by using a wave of contraction passing along itself.

peritonitis (per″ i to ni′ tis) Inflammation of the peritoneum.

peritonsillar (per″ i ton′ si lar) Around the tonsil.

phagocyte (fag′ o sīt) Any cell that ingests something else.

phagocytosis (fag′ o si to′ sis) The engulfing of microorganisms, cells, and foreign particles by phagocytes.

phagomania (fag″ o ma′ ne ah) An abnormal craving for food; obsessive preoccupation with eating.

phalanges (fah lan′ jēz) Bones of the fingers or toes.

phalangitis (fal′ an ji tis) Inflammation of one or more bones of the fingers or toes.

pharyngeal (fah rin′ je al) Pertaining to the throat.

pharyngitis (far″ in ji tis) Inflammation of the throat.

pharyngocele (far ring′ go sēl) Hernial protrusion of the pharynx.

pharyngodynia (fah ring″ go din′ e ah) Pain in the throat; sore throat.

pharyngomycosis (fah ring″ go mi ko′ sis) Any fungal infection of the pharynx.

pharyngopathy (far″ ing gop′ ah the) Any disease of the pharynx.

pharynx (far′ inks) The throat.

phlebectomy (fle bek′ to me) Removal of a vein or a segment of a vein.

phlebitis (fle bī′ tis) Inflammation of a vein.

phlebosclerosis (fle″ bō skle ro′ sis) Fibrous thickening of the walls of veins.

phlebostasis (fle bos′ tah sis) Controlling or slowing the flow of blood in a vein.

phlebotomy (fle bot′ to me) The incision of a vein.

phobia (fo′ be ah) Any persistent fear.

phonic (fon′ ik) Pertaining to the voice.

photodermatitis (fo″ to der″ mah ti′ tis) An abnormal skin reaction produced by light.

photoreceptor (fo″ to re sep′ tor) A nerve ending found in the eye that detects light.

phrenic (frēn′ ik) Pertaining to the diaphragm; pertaining to the mind.

phrenitis (fre ni′ tis) Inflammation of the diaphragm.

phrenoplegia (fre″ no ple′ je ah) Paralysis of the diaphragm.

phrenoptosis (fren″ op to′ sis) Downward displacement of the diaphragm.

pilus (pi′ lus) A hair.

pituitary (pi tu′ i ter″ e) The hypophysis, a small oval body at the base of the brain.

placenta (plah sen′ tah) An organ joining mother and offspring prior to birth.

plane (plain) A flat surface; a specific level; to rub away or abrade.

plantar (plan′ tar) Pertaining to the sole of the foot.

plaque (plak) Any patch or flat area.

pleura (ploor′ ah) Serous membrane investing the lungs and lining the walls of the thoracic cavity.
parietal p., pleura that lines the walls of the thoracic cavity.
visceral p., pleura that surrounds the lungs.

pleural (ploor′ al) Pertaining to the pleura (membrane).
p. cavity, the space between the parietal and visceral pleurae.

pleurisy (ploor′ i see) Inflammation of the pleura (membrane).

pleuritis (ploor ri′ tis) Inflammation of the pleura (membrane), or pleurisy.

pleurodynia (ploor″ o din′ e ah) Pain of the pleura (membrane); pleurisy.

pleuropneumonia (ploor′ o nu mōn ne ah) Pain of the pleura (membrane) complicated by pneumonia.

pneumectomy (nu mek′ to me) Removal of lung tissue.

pneumocardial (nu″ mo kar de al) Pertaining to the lungs and heart.

pneumocentesis (nu″ mo sen te′ sis) Surgical puncture of a lung.
pneumoconiosis (nu″ mo ko″ ne o′ sis) Any lung condition due to permanent deposit of substantial amounts of dust particles in the lung.
pneumohemothorax (nu″ mo he″ mo tho′ raks) Gas or air and blood in the pleural cavity.
pneumomalacia (nu″ mo mah la′ she ah) Softening of lung tissue.
pneumomelanosis (nu″ mo mel′ ah no′ sis) Black condition of the lung due to inhaled coal dust, soot, or other substance; pneumoconiosis.
pneumonectomy (nu″ mo nek′ to me) Surgical removal of all or part of a lung.
pneumonia (nu mo′ ne ah) Inflammation of the lung; pneumonitis.
pneumonitis (nu″ mo ni′ tis) Inflammation of the lung; pneumonia.
pneumothorax (nu″ mo tho′ raks) Air or gas in the pleural space.
podagra (pod″ a′ gra) Severe foot pain.
poikilocyte (poi′ ki lo sīt) An abnormally shaped red blood cell.
poikilocytosis (poi″ ki lo si to′ sis) The presence of abnormally shaped red blood cells.
polyarthritis (pol″ e ar thri′ tis) Inflammation of several joints.
polycystic (pol″ e sis′ tik) Containing many cysts.
polycythemia (pol″ e sīt he′ me ah) An increase in the total mass of the blood.
p. vera, a disease of unknown cause marked by an increase in red cell mass and blood volume.
secondary p., any increase in the total red cell mass other than polycythemia vera.
polydipsia (pol″ e dip′ se ah) Excessive thirst.
polydysplasia (pol″ e dis plaz e ah) Faulty development in tissues and organs or systems of organs.
polymorphonuclear (pol″ e mor″ fo nu′ kle ar) Having a nucleus that is so divided that it appears to be multiple.
polyneuritis (pol″ e nu ri′ tis) Inflammation of many nerves simultaneously.
polyneuropathy (pol″ e nu rop ah the) A disease involving several nerves.
polyp (pol′ ip) Any growth or mass protruding from a mucus membrane.
polyuria (pol″ e u′ re ah) Excessive urination.
pons (ponz) The part of the central nervous system located between the medulla oblongata and the mesencephalon and ventral to the cerebellum.
posteriad (pos ter′ e ad) Toward the posterior part of the body.
posterior (pos ter′ e or) Situated behind.
posteroexternal (pos″ ter o ek ster′ nal) Situated on the outside of a posterior part.
posterolateral (pos″ ter o lat′ er al) Situated on the side and toward the posterior aspect.
posteromedial (pos″ ter ro me′ de al) Situated in the middle of the back side.
posterosuperior (pos″ te ro soo per′ e or) Situated behind and above.
postesophageal (post e sof″ ah je al) Behind the esophagus.
postmortem (pōst mor′ tem) Occurring or performed after death.
postnatal (pōst na′ tal) Occurring after birth.
postpartum (pōst par′ tum) After childbirth.
precancerous (pre kan′ ser us) Used to describe abnormal growths or cells that are likely to become cancerous.
prenatal (pre na′ tal) Referring to the time before birth.
prepartal (pre′ part al) Occurring before or just previous to labor.
prepuce (pre′ pus) The foreskin of the penis.
primigravida (pri″ mi grav′ i dah) A woman who is pregnant for the first time.
primipara (pri mip′ ah ra) A woman bearing or having a first child.
proctalgia (prok tal′ je ah) Pain in the lower rectum.
proctoclysis (prok tok′ lī sis) Slow introduction of large quantities of liquid into the rectum.
proctodynia (prok″ to din′ e ah) Pain in the rectum.
proctoplegia (prok″ to ple′ je ah) Paralysis of the rectum.
proctoptosis (prok″ top to′ sis) Sagging of the rectum.
proctorrhagia (prok″ to ra′ je ah) Hemorrhage from the rectum.
proctorrhaphy (prok tor′ ah fe) Suture of the rectum for the purpose of repair.
progesterone (pro jes′ te rōn) The hormone produced by the corpus luteum in the ovaries, adrenal cortex, and placenta.
prognosis (prog no′ sis) Prediction of the probable outcome of a disease.
prolapse (pro laps′) Drooping, sagging, or slipping forward of a body part.
prophylaxis (pro″ fi lak′ sis) Protection against disease; a preventative action.
proptosis (prop toe sis) A forward displacement.
prostate (pros′ tāt) A gland that surrounds the neck of the bladder and urethra in the male.
prostatectomy (pros″ tah tek′ to me) Surgical removal of all or part of the prostate.
prostatitis (pros″ tah ti′ tis) Inflammation of the prostate.
proteinuria (pro″ te in u′ re ah) The presence of protein in urine.

proteuria (pro″ te u′ re ah) Protein in the urine; proteinuria.
protoplast (pro″ to′ plast) The first cells to form.
protozoan (pro″ to so′ on) A primitive parasitic animal consisting of a single cell.
proximal (prok′ si mal) Nearest the origin or point of attachment.
pruritus ani (pure′ īt us any) Itchiness around the anus.
pseudesthesia (soo″ des the′ ze ah) An imaginary sensation.
pseudocyesis (soo′ do si e sis) False pregnancy.
pseudomania (soo″ do ma′ ne ah) False mental disorder; pathological lying.
pseudoplegia (soo′ do ple je ah) Hysterical paralysis; apparent loss of muscular power without real paralysis.
psoriasis (sor″ eye′ a sis) A chronic skin disease characterized by scaly, itchy patches.
psychopath (si′ ko path) A person who has an antisocial personality.
psychopharmacology (si″ ko fahr″ mah kol′ o je) The study of drugs that affect the mind.
psychosis (si ko′ sis) Any major mental disorder of organic and (or) emotional origin characterized by derangement of the personality and loss of contact with reality.
psychotherapy (si ko ther′ a pe) Treatment of functional nervous disorders that employs psychological methods.
ptosis (to′ sis) Prolapse of an organ or part; drooping of the upper eyelid.
puberty (pu′ ber te) The period during which the secondary sex characteristics begin to develop.
pubes (pu′ bez) The hairs growing over the pubic region; the pubic region.
pubic (pu′ bik) Pertaining to the pubis, a bone of the pelvis.
pubis (pu′ bis) The anterior portion of the hip bone.
pulmonary (pul′ mo nār″ e) Pertaining to the lungs.
p. edema, effusion of fluid into the air spaces and tissue spaces of the lungs.
pulmonic (pul mon′ ik) Pertaining to the lungs.
pulse (pulz) The rhythmic expansion of an artery that may be felt with a finger at any of a number of pressure points.
p. rate, the number of pulsations of an artery per minute.
pus (pus) A product of inflammation composed of leukocytes, cellular debris, and fluid.
pyelitis (pi″ e li′ tis) Inflammation of the renal pelvis.
pyelography (pi″ e log′ rah fe) Radiography of the renal pelvis and ureter after injection of a contrast medium.
pyelonephritis (pi″ e lo ne fri′ tis) Inflammation of the kidney and its accompanying renal pelvis.
pyeloplasty (pi″ e lo plas″ te) Surgical repair of the renal pelvis.
pylorus (pi″ lo′ rus) The opening between the stomach and duodenum.
pyodermatitis (pi″ o der″ mah ti′ tis) A skin infection producing pus.
pyogenesis (pi″ o jen′ e sis) Formation of pus.
pyogenic (pi″ o jen′ ik) Producing pus.
pyorrhea (pi″ o re′ ah) A discharge of pus.
pyothorax (pi″ o tho′ raks) Accumulation of pus in the chest cavity.
pyrexia (pi rek′ se ah) A fever or febrile condition.
pyromania (pi″ ro ma′ ne ah) An abnormal preoccupation concerning fire.
pyuria (pi u′ re ah) The presence of pus in the urine.

quadriplegia (kwod″ ri ple′ je ah) Paralysis of all four extremities.

rachialgia (ra″ ke al′ je ah) Pain in the spine.
rachiodynia (ra″ ke o din′ e ah) Pain in the spinal column.
rachioplegia (ra″ ke o ple′ je ah) Spinal paralysis.
rachioscoliosis (ra″ ke o sko″ le o′ sis) Lateral curvature of the spine.
rachischisis (ra kis′ ki sis) Split spine; spina bifida.
radiopaque (ra″ de o pāk) Impervious to x-ray or other forms of radiation (shows clear on film).
rale (rahl) An abnormal respiratory sound heard in some pathological conditions.
receptor (re sep′ tor) A sensory nerve ending that responds to various stimuli.
rectocele (rek′ to sēl) Hernia of the rectum with protusion of part of the rectum into the vagina.
rectoclysis (rek tok′ li sis) Proctoclysis; slow introduction of large quantities of liquid into the rectum.
rectorrhaphy (rek tor′ ah fe) Suture of the rectum for the purpose of repair.
rectum (rek′ tum) The distal portion of the large intestine.
reduction (re duk′ shun) Pulling the broken ends of a fractured bone into alignment.
closed r., restoring a fractured bone to its normal position by manipulation without surgery.
open r., exposing a fractured bone by surgery to realign it.
renal (re′ nal) Pertaining to the kidney.

r. failure, inadequate functioning of the kidneys leading to uremia.

r. pelvis, a funnel-shaped cavity in the kidney that collects urine from many nephrons.

r. tubule, that part of a nephron where the formation of urine occurs.

resection (re sek′ shun) Removal of a portion of an organ or other structure.

retrocecal (ret″ ro se′ kal) Behind the cecum.

retrocolic (ret″ ro kol′ ik) Behind the large intestine.

retroperitoneal (ret″ ro per″ i to ne′ al) Behind the peritoneum.

rheumatoid arthritis (room′ a toyd ar thri′ tis) A chronic systemic disease characterized by inflamed joints and related structures that result in crippling.

rhinitis (ri ni′ tis) Inflammation of the mucus membranes of the nose.

rhinolith (ri′ no lith) A calculus or stone in the nose.

rhinolithiasis (ri″ no li thi′ ah sis) A condition marked by the presence of nasal stones.

rhinoplasty (ri′ no plas″ te) Surgery to correct or otherwise modify the nose; nose job.

rhinorrhea (ri″ no re′ ah) A discharge from the nose; a runny nose.

roentgen (rent′ gen) The international unit of measurement of the x-ray.

rubedo (roo′ be doh) Temporary redness.

sacral (sa′ kral) Pertaining to the sacrum, the triangular bone below the lumbar vertebrae.

sacrodynia (sa″ kro din′ e ah) Pain in the sacrum, the triangular bone below the lumbar vertebrae.

sacrum (sa′ krum) The triangular bone at the base of the spine.

sagittal (saj′ it tal) Shaped like an arrow; denotes a plane that is parallel to the midsagittal line vertically dividing the body into right and left portions.

saliva (sah li′ vah) The clear alkaline viscid secretion from the salivary glands.

salpingectomy (sal″ pin jek′ to me) Excision of a uterine tube.

salpingitis (sal″ pin ji′ tis) Inflammation of a uterine tube.

salpingocele (sal ping″ go sēl) Hernial protrusion of a uterine tube.

salpingocyesis (sal ping″ go si e′ sis) The condition in which a fertilized egg has implanted in a uterine tube; ectopic pregnancy.

salpingopexy (sal ping′ go pek″ se) Surgical fixation of a uterine tube.

salpingorrhaphy (sal″ ping′ go raf″ e) Suture of the uterine (fallopian) tube.

salpingostomy (sal″ ping gos′ to me) Formation of an opening into a uterine tube for drainage; surgical restoration of the patency of a uterine tube.

sarcoma (sar ko′ mah) A tumor, often malignant, composed of substance like embryonic tissue.

scan (skan) A representation of the gamma rays emitted by a radioactive isotope, revealing its concentration in a specific organ or tissue.

scapulothoracic (skap u lo tho ras′ ik) Pertaining to the shoulder blade and chest.

schistothorax (skis to tho rax) Splitting the thorax.

schizophrenia (skit″ so fre′ ne ah) A type of psychosis characterized by loss of contact and degeneration of the personality.

schizonychia (skiz″ o nik′ e ah) Split fingernails.

sclerosis (skle ro′ sis) Hardening of the nervous or circulatory systems.

sclerotic (skle rot′ ik) Hardening; hard.

scoliosis (sko″ le o′ sis) Lateral curvature of the vertebral column.

scrotum (skro′ tum) The pouch that contains the testicles and their accessory organs.

seborrhea (seb″ o re′ ah) Excessive secretion of sebum (oily material produced by sebaceous glands).

seborrheic (seb″ o re′ ik) Affected with seborrhea.

s. dermatitis, an inflammatory condition of the skin caused by overactive sebaceous glands.

sebum (se′ bum) The oily material secreted by sebaceous gland.

semen (se′ men) Fluid consisting of gland secretions and sperm discharged at ejaculation.

semicoma (sem″ e ko′ mah) A mild coma from which the patient can be aroused.

semiconscious (sem″ e kon shus) Only partially aware of one's surroundings.

seminal (sem′ i nal) Pertaining to semen.

s. fluid, semen; the fluid discharged from the penis at the time of ejaculation.

seminiferous (se″ mi nif′ er us) Channels in the testis in which spermatozoa develop.

sensory (sen′ so re) Pertaining to sensation.

s. nerve cells, cells of the afferent nervous system that pick up stimuli.

sepsis (sep′ sis) A poisoned state due to bacteria; infection.

septicemia (sep″ ti se′ me ah) A morbid condition due to the presence of bacteria and their toxins in the blood.

septum (sep′ tum) A dividing wall or partition.

nasal s., the partition between the two nasal cavities.

serosa (see ro′ sah) Any serous membrane; the chorion.
sinistroocular (sin″ is tro ok u lar) Stronger vision in the left eye.
sinoatrial (si″ no a′ tre al) Pertaining to the sinus venosus and the atrium of the heart.
s. node, a node in the wall of the right atrium that is the source of impulses that initiate the heartbeat.
sinus (si′ nus) A recess, cavity, or channel.
paranasal s., one of several cavities that communicate with the nasal cavity and are lined with a mucous membrane.
sinusitis (si nu si′ tis) Inflammation of a sinus.
somatic (so mat′ ik) Pertaining to the body.
somatogenic (so″ mah to jen′ ik) Originating in the cells of the body.
somatomegaly (so″ mah to meg′ ah le) Increased size of the body; gigantism.
somatopsychic (so″ mah to si′ kik) Pertaining to body and mind.
somatotropin (so″ mah to tro pin) Growth hormone.
somesthetic (so″ mes thet′ ik) Pertaining to body feeling or sensation.
somniferous (som′ ni fer′ us) Inducing sleep.
spasm (spazm) Twitching.
speculum (spek′ u lum) An instrument used to examine a body orifice or cavity.
spermatocidal (sper″ mah to si′ dal) Destructive to sperm.
spermatogenesis (sper″ mah to jen′ e sis) The process by which sperm are formed.
spermatozoan (sper′ mah to soon) A mature male germ cell that serves to fertilize an ovum.
spherocyte (sfe′ ro sīt) An abnormally round red blood cell.
spina bifida (spi″ nah bif′ i dah) A developmental abnormality marked by defective closure of the spine.
spine (spīn) The vertebral column that encases the spinal cord.
spirilla (spi ril′ ah) Spiral-shaped bacteria.
spleen (splēn) A large organ situated in the upper left part of the abdominal cavity that serves as a blood reservoir and destroys erythrocytes at the end of their usefulness.
splenectomy (sple″ nek′ to me) Removal of the spleen.
splenokeratosis (sple″ no kar at o sis) Hardening of the spleen.
splenomegaly (sple″ no meg′ ah le) Enlargement of the spleen.
splenopathy (sple nop′ ah the) Any disease of the spleen.
splenoptosis (sple′ nop to′ sis) Downward displacement of the spleen.
splenorrhagia (sple′ no ra′ je ah) Hemorrhage from the spleen.
spondylalgia (spon″ di lal′ je ah) A painful vertebra.
spondylarthritis (spon″ dil ar thri′ tis) Inflammation of joints between vertebrae.
spondylitis (spon″ di li′ tis) Inflammation of a vertebra.
ankylosing s., rheumatoid arthritis with stiffening of the spinal joints and ligaments.
sputum (spu′ tum) Material that is ejected from the trachea, bronchi, and lungs through the mouth.
staphylectomy (staf″ i lek′ to me) Excision of the uvula.
staphylitis (staf″ i li′ tis) Inflammation of the uvula.
staphylococcemia (staf″ i lo kok se′ me ah) The presence of staphylococci bacteria in the blood.
stasis (sta′ sis) A stoppage or diminution of the flow of blood or other body fluid; a state of balance between opposing forces.
steatorrhea (stea to re ah) A flow of undigested fat.
sternal (ster′ nal) Pertaining to the breast bone.
sternoschisis (ster nos′ ki sis) Congenital fissure of the sternum.
sternum (ster′ num) The breast bone forming the middle anterior wall of the thorax.
stoma (sto′ mah) A mouth-like opening that has been formed for drainage.
stomatitis (sto″ mah ti′ tis) Inflammation of the mouth.
stomatodynia (sto″ mah to din′ e ah) A painful mouth.
stomatomycosis (sto″ mah to mi ko′ sis) A fungal disease of the mouth.
stomatorrhagia (sto″ mah to ra′ je ah) Hemorrhage from the mouth.
subchondral (sub″ kon′ dral) Beneath a cartilage.
subcostal (sub″ kos′ tal) Below the ribs or a rib.
subcutaneous (sub″ ku ta′ ne us) Beneath the skin.
subdural (sub du′ ral) Between the dura mater and arachnoid.
s. hematoma, a mass of blood located beneath the dura, usually due to a head injury.
s. space, the space between the dura mater and the arachnoid.
subglossal (sub″ glos′ sal) Under the tongue.
sublingual (sub″ ling′ gwal) Situated under the tongue.
subnormal (sub″ nor′ mal) Below normal.
subphrenic (sub″ fren′ ik) Beneath or under the diaphragm.

subpubic (sub″ pu′ bik) Beneath the pubic bone.
sudoriferous (su″ do rif′ er us) Conveying perspiration.
superficial (soo″ per fish′ al) Situated on or near the surface.
superior (soo″ pe′ re or) Situated above or directly upward.
supracostal (soo″ prah kos′ tal) Above or outside the ribs.
supradrenal (soo″ prah dre′ nal) Above the kidney.
suture (soo′ chure) The act of uniting a wound by stitching; a type of joint in which the opposed bones are closely united.
symphysis (sim″ phy sis) A type of joint in which connected bones are firmly united.
sympathomimetic (sim″ pah tho mi met′ ik) Adrenergic; mimicking the effects or impulses of sympathetic nerves.
synalgia (sin′ al je ah) Pain experienced in one place as a result of soreness or injury in another.
synapse (sin′ aps) The site of junction between two neurons.
syndactyly (sin″ dak′ tilly) Adjacent digits are attached to each other by a membraneous web.
syndrome (sin drōm) A set of symptoms that occurs together and collectively indicates a particular disease.
systole (sis′ to le) The contraction or period of contraction of the heart, especially the ventricles.

tachycardia (tak″ e kar′ de ah) Fast heartbeat.
tachyphagia (tak″ e fa′ je ah) Rapid eating.
tachyphasia (tak″ e fa′ ze ah) Fast speech.
tachypnea (tak″ ip ne′ ah) Rapid breathing.
talipes (tal″ ip ees) Joints of the foot.
tarsal (tahr′ sal) Pertaining to the tarsus of an eyelid or to the instep; any of the bones of the tarsus.
tarsoptosis (tahr″ sop to′ sis) Falling of the tarsals; fallen arch.
tarsus (tahr′ sus) The seven bones composing the articulation between the foot and the leg; the cartilaginous plates of the eyelids.
tegument (teg′ u ment) Skin or covering.
tendon (ten″ dun) A fibrous cord by which a muscle is attached.
tendonitis (ten″ do ni′ tis) Inflammation of tendons and tendon muscle attachments.
tenesmus (ten″ es mas) Straining to defecate.
tenomyoplasty (ten″ o mi′ o plas″ te) Surgical repair of a tendon and muscle.
tenotomy (ten ot′ o me) Cutting of a tendon.
tensor (ten sore) Any muscle that stretches or tenses some part of the body.
teratoma (ter′ a tom ah) An unusual tumor of malformed tissues, none of which is native to the area in which it occurs.
testalgia (tes tal′ je ah) Testicular pain.
testectomy (tes tek′ to me) Surgical removal of a testicle.
testicular (tes tik′ u lar) Pertaining to a testicle.
testis (tes′ tis) The male gonad where sperm are formed.
testosterone (tes tos′ te rōn) A hormone secreted by the testes that brings about male secondary sex characteristics.
tetany (tet′ ah ne) A nervous condition characterized by intermittent or continuous tonic muscular contractions involving the extremities.
thalamus (thal′ ah mus) The largest subdivision of the diencephalon located in the brain.
thelium (theel e um) Nipple.
thermal (ther mal) Pertaining to heat.
thermolysis (ther mol′ i sis) Destruction by heat.
thermoplegia (ther″ mo ple′ je ah) Heatstroke or sunstroke.
thoracentesis (tho″ rah sen te′ sis) Surgical puncture of the chest wall into the perietal cavity for aspiration of fluids.
thoracic (tho ras′ ik) Pertaining to the chest.
thoracocentesis (tho″ rah ko sen te′ sis) surgical puncture of the chest wall for aspiration of fluids.
thoracodynia (tho″ rah ko din′ e ah) Pain in the chest.
thoracoplasty (tho″ rah ko plas′ te) Surgical removal of ribs, allowing the chest wall to collapse a diseased lung.
thoracotomy (tho″ rah kot′ o me) Surgical incision of the wall of the chest.
thorax (tho′ raks) Chest; the part of the body that is encased by the ribs.
thrombectomy (throm bek′ to me) Surgical removal of a blood clot.
thrombocyte (throm′ bo sīt) A blood platelet.
thrombocytopenia (throm″ bo si′ to pe′ ne ah) A decrease in the number of platelets in circulating blood.
thrombogenesis (throm″ bo jen′ e sis) Origin of a blood clot; clot formation.
thrombolymphangitis (throm″ bo lim″ fan ji′ tis) Inflammation of lymph vessel due to a blood clot.
thrombolysis (throm bol′ i sis) Dissolution of a blood clot.
thrombolytic (throm″ bo lit′ ik) Dissolving or breaking up a blood clot.
thrombopenia (throm″ bo pe′ ne ah) A deficiency in the number of platelets in circulating blood.
thrombophlebitis (throm′ bo fle bi′ tis) Inflammation of a vein due to a blood clot.

thrombosis (throm bo′ sis) The presence of a blood clot.

thrombus (throm′ bus) A blood clot formed in a blood vessel.

thymic (thi′ mik) Pertaining to the thymus.

thymoma (thi mo′ mah) Tumor derived from elements of the thymus.

thymus (thi′ mus) A gland-like body in the anterior mediastinal cavity that usually reaches its maximum development during childhood and then undergoes involution.

thyrochondrotomy (thi″ ro′ kond rot o me) Surgical incision of the thyroid cartilage.

thyroidectomy (thi″ roi dek′ to me) Surgical removal of the thyroid gland.

thyroiditis (thi″ roi di′ tis) Inflammation of the thyroid gland.

thyroma (thi ro′ mah) A tumor of the thyroid gland.

thyrotoxicosis (thi″ ro tok″ si ko′ sis) A morbid condition due to excessive thyroid secretion.

thyrotropic (thi″ ro trop′ ik) Capable of stimulating the thyroid gland.

thyrotropin (thi ro′ trōp′ in) A hormone of the anterior pituitary that stimulates the thyroid.

tibia (tib′ e ah) The inner and larger bone of the leg below the knee.

tibialgia (tib″ e al′ je ah) Pain in the tibia.

tibiofemoral (tib″ e o fem′ or al) Pertaining to the tibia and the femur.

tinea (tin′ e ah) A fungal disease of the skin; ringworm.

tinnitus (tin i tus) Sensation of noises in the ear, ranging from hissing to roaring sounds.

tomograph (to′ mo graf) An apparatus for moving the x-ray tube through an arc during exposure to show a plane of tissue.

tomography (to mog′ rah fe) Body-section roentgenography in an arc.

CAT scan, computerized (transverse) axial tomography is a technique that utilizes a narrow beam of x-rays to obtain a three-dimensional view of body parts.

CT scan, computed tomography is a radiological technique in which transmission patterns are recorded by electronic detectors and stored in a computer that reconstructs a three-dimensional view of internal structures of the body.

tonsil (ton′ sil) A small, rounded mass of lymphoid tissue found in the throat.

tonsillectomy (ton″ sil lek′ to me) Excision of the tonsils.

tonsillitis (ton″ sil i tis) Inflammation and enlargement of a tonsil.

tonsilloadenoidectomy (ton″ sil o ad″ e noi dek′ to me) Excision of lymphoid tissue from the throat and nasopharynx (T&A).

tonsillotomy (ton″ sil ot′ o me) Incision of a tonsil.

topical (top′ e kal) Pertaining to a particular area; local.

toxemia (tok se′ me ah) A general intoxication due to absorption of bacterial toxins; a group of pathological conditions occurring in pregnant women.

toxic (tok′ sik) Poisonous; pertaining to poisoning.

toxicity (tok sis′ i te) The degree of virulance of a toxic microbe or poison.

toxicoderma (tok″ si ko derm ah) Skin disease resulting from a poison.

toxicosis (tok″ si ko′ sis) Any disease condition due to poisoning.

toxin (tok′ sin) A substance that is highly poisonous for other living organisms.

toxoid (tok′ soid) A toxin treated in a way that destroys its damaging properties without damaging its ability to stimulate antibody production.

trachea (tra′ ke ah) The windpipe.

tracheal (tra′ ke al) Pertaining to the trachea.

tracheorrhagia (tra″ ke o ra′ je ah) Hemorrhage from the trachea.

tracheostomy (tra″ ke os′ to me) Surgical formation of a new opening into the windpipe from the neck.

tracheotome (tra′ ke o tōm) An instrument used for incision of the trachea.

tracheotomy (tra″ ke ot′ o me) Surgically cutting into the windpipe.

transfusion (trans fu′ zhun) The introduction of blood directly into the bloodstream of an individual.

t. reaction, an adverse reaction to blood received in a transfusion.

transthoracic (trans″ tho ras ik) Through the chest cavity or across the chest wall.

transurethral (trans″ u re′ thral) Through the urethra.

t. resection, resection of the prostate by means of an instrument passed up through the urethra.

transverse (trans″ vers′) Extending from side to side; at right angles to the long axis; divides the body into upper and lower portions.

trauma (traw′ mah) Any wound or injury resulting from impact.

trichocardia (trik″ o kar′ de ah) A hairy appearance of the heart due to pericarditis.

trichoid (trik′ oid) Resembling hair.

trichophagy (trik o fah je) Eating hair.

trichorrhexis (trik″ o rek′ sis) Breaking off hair.

trilodothyronine (tri″ lo″ do thi′ ro nēn) One of the thyroid hormones.

tricuspid (tri kus pid) Having three points or cusps; pertaining to the tricuspid valve of the heart.

tripara (tri′ pah rah) A woman who has given birth to three children.

trophopathy (tro fop′ ah the) Any abnormal state of nutrition.

tubal ligation (too′ bal ly gay′ shun) Cauterization and(or) tying off the uterine tubes to prevent passage of eggs and pregnancy.

tubule (too būl) A small tube.
renal t., the terminal channels of the nephrons in which urine is formed.
seminiferous t., one of several small channels of the testes in which spermatozoa develop.

tunica (too′ ni kah) A general term for a membrane or other structure covering or lining a body part or organ.
t. adventitis, the outer coat of many tubular body structures.
t. intima, the innermost coat of blood vessels.
t. media, the middle coat of blood vessels.

tympanum (tim′ pan um) The chamber where the eardrum is located.

ulcer (ul′ ser) A local defect or excavation of the surface of an organ or tissue, produced by sloughing of necrotic inflammatory tissue.
decubitus u., a skin defect caused by prolonged pressure from lying too still in bed; bed sore.
duodenal u., ulcer of the duodenum.
peptic u., a loss of tissue lining the lower esophagus, the stomach, or the duodenum.

ulna (ul′ nah) The inner and larger bone of the forearm.

ulnoradial (ul″ no ra de al) Pertaining to the ulna and the radius, both bones of the lower arm.

ultrasound (ul′ trah sownd) Mechanical radiant energy with a frequency greater than 20,000 cycles per second.

umbilicus (um bil′ i kus) The navel.

unilateral (u″ ni lat′ er al) Pertaining to only one side.

unipara (u nip′ ah ra) A woman who has given birth to one child.

urea (u re′ ah) The chief nitrogenous constituent of urine.

uremia (u re′ me ah) An accumulation of toxic products in the blood due to inadequate functioning of the kidneys.

ureter (u re′ ter) The tubular organ through which urine passes from the kidney to the bladder.

ureterocele (ūr e′ ter o sēl″) Hernia of the ureter.

ureteropyelitis (u re″ ter o pi e li′ tis) Inflammation of a ureter and renal pelvis.

urethra (u re′ thrah) The passage by which urine is discharged from the bladder to the exterior.

urethritis (u″ re thri′ tis) Inflammation of the urethra.

urethrocele (u re′ thro sēl) Herniation of the urethra.

urethrocystitis (u re″ thro sis ti′ tis) Pertaining to the urethra and bladder.

urethrorectal (u re″ thro rek′ tal) Pertaining to the urethra and rectum.

urethrorrhagia (u re″ thro ra′ je ah) Hemorrhage from the urethra.

urethrorrhea (u re″ thro re′ ah) Discharge from the urethra.

urethrotomy (u″ re throt′ o me) Incision of the urethra.

urinalysis (u″ ri nal′ i sis) Examination of urine.

urologic (u″ ro loj′ ik) Pertaining to the urinary system.

urticaria (ur″ ti ka′ re ah) Hives, a vascular reaction of the skin marked by transient appearance of wheals (raised, reddened areas).

uterine tube (u′ ter ine) One of two small tubes attached to either side of the uterus and leading to an ovary.

uterus (u′ ter us) The hollow muscular organ of the female in which the embryo develops.

uvula (u′ vu lah) A fleshy mass that hangs down from the soft palate.

vagina (vah ji′ nah) The birth canal of the female; the organ that receives the penis in copulation.

vaginal (vaj′ in al) Pertaining to the vagina.

vaginitis (vaj′ i ni tis) Inflammation of the vagina.

varicocele (var′ e co′ sēl) Swelling of veins in the testicle.

vascular (vas′ ku lar) Pertaining to the blood vessels; often indicating a copious supply of blood.

vas deferens (vas def′ er enz) The excretory duct of the male in which sperm leave the testes.

vasectomy (vah sek′ to me) Excision of the vas deferens, usually with cauterization, to result in intentional sterility.

vasoconstriction (vas″ o kon strik′ shun) Diminution of the size of a blood vessel.

vasodilatation (vas″ o dil ah ta′ shun) A state of increased diameter of blood vessels.

vasodilation (vas″ o di la shun) Stretching or dilation that results in increased diameter of the blood vessels.

vasomotor (vas o mo′ tor) Affecting the diameter of blood vessel walls by muscular control.

vasostomy (vah sos′ to me) Surgical formation of an opening into the vas deferens.

vasotomy (vah sot′ o me) Incision in or cutting of the vas deferens.

vein (vain) A vessel of the circulatory system in which blood returns to the heart.
varicose v., distended vein, often in the legs, as a result of sluggish flow of blood and defective valves in the vein.

vena cava (ve′ nah ka′ vah) Two large veins that carry blood to the right side of the heart.
inferior v.c., the venous trunk for the lower limbs and for pelvis and abdominal viscera.
superior v.c., the venous trunk that drains blood from the head, neck, upper limbs, and thorax.

venous (ve′ nus) Pertaining to a vein.

ventral (ven′ tral) Pertaining to the abdomen; situated on the belly surface; opposite of dorsal.

ventricle (ven′ trik′ l) A small cavity or chamber.

ventriculitis (ven trik″ u li′ tis) Inflammation of a ventricle, usually a cerebral ventricle.

ventriculography (ven trik″ u log′ rah fe) Radiography of the cerebral ventricles.

venular (ven′ u lar) Pertaining to a venule (a minute vein).

venule (ven ūl) A minute vein; small vessels that collect blood from the capillaries and join to form veins.

vertebra (ver′ te brah) Any one of the 33 bones of the spinal column.

vertebrectomy (ver″ te brek to me) Excision of a vertebra.

vertebrochondral (ver″ te bro kon′ dral) Pertaining to a vertebra and cartilage.

vertigo (vert i go) Dizziness.

vesicle (ves′ i kle) A small bladder or sac containing liquid.
seminal v., one of a pair of pouches attached to the posterior urinary bladder.

vesicule (ves′ i kule) A blister or small bladder.

virulence (vir′ u lens) The degree of pathogenicity of a microorganism.

virus (vi′ rus) One of a group of minute microorganisms that have the ability to replicate only within living host cells.

visceral (vis′ er al) Pertaining to large internal organs.

viscus (vis′ kus) Any large interior organ of the body.

void (voyd) To expel urine.

volvulus (vol′ vue lus) A twisting of the intestines.

wart (wort) An epidermal tumor.

wheal (wheel) A localized area of edema of the skin.

wheeze (wheez) A whistling sound made during respiration.

xanthoderma (zan″ tho der′ mah) A yellow coloration of the skin.

xanthosis (zan tho′ sis) Any yellow condition.

xanthous (zan′ thus) Yellow.

xeroderma (ze″ ro der′ mah) A disease characterized by rough, dry skin.

Appendix Three Abbreviations

There are many abbreviations used in medical communications and there are some that are unique to a specific medical community. Many hospitals have a list of acceptable "approved" abbreviations to be used in their records and this list tends to govern what is used by others outside each hospital. The following list is composed of only the more common abbreviations. It is not a definitive list and will not always indicate precisely what the writer may mean. For example, the abbreviation *PVC* is often used in the medical community to signify *Premature Ventricular Contraction.* However, *PVC* is also used by the plastics industry for the material, *polyvinyl chloride*, commonly used in the manufacture of catheters and other plastics found in some medical devices.

Abbreviations for chemicals and academic degrees are not included in this list, nor are abbreviations included for unusual or nonmedical terms like the latter definition of *PVC.* Usually the context in which the abbreviation is used will give a strong clue to its meaning.

This is an important part of the medical language and it requires rote memorization or paired association to develop recall. We suggest that you read the list in its entirety and then cover the right side of the first page with a card. Say the abbreviation and then try to guess its meaning. Do not be concerned about upper- or lower-case letters, punctuation, or the little hatbars (the lines above certain letters). Repeat the process and each time discard the ones you get correct until you are down to the last few. Leave these for a while and later return to the list, repeating the process until you have mastered them to your satisfaction.

Table of Abbreviations

Abbreviation	Meaning
$\bar{a}$	Before
$\overline{aa}$	Of Each
Ab	Antibody
ABE	Acute Bacterial Endocarditis
ACT	Acute Crisis Team
ACU	Acute Care Unit
ad lib	As Much As Wanted
ADR	Adverse Drug Reaction
Ag	Antigen
AIDS	Acquired Immune Deficiency Syndrome
AMI	Acute Myocardial Infarction

Abbreviation	Meaning
AMA	Against Medical Advice; American Medical Association
AOM	Acute Otitis Media
ARD	Acute Respiratory Distress
ARF	Acute Renal Failure
ASHD	Arteriosclerotic Heart Disease
ASCVD	Atherosclerotic Cardiovascular Disease
AV	Atrioventricular; Arteriovenous
BBT	Basal Body Temperature
BCLS	Basic Cardiac Life Support
b.i.d.	Twice Daily
BLS	Basic Life Support
BM	Bowel Movement; Basal Metabolism; Body Mass
BMR	Basal Metabolic Rate
BP	Blood Pressure; Bypass
BR	Bed Rest
BRP	Bathroom Privileges
BS	Bowel Sounds; Breath Sounds
BT	Bleeding Time; Body Temperature
BTB	Breakthrough Bleeding
$\bar{c}$	With
Ca	Cancer
CA	Coronary Artery; Chronological Age
CAD	Coronary Artery Disease
CAT SCAN	Computerized Axial Tomography Scan
CBC	Complete Blood Count
CBF	Cerebral Blood Flow
CBR	Complete Bed Rest
CCU	Coronary Care Unit
CF	Cystic Fibrosis
CHD	Coronary Heart Disease; Congenital Heart Disease
CHF	Congestive Heart Failure
CIHD	Chronic Ischemic Heart Disease
CNB	Cutting Needle Biopsy
CNS	Central Nervous System
CO	Cardiac Output; Carbon Monoxide
C/O	Complaints of . . .
COPD	Chronic Obstructive Pulmonary Disease
CP	Cerebral Palsy; Chronic Pain; Chemically Pure
CPR	Cardiopulmonary Resuscitation
C-section	Cesarean section
CSF	Cerebrospinal Fluid
DBP	Diastolic Blood Pressure
D/C	Discontinue; Discharge the Patient
D&C	Dilation and Curettage
DES	Diethylstilbestrol
DI	Diabetes Insipidus
DKA	Diabetic Ketoacidosis
DM	Diastolic Murmur; Diabetes Mellitus
DOA	Dead On Arrival
DTs	Delirium Tremens
Dx	Diagnosis
ECF	Extracellular Fluid
ECC	Emergency Cardiac Care
ECG OR EKG	Electrocardiogram
ECM	Extracellular Material
EEG	Electroencephalogram
(E)ENT	(Eye), Ear, Nose, Throat
EMG	Electromyogram

Abbreviation	Meaning
ER	Emergency Room
ESRD	End-Stage Renal Disease
FAS	Fetal Alcohol Syndrome
FBS	Fasting Blood Sugar
FHx	Family History
Fx	Fracture
GI	Gastrointestinal
GU	Genitourinary
h.	Hour
Hb or Hgb	Hemoglobin
HBP	High Blood Pressure
H/H	Hemoglobin/Hematocrit
HCT	Hematocrit
HDL	High-Density Lipoprotein
HEENT	Head, Ears, Eyes, Nose, Throat
HPI	History Present Illness
HR	Heart Rate
Hx	History
ICF	Intracellular Fluid
ICP	Intracranial Pressure
ICU	Intensive Care Unit
ID	Identification; Initial Dose; Intradermal
IHD	Ischemic Heart Disease
IOP	Intraocular Pressure
IUD	Intrauterine Device (Contraceptive)
LBW	Low Birth Weight
LDL	Low Density Lipoprotein
LLQ	Left Lower Quadrant
LOC	Loss Of Consciousness
LS	Left Septum
MED	Minimal Effective Dose
MI	Myocardial Infarction; Mitral Insufficiency
NBM	Nothing By Mouth; No Bowel Movement
n/l	Normal Limits
NOS	Not Otherwise Specified
NPO	Nothing By Mouth
N&T	Nose And Throat
OD	Overdose; Right Eye
OPD	Outpatient Department
OR	Operating Room
OS	Left Eye
OTD	Out The Door = Discharge
OU	Both Eyes
p	After
p.c.	After meals
PE	Physical Exam
PID	Pelvic Inflammatory Disease
PMH	Post Medical History
PMS	Premenstrual Syndrome
PNS	Peripheral Nervous System
PO_2	Oxygen Pressure
POD	Postoperative Day
p.r.n.	As Required
q	Every
qd, qid	Every Day, 4 Times/Day
qod	Every Other Day
QO_2	Oxygen Consumption
RBC	Red Blood Cell (Count)

Abbreviation	Meaning
ROM	Range Of Motion
RT	Room Temperature; Radiotherapy; Respiratory Therapy
s̄	Without
SCD	Sudden Cardiac Death
SH	Social History
SIDS	Sudden Infant-Death Syndrome
SOB	Shortness of Breath
SP	Systolic Pressure
SubQ or SQ	Subcutaneous
stat.	Immediately
STD	Sexually Transmitted Disease
T	Temperature; Tension
T&A	Tonsilladenoidectomy
TBW	Total Body Weight
TIA	Transient Ischemic Attack
t.i.d.	Three Times a Day
TLC	Tender Loving Care; Total Lung Capacity
Ty	Type
UG	Urogenital
UTI	Urinary Tract Infection
VO_2 MAX	Maximal Oxygen Uptake (Volume)
VW	Vessel Wall
WBC	White Blood Cell (Count)
WNL	Within Normal Limits
Y/O	Years Old

Symbols

℥	Ounce
f℥	Fluid ounce.
℞	Recipe; take.
C′	Complement.
μg	Microgram.
mg	Milligram.
m-	Meta-.
o-	Ortho-.
p-	Para-.
s̄s̄, ss	[L. *semis*]. One-half.
′	Foot; minute; primary accent; univalent.
″	Inch; second; secondary accent; bivalent.
μm	Micrometer.
μ	Micron.
+	Plus; excess; acid reaction; positive.
−	Minus; deficiency; alkaline reaction; negative.
±	Plus or minus; either positive or negative; indefinite.
×	Multiplied by; magnification.
=	Equals.
>	Greater than; from which is derived.
<	Less then; derived from.
≮	Not less than.
≯	Not greater than.
≦	Equal to or less than.
≧	Equal to or greater than.
≠	Not equal to.
∞	Infinity.
:	Ratio; "is to."
: :	Equality between ratios; "as."
∴	Therefore.
°	Degree.
□, ♂	Male.
○, ♀	Female.
⇌	Denotes a reversible reaction.

Terminology Trivia

Charles Drew (1904–1950) developed the technique for separating blood plasma from whole blood at the age of 32. Today, we take this technology for granted, but prior to the mid-1930s blood could not be stored and deaths due to the unavailability of blood were common. Drew's innovative talent and desire to serve the world led to his development of another concept we take for granted: the blood bank. He also directed a blood plasma project in Great Britain in 1940 and later directed the Red Cross in New York City. He received the coveted Spingarn Medal in 1944 for his contributions to humankind and his professional achievements; his research and public service saved literally thousands of people from bleeding to death.

In 1950, while traveling through North Carolina, Dr. Drew was involved in a car accident. He was taken to a local hospital where eventually he bled to death. Ironically, he was not given a blood transfusion because the hospital would not admit him. He was black.

Medical progress is often thwarted by the attitudes and lack of acceptance of the public. This tragic account serves to remind us that not many years ago social opinion dominated medical action. The public is very slow both to accept innovation and to act on behalf of its own health. Jenner's 1796 discovery of a vaccine for smallpox was not put into action until much later. Despite the high mortality rate of this dreaded disease, the first mass vaccination program against it did not take place until 1914.

Appendix Four
Medical Records and Forms

Written records have an important role in health care. Although the form of the record may vary considerably from place to place, all generally serve the same functions. Records are written, legal documents of the patient's progress and treatment. They serve the following purposes:

1. They help to coordinate care.
2. They eliminate the need for the patient to repeat information to other health workers.
3. They promote accuracy and assign responsibility for care.
4. They help avoid duplication and overlapping of patient care services.

The patient's record is an account of health status and care. It describes the patient's health, specifies diagnostic and therapeutic measures employed, and records the patient's responses to these actions. The record is kept current as long as the patient is receiving care.

Patient records serve the following functions:

Communication—Although health workers do talk to each other, the patient's record is a permanent and easily accessible form of communication that conveys meaningful care information. An accurate record also serves to clarify messages and prevent errors, such as the inadvertent administration of a duplicate medication.

Audit—The patient's record is also used to monitor both the quality of care and the related competencies of the people providing that care. When possible, this care is measured against established standards; when it is conducted by another person of the same profession, the audit is called a *peer review*. Hospitals and other organizations have audit committees that regularly monitor professional practice.

Legal documentation—The patient's record is a legal document that is considered the property of the organization keeping it. However, according to the *Patient's Bill of Rights*, the patient has a right to see it.

Statistics—Statistical information culled from records can help an agency plan for future needs. For example, admission statistics in hospitals may show which services need to be expanded or curtailed. Some statistics are kept by requirement of the law, such as birth records, death records, and reports of certain communicable diseases.

Research—Information found in records can be a valuable data source. Researchers may study diverse treatment plans of similar conditions to determine which course of action was of greatest benefit. A record may also reveal forgotten or seemingly insignificant facts that may shed light on a mysterious problem.

Education—Records provide a comprehensive view of patients, illnesses, and treatments. They are valuable educational tools and as such are used to educate people in most of the health disciplines.

Traditional Patient Records

The traditional patient record is considered source-oriented since each source of information (health worker) writes out the record. The records found in this text include an admission note, history and physical exams, patient charts, a discharge summary, an autopsy report, and a prescription form. The emphasis here is on developing skill in reading records rather than in composing them. So, read the first example and as you do, skip over the words you do not recognize or cannot immediately interpret. Then, read the report a second time and try to determine these words through the context in which they are used. For example, if the sentence refers to the abdomen, then the unrecognized word or abbreviation may be related to that area or to the condition described. In other words, there may be hints contained in the words around it. If you cannot figure it out or you are in doubt, take the time and look it up in the glossary. If it is an abbreviation, look at the alphabetical listing of abbreviations in Appendix Three.

Admission Notes

The *admission notes* contain specific data about the patient at the time of admission. Most contain the following information:

patient's name
patient's address
date of birth
name of attending physician
sex and marital status
nearest relative
occupation and employer
date and hour of admission
hospital unit
admitting diagnosis or impression
identification number

An example of the form used to record admission notes is shown in Form A.

History

The *history* is a record of the patient's health history and is written by a physician or physician assistant. The contents of the history vary depending on the chief complaint of the client; planned actions are not part of the history. If information is listed as other than progress notes or orders, it is put on a *Problem List* when a *POMR* (*P*roblem, *O*bjectives, *M*ethods, *R*eview) format is used. In the examples shown on the following pages, the hospital has guided the entries by listing the information they want and the order in which they

Form A Admission notes.

J.D.

I.D. # 84-1002-45

IMPRINT

ADMISSION NOTE

HOSPITAL REGULATION: ALL POSITIVE AND IMPORTANT NEGATIVE FINDINGS SHALL BE RECORDED

Date________ Hour________ a.m. p.m. Age____ Sex____ Weight________

Temp.________ Pulse________ Resp.________ Blood Pressure________

Patient is a ten year old WD black male named J.D. He had been involved in an auto accident approximately 35 minutes earlier. The boy's brother described that J. had been expelled from the vehicle and fell about 30 feet from it. He was apparently unconscious and on route to the ER nad some intermittent convulsive activity. Upon admission his pupils were midposition and reactive with OS > OD. Seizures were evident but s̄ true clonic activity.

Patient was making some semipurposive movements with his extremities. He was comotose with dyspnea. Optic fundi appeared normal.

Breath sounds were normal on both sides but tne left side of the thorax was dull to percussion. Slight blood discharge from mouth and evident in sputum. There was an abrasion on the left arm with a large contusion extending the full length of the left humerus.

Impression: concussion
possible skull fracture
possible hemothorax

Address: 432 South Lloyd Street
City, 55321
Phone: 555-4321
Closest relative:________________

Physician:________________

____
Signature

0753803 CONTINUE ON REVERSE SIDE 1-421-2-0879

want it. However, Form B illustrates an extensive listing of the content in a patient history. Key data to be collected from all clients are marked with an asterisk ('*'). Examples of actual patient histories are shown in Forms C, D, E, and F.

Form B The contents of a complete medical history.

I. Chief complaint of client
  A. Location
  B. Character
  C. Chronology
  D. Situational determinants
  E. Aggravating or alleviating factors
  F. Previous attempts at therapy and their effectiveness
  G. Disability resulting from this complaint
II. Social systems
  A. Social development
    *1. Age
    *2. Sex
    *3. Developmental tasks
    *4. Psychosocial personality development (Erickson's Eight Stages of Man)
    *5. Diversional, recreational interests (what to do to pass time while ill)
    *6. Roles in family, community, work, and perceived performance of them
    *7. Degree of independence-dependence
    *8. Child's favorite play activity
    *9. Socially oriented habits (include alcohol, drugs), frequency of use, and response to use
  B. Family or significant others
    *1. Others in living group
    *2. Significant others outside living group
    *3. Visiting preferences and who is able to visit
    *4. Marital status
    *5. Alterations for family's life because of ill member
    *6. Interaction patterns (observe this also)
    *7. Presence of disease in other family members
  C. Work
    *1. Occupation
    *2. Source of income
    *3. Insurance (hospitalization)
    *4. Changes in work pattern because of illness
    *5. Feelings about work and being away from productivity and routine
  D. Religion
    *1. Religious affiliation
    *2. Desire for chaplain visit
    *3. Practices or beliefs that might affect reaction to health care (proscriptions against immunization or blood transfusion, dietary laws, beliefs about disease causation, death)
  E. Education
    *1. Formal education
    *2. Satisfaction and progress with school
  F. Community
    *1. Type of housing
    *2. Contacts or previous referrals to social agencies
    *3. Availability and pattern of utilization of health care facilities (physician, dentist), frequency and reason for visits
    *4. Immunizations (type, date)
  G. Ethnic-cultural system
    *1. Factors that may influence reaction to hospitalization, therapy, illness
    *2. Food preferences
    *3. Response to stress (e.g., pain)
  H. Environment
    *1. Effect of present environment on health status and developmental level (e.g., lighting, noise, activity, color—variation, consistency excessive or absent)
    *2. Arrangement of environment in relation to functional abilities or disabilities

---

*Key data to collect for all clients. Data not marked are collected if dysfunction is found in system.

- *3. Safety factors
  - a. Mobility (arrangement of objects in physical environment)
  - b. Use of prosthetic or supportive devices (e.g., crutches, wheelchair)
- *4. Infection control
  - a. Ready sources of infection
  - b. Barriers to infection (isolation technique, handwashing facility)

III. Psychological systems

- A. Cognition
  - *1. Level of consciousness (response to sensory stimuli)
  - *2. Orientation to time, place, person
  - *3. Mental skills
    - a. Ability to read and write
    - b. Vocabulary
    - c. Ability to comprehend and follow directions
    - d. Attention and memory span
  - *4. Intellectual development relative to chronological age (e.g., Piaget's formulation)
  - *5. Understanding of and reaction to health concern and goals of medical-nursing therapy
  - *6. Desired information about present tests and treatment
  - *7. Previous experience with and reaction to illness and hospitalization
  - *8. Name child or adolescent prefers
- B. Emotion
  - *1. Quality of mood, expression, intensity of reaction
  - *2. Activity level (active, sluggish, hyperactive)
  - *3. Effect of illness on life and expectation of future effects
  - *4. Feelings about hospitalization
  - *5. Coping patterns in stressful situations (describe stressful situations); availability, need for, and effectiveness of internal-external support systems
  - *6. Special concerns or fears
  - *7. Patterns of relating to others (e.g., verbal, congenial)
  - *8. Self-concept (body image before and in relation to current health problem)
  - *9. Comfort, rest and sleep patterns (hours, time, nap periods, feeling of being rested) before and since illness
  - *10. Aids used to sleep
  - *11. Presence of pain or discomfort (location, duration, degree, character, precipitating factors, change in pattern)
  - *12. Use of aids to relieve pain

IV. Biological systems

- A. Gas transport and exchange
  - 1. Cardiovascular
    - *a. Past or present disease of cardiovascular system
    - *b. Syncope
    - *c. Dizziness
    - *d. Fatigue, activity tolerance
    - *e. Chest pain
      - (1) Type
      - (2) Pattern
      - (3) Precipitating factors
      - (4) Relief measures
    - *f. Subjective feeling of warmth or coldness of body parts
    - *g. Medications taken to affect CV system
    - *h. Edema of body parts
  - 2. Respiratory
    - *a. Past or present diseases of respiratory system
    - *b. Cough
      - (1) Frequency
      - (2) Duration
    - *c. Sputum
      - (1) Color
      - (2) Odor
      - (3) Amount
    - *d. Shortness of breath
      - (1) Precipitating factors
      - (2) Frequency
      - (3) Effect on activity
    - *e. Allergies
    - *f. Smoking
      - (1) Amount
      - (2) Duration
      - (3) Attempts and success at stopping
    - *g. Medications taken to affect respiratory system
    - h. Orthopnea
    - i. Hemoptysis
    - j. Fever
    - k. Frequency of colds and sore throat
    - l. Activity tolerance
    - m. Factors affecting breathing
      - (1) Emotion
      - (2) Pollution
      - (3) Position

B. Nutrition and elimination
  1. Gastrointestinal
    *a. Past or present disease of GI system
    *b. Dietary habits
      (1) Amount of basic four food groups
      (2) Amount of fluid intake daily
      (3) Likes
      (4) Dislikes
      (5) Number of meals and snacks
      (6) Time of meals
      (7) Assistance needed with eating
      (8) Alcohol intake
    *c. Appetite, thirst, stability of weight
    *d. Factors related to ingestion
      (1) Nonoral intake
      (2) Chewing
      (3) Swallowing
      (4) Oral hygiene habits
    *e. Factors related to digestion
      (1) Ease
      (2) Nausea
      (3) Vomiting
      (4) Belching
      (5) Pain in abdomen
    *f. Bowel elimination pattern
      (1) Time and frequency of bowel movements
      (2) Degree of child's independence in toileting
      (3) Words used by child regarding elimination
      (4) Character of stools
      (5) Ease (constipation, diarrhea)
      (6) Hemorrhoids
      (7) Passage of gas, blood
    *g. Abdominal pain and character
    *h. Medicines taken to alter digestion and metabolism of foods
  2. Urinary
    *a. Past or present diseases of urinary system
    *b. Fluid intake
    *c. Urination pattern
      (1) Amount
      (2) Color
      (3) Odor
      (4) Frequency, night or day urgency
      (5) Dysuria
    *d. Vaginal or urethral discharge
    *e. Degree of independence in toileting
    *f. Edema

C. Sensorimotor
  1. Musculoskeletal
    *a. Past or present diseases of musculoskeletal system
    *b. Abnormal innervation to muscles (paralysis, weakness, spasticity)
    *c. Activity endurance
    *d. Method of ambulation
      (1) Assistance needed with dressing, hygiene,
      (2) Safety measures needed
    *e. Range of motion limitation
    *f. Muscle weakness
    *g. Medicines taken to affect musculoskeletal subsystem
  2. Nervous
    *a. Past or present diseases of nervous system
    *b. Visual status
      (1) Acuity
      (2) Deficits and corrective devices
    *c. Auditory status
      (1) Deficits and corrective devices
      (2) Unusual sensations (ringing, buzzing, vertigo, pain)
    *d. Olfactory status
    *e. Taste status
    *f. Tactile status (ability to discriminate sharp-dull, light-firm, heat-cold sensations)
    *g. Mobility (coordination, balance)
    *h. Medicines taken to affect nervous system

D. Protective mechanisms
  1. Integument
    *a. Past or present diseases of integumentary system
    *b. Factors predisposing to skin breakdown
    *c. Personal hygiene
      (1) Bathing (kind, type, frequency)
      (2) Frequency, time of shaving
      (3) After bath skin care
    *d. Medicines taken to affect integumentary system
  2. Immune mechanism
    *a. Past or present allergy

- *b. Past or present sensitivities to drugs or other agents (pollens, insect bites)
- *c. Past or present high susceptibility to infection

E. Endocrine mechanisms
- *1. Abnormal function of endocrine gland(s) and effect; past or present diseases
- *2. Growth patterns
- *3. Medicines taken to affect endocrine system

F. Sexuality and reproduction
- *1. Past or present alterations of reproductive system
- *2. Reproductive data
  - a. Number of pregnancies
  - b. Live births
  - c. Living children
  - d. Family planning (methods used)
  - e. Menstrual pattern
  - f. Menopause (age of onset and associated factors)
- *3. Breast self-examination routine
- *4. Frequency of Pap smears
- *5. Sexual libido and performance
- *6. Level of sexual development
- *7. Attitudes toward own sexuality
- *8. Medicine taken to affect reproductive system

Form C Example of patient history.

98765-431-84

Mr. A.B.

9/4/84 4/11/37

IMPRINT

HISTORY

HOSPITAL REGULATION: ALL POSITIVE AND IMPORTANT NEGATIVE FINDINGS SHALL BE RECORDED

ORDER OF RECORDING

1. Chief Complaint
2. History of Present Illness
3. History of Past Illness
   a) childhood
   b) adult
   c) operations
   d) injury
4. Systemic Review
   a) General
   b) Skin
   c) Head-Eyes Ears-Nose Throat
   d) Neck
   e) Respiratory
   f) Cardiovascular
   g) Gastro-intestinal
   h) Genito-urinary
   i) Gynecological
   j) Locomotor
   k) Neuropsychiatric
   l) Allergic Conditions
   m) Immunization
5. Family History
6. Social History

Date 4 September 1984 Hour 3:00 p.m. a.m. p.m.

Chief Complaint: "Pain in my stomach and just feeling sick"

History of Present Illness: AB presented to County Hospital this morning at 10:00 a.m. with a three year history of intermittent episodes of "crampy" pain in the epigastrium and right upper quadrant. The pain is diffuse without radiation and ranks 3 on a scale of 0-10, 10 worst. The pain is related to eating of meals, occurring approximately two hours after the beginning of a meal and is worst with a fatty diet. There are no other associations with time of year or month. The most recent attack of pain came three days ago, 1 September 1984, and has not let up since, also made worse two hours after a meal. This morning at 8:00 a.m. after the patient's 6:00 a.m. breakfast, the pain worsened and became associated with nausea and a few minutes later with vomiting. Because of this concern over this pain, and new symptoms, AB had his wife drive him to the County Hospital Emergency room. Other pertinent facts of AB's medical condition: he is a sickle cell trait heterozygote diagnosed in 1970 age 33 after a prolonged "ill feeling"; he is a hypertensive, well controlled on diuretic Furosemide 80 mg twice a day.

History of Past Illness:
Measles without complications age 12, 1949
Mumps with unilateral right sided orchitis age 17, 1954
No history of Rheumatic fever
Prolonged ill feeling diagnosed as anemia with etiology of sickle cell trait - age 33, 1970
Hypertensive diagnosed on routine physical for work, age 35, 1972
Right sided wrist fracture from a raquet ball accident, age 28, 1965

Review of Systems:
No history of weight loss, change of diet or appetite not associated with pain episodes. No changes in sleep patterns. No changes in skin, nails or hair. No enlarged lymph nodes, no pain in joints, no recent bleeding or dizziness. No changes in bowel or bladder function, or habits.

Family Medical History:
Mother and father still living. Mother had gall bladder removed 3 years ago. Father has high blood pressure and chronic anemia, and a stroke in 1963. One older brother, 7/13/35 and sister 1/27/45 alive and well. Children, three boys 3/20/62, 9/29/64 and 5/26/67 alive and well. No family history of diabetes or cardiovascular disease.

Social History: AB is a full-time worker at C.D. Municipal Utilities where he has a desk job, which involves travel across the country, but not into foreign countries. He eats regular meals, low salt, balanced three times a day except with this pain. He exercises regularly four times a week running 5 miles in approximately 35-40 minutes. AB is a non-smoker and drinks socially approximately 3 beers/week.

Signature of Attending Physician

0742805 **HISTORY** 1-421-2-0879

Form D Example of patient history.

87698-963-84

Mrs. C.D.

9/5/84 10/3/84

IMPRINT

HISTORY

HOSPITAL REGULATION: ALL POSITIVE AND IMPORTANT NEGATIVE FINDINGS SHALL BE RECORDED

Date 5 September 1984 Hour 1:40 p.m. a.m. p.m.

ORDER OF RECORDING

1. Chief Complaint
2. History of Present Illness
3. History of Past Illness
   a) childhood
   b) adult
   c) operations
   d) injury
4. Systemic Review
   a) General
   b) Skin
   c) Head-Eyes Ears-Nose Throat
   d) Neck
   e) Respiratory
   f) Cardiovascular
   g) Gastro-intestinal
   h) Genito-urinary
   i) Gynecological
   j) Locomotor
   k) Neuropsychiatric
   l) Allergic Conditions
   m) Immunization
5. Family History
6. Social History

CC: "Fell and cut my chin"

HPI: At home, patient experienced dizziness and fell, striking chin on coffee table, causing small laceration. No associated LOC, N/V, headache, angina. No previous history of LOC, seizures, CVA, or T/A. S/P mitral valve replacement, on coumadin. DM on insulin (adult type), COPD x20 years requiring nasal O_2.

PMH: Measles +, Mumps +, RF + with three months in hospital at age 14.
Total hip R replacement in 1979, after a fall on ice.
G3P3 vaginal delivery x3.
NKA
Meds: Coumadin 10 mg qd po
NPH insulin 80 units SQ qd at breakfast
nasal O_2 at 2 L/min
ASA 500 mg tid p.o. prn arthritis pain
vitamin pill qd p.o.

ROS: Multiple age spots on hands, crepitus of both hands
↓hearing both sides, sleeps better on three pillows

FMH: Father died of heart attack age 67
Mother died of old age
Sister died in childbirth
3 children A&W

SH: Living in nursing home with few visitors, husband died two years ago.
EtOH chronic 2 pints whiskey/day
Smokes 3 ppd x30 years

Signature of Attending Physician

0742805 **HISTORY** 1-421-2-0879

Form E Example of patient history.

72146-078-84

Mr. D.E.

9/5/84 1/14/72

IMPRINT

HISTORY

HOSPITAL REGULATION: ALL POSITIVE AND IMPORTANT NEGATIVE FINDINGS SHALL BE RECORDED

Date 5 September 1984 Hour 2:40 p.m. a.m. p.m.

ORDER OF RECORDING

1. Chief Complaint
2. History of Present Illness
3. History of Past Illness
   a) childhood
   b) adult
   c) operations
   d) injury
4. Systemic Review
   a) General
   b) Skin
   c) Head-Eyes Ears-Nose Throat
   d) Neck
   e) Respiratory
   f) Cardiovascular
   g) Gastro-intestinal
   h) Genito-urinary
   i) Gynecological
   j) Locomotor
   k) Neuropsychiatric
   l) Allergic Conditions
   m) Immunization
5. Family History
6. Social History

CC: MVA - History from mother

HPI: Sitting in passenger seat without seat belt when car crossed the median and struck another car head on. DE was found 50 feet to the right of his car in median. Brought in by ambulance comatose, with neck collar, intubated and bagged @20/min 100 % O_2. Vitals in field Pulse 140, Blood Pressure 80/40, R Ø.

PMH: NKA
No meds - may be taking drugs from school friends - pot, coke?
RF ⊖

ROS: N/C

FMH: Mother DM

SH: Lives with mother, father and one sister
Going to school at County Junior High
EtOH ⊖
Smokes ⊖

Signature of Attending Physician

0742805 **HISTORY** 1-421-2-0879

Form F Example of patient history.

27874-362-84

Mrs. E.F.

9/5/84 2/7/52

IMPRINT

HISTORY

HOSPITAL REGULATION: ALL POSITIVE AND IMPORTANT NEGATIVE FINDINGS SHALL BE RECORDED

ORDER OF RECORDING

1. Chief Complaint
2. History of Present Illness
3. History of Past Illness
   a) childhood
   b) adult
   c) operations
   d) injury
4. Systemic Review
   a) General
   b) Skin
   c) Head-Eyes Ears-Nose Throat
   d) Neck
   e) Respiratory
   f) Cardiovascular
   g) Gastro-intestinal
   h) Genito-urinary
   i) Gynecological
   j) Locomotor
   k) Neuropsychiatric
   l) Allergic Conditions
   m) Immunization
5. Family History
6. Social History

Date 5 September 1984 Hour 3:15 p.m. a.m. p.m.

CC: "Pain in my stomach, then vomiting blood."

HPI: E.F. First noted a pain in her stomach three years ago and attributed it to spicy foods. At that time, she took antacids and it went away. This morning before breakfast she felt the pain more severely, and as she does every 3-4 days, she took antacids and ate her breakfast. Mid-way through her cereal, she became nauseous and vomited approximately one cup of bright red blood with food. At 10:00 a.m. this morning she again vomited about one cup blood. No history of dizziness, diarrhea, SOB previous episodes of hematemesis or stool.

HDI: Measles -, Mumps -, RF -
No injury or hospitalization other than normal vaginal deliveries.
G3P3
NKA
Meds: antacid tablets 2, p.o. prn stomach pain
ASA occasionally with headache

ROS: wears glasses
deviated septum
hard time getting to sleep without daytime sleepiness

FMH: - ulcers, - blood dipcrasias - coagalopathies
Father has colon Co with polyposis
- DM, - CHD, - ASCUD

SH: Smokes 2 ppd/30 years
EtOH "heavy" 3-4 pints over 2 days
Housewife with children 12, 10, 7 years old

Signature of Attending Physician

0742805 **HISTORY** 1-421-2-0879

Physical Examination

The *physical examination* report is completed by the person conducting the examination. This may be a physician, physician assistant, or nurse practitioner. The examples shown on the following pages (Forms G, H, I, J, and K) are authentic. Note that each physical examination form guides the entries down the left margin and by so doing gives the order of the entries. Also note that there is a marked difference in the quality of their composition. They were selected for inclusion here to illustrate the reporting variability that exists.

Read them, but do not expect to completely understand them the first time through. They are interesting, so do not struggle with them, just read and interpret as you go.

Some abbreviations commonly found in physical examination reports are:

PMH—past medical history
FH—family history
RS—review of systems
PE—physical examination
WD—well developed
WN—well nourished
VS—vital signs
BP—blood pressure
ER—emergency room
HEENT—head, ears, eyes, nose, and throat
EOM—extraocular movement; movement of eyes grossly
ENT—ear, nose, throat
WNL—within normal limits
PERRLA—pupils equally round and react to light and accommodation
NPO—non per os: nothing by mouth, including water
PO2—oxygen pressure
SOB—shortness of breath

Form G Example of physical examination report.

98765-431-84

Mr. A.B.

9/4/84 4/11/37

IMPRINT

PHYSICAL EXAMINATION

HOSPITAL REGULATION: ALL POSITIVE AND IMPORTANT NEGATIVE FINDINGS SHALL BE RECORDED

ORDER OF RECORDING

1. General
2. Skin
3. Eyes
4. Ears
5. Nose
6. Mouth
7. Throat
8. Neck
9. Chest
10. Heart
11. Abdomen
12. Genitalia
13. Lymphatic
14. Blood Vessels
15. Locomotor
16. Extremities
17. Neurological
18. Rectal
19. Vaginal
20. Diagnosis
21. Signature

Date 4 September 84 Hour 3:00 p.m. a.m./p.m. Age 47 Sex M Weight 138#

Temp. 100^{2} Pulse 62 Resp. 14 Blood Pressure 138/88

General: Well developed, well nourished black male appearing younger than his stated age, supine in pain with legs drawn up.

Skin: Without erythema or edema, normal male hair distribution.

Eyes: Pupils equal; round, responsive to light and accommodation, no hypertensive changes, extraocular movements intact.

Ears: air conduction greater than bone conduction, both sides tympanic membrane both sides clear, normal wax.

Nose: Without inflammation, swelling or blood.

Mouth: Upper dentures, no inflammation or masses

Neck: range of motion in tact, no lymph nodes palpable, thyroid not palpable.

Chest: Lungs clear to auscultation and percussion. Symmetrical diaphram movement by percussion.

Heart: Regular rate and rhythm, first and second Heart sounds present, normal physiological splitting of second heart sound without murmur gallop or rub.

Pulses: (Scale 1+ to 4+) carotid++, radial ++, ulnar +, branchial ++, femoral ++, popliteal +, dorsalis pedis ++, posterior tibial +, symmetrically. No bruits carotid or femoral.

Abd.: Bowel sounds normoactive, tenderness to deep palpation in right upper quadrant without rebound. No palpable masses, liver 12 cm by percussion with a smooth edge. Spleen not felt.

Ext.: Range of motion intact, no femoral or axillary lymph nodes noted. Without cyanosis, clubbing or edema.

GU: normal male uncircumcised, bladder not distended, right testicle smaller than normal.

Rectal: Prostate not enlarged, uniform density without local areas of hardness, no masses felt, stool present in anal vault, occult and gross blood not present.

Signature

0753803 CONTINUE ON REVERSE SIDE **PHYSICAL EXAMINATION** 1-421-2-0879

Form H Example of physical examination report.

98765-431-84

Mr. A.B.

9/4/84 4/11/37

IMPRINT

PHYSICAL EXAMINATION

HOSPITAL REGULATION: ALL POSITIVE AND IMPORTANT NEGATIVE FINDINGS SHALL BE RECORDED

Date 4 September 84 Hour 3:00 p.m. a.m./p.m. Age 47 Sex M Weight 138#

Temp._____ Pulse_____ Resp._____ Blood Pressure_____

Continued

Neurological: awake, alert, oriented to time, person and place, in pain but speech normal, good muscular strength, cranial nerves II through XII intact, normal sensory perception to pain and vibration. Finger to nose test and heel to shin test intact. Superficial long tract reflex responds in a plantar direction.

Diagnosis: Pain due to cholangitis, probably associated with cholecystitis and cholelithiasis.

ORDER OF RECORDING

1. General
2. Skin
3. Eyes
4. Ears
5. Nose
6. Mouth
7. Throat
8. Neck
9. Chest
10. Heart
11. Abdomen
12. Genitalia
13. Lymphatic
14. Blood Vessels
15. Locomotor
16. Extremities
17. Neurological
18. Rectal
19. Vaginal
20. Diagnosis
21. Signature

____
Signature

0753803 CONTINUE ON REVERSE SIDE **PHYSICAL EXAMINATION** 1-421-2-0879

Form I Example of physical examination report.

87698-953-84

Mrs. C.D.

9/5/84 10/3/4

IMPRINT

PHYSICAL EXAMINATION

HOSPITAL REGULATION: ALL POSITIVE AND IMPORTANT NEGATIVE FINDINGS SHALL BE RECORDED

ORDER OF RECORDING

1. General
2. Skin
3. Eyes
4. Ears
5. Nose
6. Mouth
7. Throat
8. Neck
9. Chest
10. Heart
11. Abdomen
12. Genitalia
13. Lymphatic
14. Blood Vessels
15. Locomotor
16. Extremities
17. Neurological
18. Rectal
19. Vaginal
20. Diagnosis
21. Signature

Date 5 September 84 Hour 2:00 p.m. a.m. p.m. Age 70 Sex ____ Weight 98#

Temp. 96^8 Pulse 96 Resp. 8 Blood Pressure 164/104

Gen: frail LOL in NAD, long laying supine relaxed

Skin: Pink warm, without edema, laceration 2 cm Ⓡ chin, 1 cm from midline

Eyes: PERPEA, no DM △ , EOMI

Ears: ↓ hearing both sides, AC > BC both sides, TM clear

Nose: without inflammation, dry mucosa, deviation to Ⓛ

Mouth: edentulous with dentures, no inflammation, odor of EtOH.

Neck: limited ROM with crepitus, no nodes, thyroid firm

Chest: bibasalar roles 1+, very resonant to percussion

Heart: RRR, S_1 clicks (mechanical) S_2 normal slight systolic flow murmur II/VI

Pulses: C+, R+, V-, B+, F+, P-, DP+, PT- both sides no bruit C.F.

Abd.: protuberant with normoactive BS, transmitted heart sounds. Liver palpable, 10 cm by percussion, spleen not felt.

Ext.: Limited ROM Ⓛ with crepitus, R without crepitus but painful. No DM△ or ulcers.

GU: normal female, dry mucosa, no masses

Rectal: no masses, no stool, heme +

Neuro: awake, but at times distant, oriented x2, good strength but motion limited on Ⓛ . CN II - XII intact. ↓ sensory on Ⓛ Ⓛ Babinski. F → N, H → S tremorous but grossly intact. Speech at times slurred.

Diag: TIA 2° to emboli formed on mitral valve

____
Signature

0753803 CONTINUE ON REVERSE SIDE **PHYSICAL EXAMINATION** 1-421-2-0879

Form J Example of physical examination report.

72146-078-84

Mr. D.E.

9/5/84 1/14/72

IMPRINT

PHYSICAL EXAMINATION

HOSPITAL REGULATION: ALL POSITIVE AND IMPORTANT NEGATIVE FINDINGS SHALL BE RECORDED

ORDER OF RECORDING

1. General
2. Skin
3. Eyes
4. Ears
5. Nose
6. Mouth
7. Throat
8. Neck
9. Chest
10. Heart
11. Abdomen
12. Genitalia
13. Lymphatic
14. Blood Vessels
15. Locomotor
16. Extremities
17. Neurological
18. Rectal
19. Vaginal
20. Diagnosis
21. Signature

Date 5 September 84 Hour 2:50 p.m. a.m./p.m. Age 12 Sex M Weight 135#

Temp. 95⁶ Pulse Thready 120 Resp. Bagged 20 Blood Pressure 90/50

General: WDWN male while adolescent of adult proportion. Multiple lacerations on face, displaced Ⓡ shoulder and Ⓡ rib fractures with indentation, head covered in blood.

Skin: Pale, shrunken with bleeding from multiple sites.

Eyes: Ⓡ Pupil fixed and dialated, Ⓛ pinpoint, No EOM corneal reflex ⊕ both sides.

Ears: Blood in external canal

Nose: Displaced to Ⓛ grossly with blood in vestibule

Mouth: Jaw displaced to Ⓛ without fx of mandible

Throat: ET tube in place

Neck: Neck collar, no deviation of teacher, no deformity, JVD ⊕

Chest: Lungs clear to auscultation

Heart: Weak beat RRR, S_1 and S_2 muffled.

Abd.: ⊖ BS, no masses

Pulses: C+, F+, R-, V-, DP-, PT-

EXT.: R humeral head displaced

Rectal: heme ⊖ , no masses

Neurological: Comatose, not responsive to pain, decorticode posture. Babinski Ⓛ , plantar response Ⓡ .

Diagnosis: Hemorrhage with hypovolemic hypotension
Cranial Damage - possibly epidural or dubdural
Pericardiac tamponade

Signature

0753803 CONTINUE ON REVERSE SIDE **PHYSICAL EXAMINATION** 1-421-2-0879

Form K Example of physical examination report.

27874-362-84

Mrs. E.F.

9/5/84 2/7/52

IMPRINT

PHYSICAL EXAMINATION

HOSPITAL REGULATION: ALL POSITIVE AND IMPORTANT NEGATIVE FINDINGS SHALL BE RECORDED

ORDER OF RECORDING

1. General
2. Skin
3. Eyes
4. Ears
5. Nose
6. Mouth
7. Throat
8. Neck
9. Chest
10. Heart
11. Abdomen
12. Genitalia
13. Lymphatic
14. Blood Vessels
15. Locomotor
16. Extremities
17. Neurological
18. Rectal
19. Vaginal
20. Diagnosis
21. Signature

Date 5 September 84 Hour 3:30 p.m. a.m./p.m. Age 32 Sex F Weight 124#

Temp. 101^2 Pulse 86 Resp. 18 Blood Pressure 132/82

General: WDWN white female looking tired and older than her stated age, looks sick.

Skin: Pale but warm, normal female hair.

Eyes: PERRLA, EOMI, fundi orange A/V = 3/4

Ears: Excessive wax occluding both TM, AC BC both sides.

Nose: Flow R L, without hemorrhage, without inflammation, without

Mouth:

Neck: ROMI, submandibular nodes 2 cm diameter

Chest: Diaphram symmetrical, R dull to percussion BS sounds.

Heart: RRR S_1 and S_2 normal

Pulses: C++, B++, R++, V+, F++, P-, DP++, PT+ sym. no bruits C,F.

Abd.: BS hyperactive, pain sub xyphoid

Ext.: ROMI, warm hands, cold feet

Rectal: Good sphincter tone, occult blood +

Neuro: Awake, alert, oriented x^3, good speech, strength good, gait good, CN II XII intact. Normal sensory. Plantar response.

Diagnosis: Gastric ulcer with hypo, R/O EtOH gastritis
R pneumonia 2 to aspiration

Signature

0753803 CONTINUE ON REVERSE SIDE **PHYSICAL EXAMINATION** 1-421-2-0879

Patient Charts

Patient charts usually contain seven parts:

admission notes
face sheet
physician's orders
history
physical examination
nurses' notes
other special records such as progress notes

The admission notes, history and physical exam have already been discussed.

The *face sheet* is the front page of the chart. It is a list of pertinent information, such as any allergies the client may have.

The *physician's orders* give directions and actions to be taken with the patient. The physician should date and sign each order or set of orders. When a physician phones in an order, it is entered on the chart with time and date and signed by the nurse receiving it. The physician countersigns it within forty-eight hours.

The *nurses' notes* are records of nursing interventions and their assessments of patients and evaluations of the effectiveness of their efforts. These records include:

1. Observational assessments of the patient.
2. Nursing interventions ordered by the physician.
3. Interventions initiated by the nurse.
4. Evaluations of the interventions.
5. Actions taken by other health care givers.

Special reports and records include progress notes, radiographic reports, physical therapist's reports, occupational therapist's reports, laboratory findings, reports of surgery, anesthesia records, and when appropriate, an autopsy report.

Examples of the types of information found on patient charts can be seen on Forms L, M, N, O and P.

Other Records

Every admission to a hospital must be accompanied by a discharge summary. This record brings closure to patients' hospitalization and describes their condition at the time of discharge. It usually includes a final diagnosis, a chief complaint, and a summary of the patient's history—present illness, past and family illnesses, review of systems, and physical examination. An example of a discharge summary is found on Form Q.

Form L Example of patient chart report.

X-MATCH

DATE	MEDICATIONS	TIME	DATE	I.V.S
JULY 4	MYLANTA 15cc q. 2 h.	06-08-10 12-14-16		
"	HALDOL 1 mgm. T. I. D.	08-14-20		
"	FROSST 292 - CRUSHED FOR PAIN	P. R. N.		
"	SLIDING SCALE TORONTO INSULIN			
	5% GIVE 12 UNITS			
	3% " 10 UNITS			
	2% " 8 "			TREATMENTS/PROCEDURES
	2%-0 " 0 "		JULY 4	CLINITEST T. I. D + H. S. – 07-11 17-H.S.
JULY 11	AZOGANTRISIN $\dot{\bar{i}}$ Q. I. D.	06-11 16-22	JULY 8	IRRIGATE FOLEY CATH. DAILY ·/c N. S
	H.S. MED.			
JULY 4	DALMANE 30 mgm.	H.S.		
JULY 14	AMITRIPTYLINE (ELAVIL) 25 mgm.	H.S.		

NAME | ROOM | DOCTOR | 015

- -

DATE	No.	PROBLEM LIST	RESOLVED	DATE	OTHER RELEVANT DATA (Include x-rays and tests)
JULY 17	#1	PT. STILL VERY DEPRESSED			DATE OF BIRTH
	#2	L-SIDED WEAKNESS		JULY 17	CHEST PHYSIO.
	#3	COMMUNICATION PROBLEMS		JULY 14	BARIUM MEAL ✓
					HEALTH CARE CONSULTANTS
DATE REVIEWED					

Form M Example of patient chart report.

DIET	FLUIDS	ACTIVITY	SAFETY	SPECIAL CONSIDERATIONS:
☒ Regular	☐ I. & O.	☐ Up ad lib	Side Rails	
☐ Soft	☐ ....Am't Daily	☐ B.R.P.	☒ Constant	
☐ Fluid	☐ I.V.	☐ Amb c asst	☐ Night Only	
☐ Clear Fluid	☐ Preferred Fluids	☐ Walker	Other	
☐ N.P.O.	**ELIMINATION**	☒ Chair T·I·D	**PROSTHESIS**	
☐ Other	☐ B.R.	☐ Dangle	☐ Glasses	
FEEDING	☒ Commode	☐ Bed rest	☐ Hearing Aid	
☒ Self ·/c SOME ASSISTANCE	☐ Ostomy	**HYGIENE**	☐ Dentures	
☐ Assist	☐ Incontinent	☒ Self ·/c SOME ASSISTANCE	☐ Other - Specify	**ALLERGIES**
	☐ Condom	☐ Partial	**V. S. FREQUENCY**	
	☐ Catheter	☐ Bed	☒ B.P. O·D @ 0800	
	Size #16 Date JULY 6 30cc BALOON	☐ Tub	☒ T.P.R. O·D @ 0800	
	☐ Other Specify	☐ Shower	☐ Other – Specify	
		☐ Mouth Care		

DISCHARGE AND REHAB. PLANS: DATE REVIEWED

DATE	PROBLEM AND SHORT TERM GOAL	APPROACH
JULY 17	#1 PT. WILL BE LESS DEPRESSED, PARTICIPATE MORE IN A·D·L· — ↑ HER SELF-ESTEEM	① SHOW CARING BY BEING PATIENT AND UNDERSTANDING. ② BE CONSISTENT IN INVOLVING HER AS MUCH AS POSSIBLE IN A·D·L - AND PRAISE HER WHEN SHE ACCOMPLISHES THEM. ③ MAINTAIN A ROUTINE OF CARE + EXPECT HER TO DO HER SHARE.
JULY 17	#2 PT. WILL BE ABLE TO PARTICIPATE AS MUCH AS POSS. IN A·D·L AND BE AWARE OF POSITIONING OF Ⓛ LIMBS	① ASSIST PT. WHENEVER NECESSARY ② EXPECT PARTICIPATION IN A·D·L· ③ KEEP PT. AWARE OF LEFT LIMB POSITIONS.
JULY 17	#3 PT. WILL UNDERSTAND PROCEDURES ETC.	① GET INTERPRETER WHEN NEC. ② SPEAK SLOWLY

Next of Kin: HUSBAND - FOO YUNG TOY			S.I.	Isolation	
Occupation: HOUSEWIFE			Surgery: JULY 4 - ESOPHAGOSCOPY		
Age: 63	Religion: NONE	Mar. Status: M.	Adm. Date: JUNE 21/85	Diagnosis: ① ACID INGESTION ② DIABETES ③ OLD (LT) C·V·A·	
Name			Hosp. No.	Accom. Ⓦ P SP	Doctor	016

Form N Example of patient chart report.

H. D. = Hospital Day

P. O. D. = Post Operative Day

GRAPHIC OBSERVATION RECORD

	DATE 7-10-83	DATE 7-11-83	DATE 7-12-83	DATE 7-13-83	DATE 7-14-83
H.D.	1	2	3	4	5
P.O.D.			1	2	3

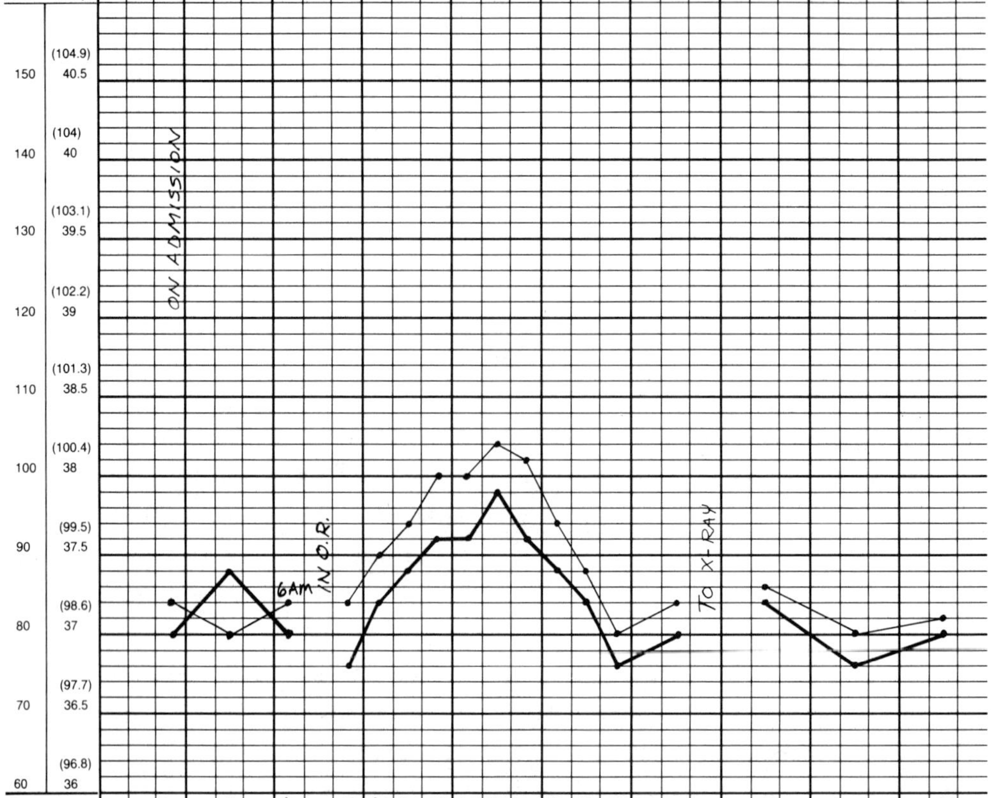

Respirations:

Date	A.M. 4	A.M. 8	A.M. 12	P.M. 4	P.M. 8	P.M. 12
7-10-83			20		16	
7-11-83	20		18	20	20	24
7-12-83	24	24	20	16	16	18
7-13-83	20				20	
7-14-83		16			20	

	7-10-83				7-11-83				7-12-83				7-13-83				7-14-83			
Fractionals Time:			4P	9P	6A	11A	4P	9P	7A	11A	4P	9P	7A	11A	4P	9P	7A	11A	4P	9P
Sugar/acetone long					0/0				Tr/0				0/0				0/0			
Sugar/acetone short			Tr/0	0/0		1+/0	0/0	Tr/0		1+/0	Tr/0	0/0		0/0	0/0	0/0		Tr/0	0/0	0/0
B. P. Time		12N			6AM	12N	4PM	8PM	8AM	12N	4PM	8PM	8A		8PM		8AM		8PM	
Values		120/70			124/72	118/70	120/72	120/72	128/80	128/76	124/72	120/70	118/70		120/72		118/74		118/72	
Weight	123 lbs.																			
Bowel Movement	✓				ō				✓				✓				✓			

FORM NO. 22182 (REV. 5/76)

Form O Example of patient chart report.

Nursing History Form

Admission date 4-1-84 History taken by CRS Date 4-3-84

Diagnosis Cerebrovascular lesion Date of injury/illness 3-30-84

Special circumstances of present illness paralysis left side, dysphasia, periodic disorientation

Previous hospitalization pelvic fracture 3-10-83; hysterectomy 1972

List nursing activities or omissions which were helpful or deleterious to the patient during

previous hospitalization becomes obnoxious on awakening - demands cigarettes in am

Expected result from present hospitalization will require pt to regain functioning

Is patient transient no

Family background

married ____ single ____ widowed xx divorced ____ estranged ____ common law ____

Religion Catholic

Does patient wish visitors excluded? no If so, give reason ____

Daily living habits:

Food and fluid likes and dislikes prefers soft foods - no teeth on left side

Sleeping habits: preferred time of retiring and arising 10 pm; 9 am

dreams DK nightmares DK insomnia DK

Television, radio, and phone preference all times; watches TV intently

Bowel and urinary habits normal

Medicines taken regularly diuretic Known allergies pollens/foods

Female patients: Is a personal supply of pads or tampons available? N/A

Interests, hobbies, pastimes none

List wounds or special medical care N/A

Cultural factors, vocabulary, education 9th grade level, high school

Questions patient asked Where are my children? When do I get to go home?

Additional observations Acts and projects independence but thrives on visitations and attention.

*Adapted from Shaw, J. S., McLaughlin, M.: Nursing Histories in a Naval Hospital, U.S. Navy Medical News Letter. 54:43-46, 1969.

Form P Example of autopsy report.

IMPRINT

AUTOPSY REPORT

HOSPITAL REGULATION: ALL POSITIVE AND IMPORTANT NEGATIVE FINDINGS SHALL BE RECORDED

Date________ Hour________ a.m. p.m. Age____ Sex____ Weight______

FINAL PATHOLOGIC DIAGNOSES

1. Esophageal varices with thrombosis
2. Splenomegaly, 420 gm, secondary to portal hypertension
3. Chronic peptic ulcer, stomach
4. Recent surgery: suture closure of ulcer bed, stomach; pyloroplasy, vagotomy, liver biopsy, jejunostomy
5. Sclerosis of aorta and coronary arteries
6. Thrombosis of portal vein
7. Carcinoma of liver, liver cell type, with invasion of portal vein
8. Carcinoma of adrenal gland, left, secondary
9. Portal cirrhosis
10. Occlusion of right coronary artery, old
11. Fibrosis of myocardium
12. Lobar pneumonia, left lower lung
13. Cholelithiasis, calculus in common bile duct
14. Hyalinization of islets of Langerhans
15. Simple cysts of kidney
16. Arteriosclerosis of kidney
17. Old surgery: cholecystectomy and appendectomy

____
Signature

0753803 CONTINUE ON REVERSE SIDE 1-421-2-0879

Form Q Example of discharge summary.

IMPRINT

DISCHARGE SUMMARY

HOSPITAL REGULATION: ALL POSITIVE AND IMPORTANT NEGATIVE FINDINGS SHALL BE RECORDED

Date________ Hour________ a.m. p.m. Age____ Sex____ Weight________

FINAL DIAGNOSIS: Idiopathic convulsive disorder.

CHIEF COMPLAINT: This is a second admission for this 40-year-old black male with the chief complaint of blacking out.

HISTORY OF PRESENT ILLNESS: The patient was in excellent health until the day of admission when he developed tonic and clonic muscle activity with complete loss of consciousness that lasted less than 5 minutes. There was no tongue biting or incontinence of urine or stool. He returned to consciousness but with severe headaches and was confused and disoriented for 45 minutes. He was first taken to Mercy Hospital where a variety of tests were done including EKGs, 2 X which were nonrevealing. While waiting to see Dr. A., he suddenly felt nauseous accompanied by loss of consciousness and a similar but less violent episode, again followed by confusion. He was returned to the ER for admission. For the past few days prior to admission the patient had been eating very little and working very hard. He had no prior history of any seizures or head trauma, febrile or serious childhood illness. Current medication is a quaalude pill 4 times a day. The patient drank heavily until 10 years ago, one-half case of beer per day, but not since. The patient was in an auto accident 5 days prior to admission but without any head trauma. No history of diabetes.

PAST HISTORY: The patient had a varicose vein stripping 1 year ago. No allergies. Medications are as above. No blood transfusions.

REVIEW OF SYSTEMS: The patient has had a pruritic erythematous localized over the right arm for several weeks.

FAMILY HISTORY: Father CA of 77, has high blood pressure and congestive heart failure. Mother is 74 years old, has low blood pressure. Brother is 36 years old, alive and well. No family history of seizure disorders. Patient smoked 2 packs of cigarettes per day for 10 years, quit 10 years prior to admission.

PHYSICAL EXAMINATION: The patient is a well-nourished, well-developed male complaining of headache and diffuse myalgia. BP is 150/65, pulse is 96 regular, respiration 12; he is afebrile.

HEENT: Reveals no bruits. Pupils are equal and reactive. Fundi reveal sharp discs. Ears are normal.

____
Signature

0753803 CONTINUE ON REVERSE SIDE 1-421-2-0879

Prescription Forms

A prescription is an order for medications written by a licensed medical, dental, or veterinary practitioner. A prescription authorizes the purchase of a prescription drug from a licensed pharmacist. It usually contains the name and quantity of the drug, by generic or trade name, with instructions to the pharmacist regarding composition and patient use. All prescription drugs must bear this statement on their labels: CAUTION: FEDERAL LAW PROHIBITS DISPENSING WITHOUT PRESCRIPTION.

Although a physician may telephone authorization to a pharmacist to dispense drugs, the most reliable method is with a prescription form. This document (see Form R) is usually written using terminology and abbreviations that are understood by the pharmacist. (See Chapter Seventeen for a listing of abbreviations used in prescription writing.) The physician can indicate whether the name of the drug should appear on the label. There are both advantages and disadvantages to this decision. The biggest advantage is that in the case of overdose or adverse reaction, a poison control center can promptly recommend an antidote. In such an emergency situation as this, time is critical and a label that identifies the drug is faster than trying to track down the prescription through the pharmacy or through the color coding of the medication itself (capsule or pill). The greatest disadvantage to labeling the drug is the problem of self-medication and theft.

Form R Example of prescription form.

Heading Prescriber →	John Smith, M.D. – Family practice
Patient →	Name ______ Age ____ Date ____ Address ______
Superscription →	℞
Inscription →	Atropine sulfate 0.5 mg Thenobarbital 30 mg
Subscription →	D.T.D. caps #60
Refil Information →	N.E. REP ☐ LABEL ☐ ______ REP ______ times
Signature of → Prescriber	______ M.D. Never offer this prescription to a friend for a seemingly similar ailment; it is your personal prescription, prepared for your specific illness at this particular time.

Computerized Information Systems

The use of computers can speed the processing of data related to patient care and can improve the handling of records. There are many types of computer systems and equipment in use today. A networking system uses one large computer with a number of connecting computer terminals (modules). A stand-alone system is self-contained and operates much the same as a personal computer.

Large organizations, such as hospitals, use a mainframe computer located either within or outside the hospital. Mainframes have large amounts of memory and can manipulate data in a wide variety of ways. A personal password may be entered by some stand-alone systems and with almost all multiuser mainframe systems. The password or nonsense syllables are entered either directly on the keyboard or by inserting a card in a slot. This method safeguards the system from unauthorized use and charges the cost to the user if computer time is charged. Common uses of computer systems include generating worksheets, organizing and tracking patient care, recording data, and accessing actions taken or ordered by others.

Index

Index numbers have been given to word elements and the example words that follow them. These numbers have two parts separated by a decimal. For example, the index listing, **abnormal, 2.72,** is included below. The whole number (the 2 on the left side of the decimal) refers to its chapter number and the 74 (on the right of the decimal) is its sequence number. Note that 2.1 is not the same as 2.10. Index numbers appearing here are in bold type, just as they are presented in the text. Terms not given index numbers in the text are listed by page number only.

A6
B7
C8
D9
E0
F1